—What do families do when long after the terribly ill, inexorably dying person has uttered her last meaningful word, she is "salvaged" for a twilight life on machines after physicians ask, "Do you want us to do everything for your mother?"

—Should a quarter-million dollars be spent saving a 600-gram unwanted *abortus* which manages to stir and survives with scarred lungs and a damaged brain—when tens of thousands of wanted children are born without prenatal care for lack of funded programs?

—Should "cost-effectiveness" continue to be a criterion for deciding who gets care—and what kinds of treatment?

—Why is there an emerging scarcity of physicians providing basic care?

—How can we respond to the HIV epidemic when our system lacks preventive care, primary care for the poor, and facilities for long-term care?

These and other contemporary issues form a new set of ethical dilemmas for the health-care provider. Discover the issues and how they are being dealt with in this essential book.

Nancy F. McKenzie, Ph.D. has taught philosophy and ethics at Vassar College, Cornell University Medical College and the New School for Social Research. She is presently director of the health division of the Community Service Society, a social policy/social advocacy agency in New York City.

THE CRISIS
IN
HEALTH CARE
Ethical Issues

EDITED BY

Nancy F. McKenzie, Ph.D.

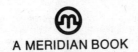

A MERIDIAN BOOK

MERIDIAN
Published by the Penguin Group
Penguin Books USA Inc., 375 Hudson Street, New York, New York 10014, U.S.A.
Penguin Books Ltd, 27 Wrights Lane, London W8 5TZ, England
Penguin Books Australia Ltd, Ringwood, Victoria, Australia
Penguin Books Canada Ltd, 2801 John Street, Markham, Ontario, Canada L3R 1B4
Penguin Books (N.Z.) Ltd, 182-190 Wairau Road, Auckland 10, New Zealand

Penguin Books Ltd, Registered Offices: Harmondsworth, Middlesex, England

First published by Meridian, an imprint of Penguin Books USA Inc.
Published simultaneously in Canada.

First Printing, April, 1990
10   9   8   7   6   5

Copyright © Nancy F. McKenzie, 1990
Foreword copyright © Dawn McGuire, 1990
All rights reserved

 REGISTERED TRADEMARK—MARCA REGISTRADA

LIBRARY OF CONGRESS CATALOGING-IN-PUBLICATION DATA

The Crisis in health care / edited by Nancy F. McKenzie.
        p.   cm.
    ISBN 0-452-01028-4
    1. Medical care—United States.   2. Medical ethics—United States.
    3. Medical policy—United States.   I. McKenzie, Nancy F.
    [DNLM: 1. Delivery of Health Care—standards—United States.
2. Ethics, Medical.   3. Health Policy—United States.   W 50 C932]
RA445.C73   1990
362.1′0973—dc20
DNLM/DLC
for Library of Congress   89-13631
                                                                        CIP

Printed in the United States of America
Set in Times Roman
Designed by Julian Hamer

BOOKS ARE AVAILABLE AT QUANTITY DISCOUNTS WHEN USED TO PROMOTE PRODUCTS
OR SERVICES. FOR INFORMATION PLEASE WRITE TO PREMIUM MARKETING DIVISION,
PENGUIN BOOKS USA INC., 375 HUDSON STREET, NEW YORK, NEW YORK 10014.

*To my students
and to the medically invisible*

Contents

Section VI   Medicine and the Quality of Dying

A. Euthanasia

B. Human Organ Procurement

Section VII   Medicine in the Age of HIV

Foreword

Medicine: A Bedside View

The medicine that today's house officers dreamed about, which they went to college and medical school and deep into debt for, no longer exists. Our young physicians are bemused and beleaguered, and they feel they have been betrayed.[1]

It is curious that the voices usually absent from discourses on medical ethics are those of the sick and their immediate caregivers, the house officers and ward physicians responsible for day-to-day care. It should not surprise, really, for our discourse is not powerful. We are each strained and vulnerable, and for the most part we are transient as well; for the sick will heal in some fashion or die, and the house officer will complete training and move on. So our status is low, we for whom this drama matters most, and the mandarins, medical and legal, find it easy to speak for us, "objectively."

I welcome, though with trepidation, the opportunity to speak for myself, a house officer, one intimate with the actual care of the very ill in their time of crisis; with trepidation, for it is a difficult and somewhat painful task, since much of what I shall say concerns conditions against which I defend myself with a sort of desperate vigor. I begin, then, with a story by Kafka, whose "fiction" can both disarm and ready one for truth.

According to Kafka, the Great Wall of China was built to protect the Empire from the People of the North. Dutifully, the wall builders laid brick on brick, night and day, wherever they were directed. So there arose many odd, discontinuous fragments of wall over the countryside. These were a pious people, and they trusted that a master plan was indeed being executed by their small labors (though some wondered, quietly, how a wall built in fragments could protect).

None actually knew the extent of the wall, how near it was to completion, nor if it would "work" for the purposes planned.

11

There was rumored to be an Office of the Command; but no one knew where it was nor who commanded. In fact, despite their dedication, no builder knew the wall as well as did the People of the North, the barbarians it was designed to keep out. They rode on their dirty ponies up and down the thousand hills, and they saw and knew everything.

Those of us who spend our days and nights on hospital wards defend and maintain the health care empire. Far from the office of the command, we can only dimly perceive its unwieldy 400-billion-dollar dimensions. So we must look to the "barbarians" for clarity, and this extraordinary anthology includes the most erudite among them. Here we find the critics and visionaries with whose help we may piece together, with discomfiting ease, the picture of an empire at war with itself. A graceless, antique empire, it is probably indefensible in its present form. The structure is feeble; the "cracks" between which people fall are fissures. Its walls are arbitrary, and the excluded become its enemies. Even its pious defenders are demoralized: by the end of a residency, too often the love of medicine and the affection for the sick have been so exploited that young physicians, like the workers on the Great Wall, are, in Kafka's words, "quite exhausted and [have] lost all faith in themselves, in the wall, in the world."

Kafka's tale ends abruptly. His narrator falls silent when he realizes that it is mortal whim, and not vision, behind such walls. The narrator is a politic and pious man. If I risk impiety in pursuing my remarks, it is not recklessly, but out of regard for my trade, and in fear of its disintegration. So I will describe the country of my experience, where I take care of sick people; it is 1989, the age of HMOS and DRGs, of "provider units" and "capitation units"; the age of the "medicolegal document"; the age of AIDS.

It is, first, a country morally imperiled, and those of us who care for patients cannot but do so in bad faith. This country and South Africa stand alone among industrial powers in having no national system of health care. Here, we have elected the commercialization of medicine rather than its socialization. The only aspect of our health policy which resembles a system is the systematic exclusion of millions. It is the fittest who benefit, not the frail, and not the vulnerable. So my work entails filtering the white noise of a moral disquietude. I live and work in the richest state in the richest country in the world, and here one-quarter of the children have no medical care. The ironies are not artfully concealed; the attention is just aimed elsewhere. To expect that the commercialization of medicine will protect the public health requires the kind of optimism that builds broken walls: the smug optimism of the unscathed.

In brief, these are the gaps and discontinuities as seen from a great height; but, like a chaotic coastline, the crazy contour repeats itself on smaller and smaller scales. So I would next describe the hospital, where on entering one acquires a peculiar sort of vision: a tunnel vision which manages to cheapen life, while making a cruel expense of "keeping alive"—some, that is. If the standard is the surgeon's knife, or transplanting the untransplantable, or "salvaging" the unsalvageable, then we deserve praise. Cut and cure is better than ever; but *care* is mediocre, when you can get it. Long after the terribly ill, inexorably dying person has uttered her last meaningful word, she is "salvaged." Too often this is not discussed with patients or their families beforehand. Then families are confronted when they are most vulnerable with a painful decision and little realistic guidance: "Do you want us to do everything for your mother?" So the fist crashes on the heart with all the *don't die* wrath of a child. The next breath is forced by machine, the person chemically paralyzed so as not to resist. This is what "doing everything" looks like here.

The 600-gram *abortus* which manages to stir and is therefore "viable" is salvaged: months in intensive care, surviving but with scarred lungs and a damaged brain; sick, unwanted, "difficult to place"; one quarter of a million dollars spent. Yet tens of thousands of wanted children are born without benefit of prenatal care for lack of funded programs. But salvage we must, for we are "obligated"; by whom or by what it is unclear, and it should be clear what obligates us to such cruelty and wastefulness.

I am not a seasoned doctor. I am not dispassionate. Contradiction nags me, suffering grieves me, waste offends me. But nagged, aggrieved, offended, impatient, I am no less a disciplined doctor. I do my job, and this is the context in which I work; this is what I see.

I see a devastating disease, the dimensions of which mock the facile claim that medicine is science and not politics. The phenomenon AIDS has exposed the social diseases which killed long before HIV: denial of health care to millions; the use of drugs to regulate a passive underclass; the easy tolerance of violence toward gay and lesbian people; the intractable racism with its myriad masks and intentions. AIDS is revealing ourselves to ourselves. The afflicted are mostly the oppressed, but, once afflicted, all become marginal, and the easy targets of bigotry. In San Francisco, gay men painstakingly acquired a modest political power before the epidemic. They organized quickly, and have been able to exercise some control at least over the medical community's response. There are AIDS wards, hospices, support for partners; there is some *care* for these men. Yet it is also true that they are well-educated, middle-class, mostly white, comfortable with power, male-identified, and male. They could be doctors, scientists, senators. They "fit" power. Nonetheless, their vigilance to some extent protects all those affected. It would not happen, as in New York, that Jorge, a Puerto Rican gay man, would spend thirty hours in an emergency room, vomiting, incontinent, febrile to 105 degrees, to be sent away without care. This reflects the lifeboat politics of a city disorganized and stressed beyond tolerance. In New York City, AIDS is mostly in the underclass, and it kills faster there. The forces which shape the medical response to this disease are first, second and third *political*. The political agenda shapes our science and it shapes our service.

Is this the vocation to which I was called? It is, and it isn't. *Ars toto requirit hominem:* the art takes all you've got to give. That part is certainly the same. I recall what compelled me to medicine: the sense of deep privilege and just good fortune that I could learn the mysteries and heal the wounds. And where I could not cure, I could nonetheless assist my patients toward their own "good" death. What is true is that while I can shock to life a dying heart, I have left many broken ones unattended. My training, technically impeccable, doesn't reach this far, and even mediocrity in this regard is above the accepted standard. Daily I deal clumsily with the most important moments in my patients' lives. The scenes which should be played before a hushed house I attend, barely, half in, half out of a psychological doorway. It may be my thirtieth working hour, or even my thirty-sixth. My beeper is bleating. My neck is in spasm, and I feel nothing except the drive to be horizontal. The light from my private life is so remote as to be doppler-shifted. I make just over minimum wage for a week that can exceed one hundred hours. My debt from training has the next decade mortgaged. Yet, despite the structural limitations, and my own, I *am* the intimate companion of *this* sick person. It is we two who meet and probe one another, sense each others' strengths and frailties, who trust one another or not. This particularity, this relationship, however disguised and tyrannized, is the level on which it makes sense to speak of healing. It is unique; it cannot be reproduced; it is not a science.

But I am trained in science, not in healing. I "treat" patients. And of the patients I have treated, I have probably helped only a third; to another third, I have at least kept my oath and done no harm. As for the rest, I have certainly added to their suffering, especially the oldest, the most frail, those with no advocate to speak out when they are silenced by disease. To these, I have "done everything," as my job obliges. And there is something darkly depleting about having so little to offer the sick.

So there is a wounding to this work. The relationship between the wounded healer and the art of healing is a very ancient one. Even Galen, father of our science, tells us he was cured of a mortal illness by Aesculapius in a dream.[2] Native healers from the Four Corners to the Sub-Sahara still must undergo a "shamanic illness" in their training, from which they recover, often after years, and become healers, or else succumb. And so do we, for three to seven years, live sleep-deprived, hypervigilant, anxious, isolated, and often secretly terribly sad. We should perhaps celebrate, then, our initiation illness, through which we may learn to use our power gracefully. However, unlike the training shaman, we do little in the way of meditation on our journey. We remain only crudely aware of our own affliction, and the most defended are the most rewarded here. The passage is endured, merely; we are reduced, but not refined. The experiences, unprocessed, weigh on us like lead. That it could be otherwise seems as improbable as alchemy.

I think patients must often sense the wounds of their doctors. But we are so protective of our role, and so defended against our vulnerabilities, that we thwart their care toward us. The expected comportment is that of studied concern, unflappable authority, taut patience. Their concern for us is inappropriate, we say. It breeches boundaries. But don't we doctors, with our hidden sores, know this: that it is part of being healed, to heal?

Where are the teachers, our guides for this passage? The list of scientists I admire is long; but when I consider healing, I see not Osler, Virchow; not even Lewis Thomas, nor Victor Sidel. I see a fat, pale baker from a story by Raymond Carver.[3]

"A Small, Good Thing" is a quietly remarkable parable of healing; not that it tries to define healing, nor to dissect the healing relationship. Its aims are simple, its vision local. The story just shows the "close work" of healing; and so restores it to its mystery and simplicity, its particularity, its breathtaking exactness.

A boy is hit by a car on his birthday. The physician, wishing to reassure—himself? the helpless parents?—insists that the boy is not "really" in a coma. He is a *nice* man, but his caring is brief, embarrassed, inept. He is not "good" at helplessness, except to conceal it. Hungry as the young parents are for nurturance, his best is to send them elsewhere for it. *Feel free to go out for a bite. It would do you good.*

When the boy dies, the physician is truly sorry. *A hidden occlusion*, he explains vaguely. *A one-in-a-million circumstance.* He embraces the couple, then hurries them to the parking lot. *He seemed full of some goodness she didn't understand.*

Throughout the hospital vigil, the couple had been getting bizarre phone calls. A man's voice would ask: *Your Scotty, I got him ready for you. Have you forgotten about Scotty?* On the night the child dies, his mother remembers the cake she had ordered for his birthday. She remembers the strange, sour baker—it had been *he*, then, calling about the cake!

She is so angry she feels crazy. Her husband drives her to the bakery in the dark of night. It is a petty, sinister little man who reluctantly opens his door to them. He is snide and contentious at first: the sixteen-dollar cake is stale. And then he hears her: *He's dead, you bastard.* The baker stops his work. He takes off his apron. He pulls up three chairs and makes a space at the table. He allows the impact of what he has done to impress upon him fully: he has added to their unspeakable suffering. He opens himself to their grief. And then he speaks, disarmed, from his heart:

Listen to me. I'm just a baker. I don't claim to be anything else. Maybe once, maybe years ago, I was a different kind of human being. I've forgotten, I don't know for sure. That don't excuse my doing what I did, I know. But I'm deeply sorry. I'm sorry for your son, and sorry for my part in this. . . . Please, let me ask you if you can find it in your hearts to forgive me?

Then the baker feeds them. They, who are more empty than they've ever been, eat fresh sweet rolls from his oven. He tells them, *There's all the rolls in the world here. Eating is a small, good thing in a time like this.*

As the three sit together in the early light, the baker also shares himself. *They nodded when the baker began to speak of loneliness, and of the sense of doubt and limitation that had come to him in his middle years. He told them what it was like to be childless all these years.* Such a gifted healer, this baker. He gives exactly what he has, and it suffices, exactly. He permits these suffering people to extend themselves, through their grief, to him, and their emptiness relents. *They listened to him. They ate what they could. They talked on into the early morning. And they did not think of leaving.*

Imagine the baker's first speech delivered by the physician. *I'm just a doctor. . . .* What he did say was, sadly, true: *I'm so very sorry, I can't tell you.* How empty we sound when, failing cure, we distrust ourselves, and reject whatever small, good thing that might be ours to offer. Full of some opaque, private goodness, we do not ask forgiveness, and we do not forgive ourselves.[4] I think it must be in the setting of forgiveness that healing becomes possible, for any of us.

But small, good things won't be coming from doctors in doorways, half-asleep. The standards must be articulated, the structure of care and training changed to accommodate the standards. To say there isn't time, or money, or the physician labor force to make *care for all* a meaningful concept, is to say there isn't the political will. The conditions we have accepted, which our values have determined, are as arbitrary as they are resistant to change; and can, nonetheless, be changed.

The anthology you hold in your hands is more than a text of medical ethics; it is about the ethics of care. It is a thoughtful, courageous, uncompromising collection, which helps us rethink what we value and accept, and meet close up the casualties. Its focus is on the medically unserved: children, the homeless, the uninsured, those stricken with socially unacceptable disease.

Those the health care system fails are acknowledged here, and the values which such failures reflect are teased out of the debris of excuses, and placed in economic and political perspective. This will create unease; for the Kantian editor of this collection insists that, ill or well, we either choose values or have them inflicted upon us by the dominant ideology. "Medical ethics" implies an active interest in, and responsibility for, transforming medicine such that an ethics of care becomes possible. This work belongs to all of us, for we are healers, all. And it remains, despite this painful stage, the best work I can imagine.

—DAWN McGUIRE, MD
San Francisco, July 1989

NOTES

1. J.E. Hardison. "The House Officer's Changing World," *New England Journal of Medicine* 1986; 314: 1713-5.
2. Galen, "On His Own Books," from Arthur J. Brock, *Greek Medicine*, JM Dent and Sons, London, 1929. p. 177.
3. Raymond Carver, "A Small, Good Thing," from *Cathedral*, Alfred A. Knopf, Inc., 1983.
4. Cf. David Hilfiker. Facing Our Mistakes, *New England Journal of Medicine* 1984; 310:118–22.

SECTION I

THE SOCIAL DISTRIBUTION OF HEALTH CARE

Uninsured and Underserved: Inequities in Health Care in the United States

Karen Davis and Diane Rowland

THE United States has one of the highest quality and most sophisticated systems of medical care in the world. Most Americans take for granted their access to this system of care. In times of emergency or illness, they can call upon a vast array of health resources—from a family physician to a complex teaching hospital—assured that they will receive needed care and that their health insurance coverage will pick up the tab for the majority of bills incurred.

For a surprisingly large segment of the United States population, however, this ease of access to care does not exist. At any point in time, over 25 million Americans have no health insurance coverage from private health insurance plans or public programs (Kasper et al. 1978). Without health insurance coverage or ready cash, such individuals can be and are turned away from hospitals even in emergency situations (U.S. Congress. House. Committee on Energy and Commerce 1981). Some neglect obtaining preventive or early care, often postponing care until conditions have become life-threatening. Others struggle with burdensome medical bills. Many come to rely upon crowded, understaffed public hospitals as the only source of reliable, available care.

The absence of universal health insurance coverage creates serious strains in our society. These strains are felt most acutely by the uninsured poor, who must worry about family members—a

From *Milbank Quarterly:* Health and Society, Vol. 61, No. 2, 1983. Reprinted by permission of the *Milbank Quarterly*, Milbank Memorial Fund.

sick child, an adult afflicted with a deteriorating chronic health condition, a pregnant mother—going without needed medical assistance. It strains our image as a just and humane society when significant portions of the population endure avoidable pain, suffering, and even death because of an inability to pay for health care. Those physicians, other health professionals, and institutions that try to assist this uninsured group also incur serious strain. Demands typically far outstrip available time and resources. Strain is also felt by local governments whose communities include many uninsured persons, because locally funded public hospitals and health centers inevitably incur major financial deficits. In recent years, many of the public facilities that have traditionally been the source of last-resort care have closed, thereby intensifying the stresses on other providers and the uninsured poor.

As serious as these strains have been in the last five years, the years ahead promise to strain the fabric of our social life even more seriously. Unemployment levels today are the highest since the Great Depression. With unemployment, the American worker loses not only a job but also health insurance protection. As unemployment rises and the numbers of the uninsured grow, fewer and fewer resources are available to fill the gaps in health care coverage. Major reductions in funding for health services for the poor and uninsured have been made in the last year; further reductions are likely. Deepening economic recession, high unemployment, and declining sales revenues are strapping the fiscal resources of state and local governments. Their ability to offset federal cutbacks seems limited. Nor can the private sector be expected to bridge this gap. The health industry is increasingly becoming an entrepreneurial business endeavor—with little room for charitable actions.

It is especially timely, therefore, to review what we know about the consequences of inadequate health insurance coverage for certain segments of our population. The first section of this paper presents information on the number and characteristics of the uninsured, while the second section describes patterns of health care utilization by the uninsured. The third section assesses the policy implications of these facts and offers recommendations for future public policy to ensure access to health care for all.

Who Are the Uninsured?

The 1977 National Medical Care Expenditure Survey (NMCES) provides extensive information on the health insurance coverage of the U.S. population. Six household interviews of a nationwide sample of over 40,000 individuals were conducted over an 18-month period during 1977 and 1978. By following the interviewed population for an entire year, NMCES provided a comprehensive portrait of health insurance coverage, including changes in health insurance status during the course of that year.

Although the scope of the NMCES survey provides extensive information on the characteristics and utilization patterns of the uninsured, it should be noted that the profile of the uninsured presented here describes the portion of the population without insurance in 1977. Recent changes in health insurance coverage due to unemployment and cutbacks in eligibility for Medicaid have increased the size of the nation's uninsured population, but are not reflected in the statistics in this paper.

In the NMCES results, individuals classified as insured are those who were covered throughout the year by Medicaid, Medicare, the Civilian Health and Medical Program of the Uniformed Services (Champus), Blue Cross/Blue Shield or commercial health insurance, or who were enrolled in a health maintenance organization. Differences in scope of coverage among the insured were not available, although further analysis of the NMCES data will address this issue. Therefore, many individuals in the insured category may have actually had very limited health insurance coverage, leaving them basically uninsured for most services. For example, many individuals classified as insured have coverage for inpatient hospital care, but are not covered and are, therefore, essentially uninsured for primary care in a physician's office. In contrast, insured individuals also include those enrolled in a health maintenance organization offering comprehensive coverage for both inpatient and ambulatory care.

The uninsured fall into two groups: the always uninsured and the sometimes uninsured. The always uninsured are individuals without Medicare, Medicaid, or private insurance coverage for the entire year. Individuals using Veterans Administration hospitals and clinics or community health centers are classified as uninsured unless they have third-party coverage. The sometimes uninsured are those who were covered by public or private insurance part of the year but were uninsured the remainder of the year. The sometimes uninsured include the medically needy individuals who qualify for Medicaid coverage during periods of large medical expenses, but are otherwise uninsured. Changes in insurance status during the year are generally the result of loss of employment, change in employment, change in income or family situation that alters eligibility for Medicaid, or loss of private insurance when an older spouse retires and becomes eligible for Medicare.

A snapshot view of the uninsured at a given point in time understates the number of people who spend some portion of the year uninsured. At any one time, there are over 25 million uninsured Americans, but as many as 34 million may be uninsured for some period of time during the year. Approximately 18 million are without insurance for the entire year, and 16 million are uninsured for some portion of the year (Wilensky and Walden 1981; Wilensky and Berk 1982).

The 34 million uninsured are persons of all incomes, racial and ethnic backgrounds, occupations, and geographic locations. In some cases whole families are uninsured, while in others coverage is mixed depending on employment status and eligibility for public programs (Kasper et al. 1978). However, the poor, minorities, young adults, and rural residents are more likely than others to be uninsured. As noted in Table 1, over one-quarter of all blacks and minorities are uninsured during the year—a rate 1½ times that of whites. This disparity holds across the demographic and social characteristics of the uninsured (Wilensky and Walden 1981; Institute of Medicine 1981).

Age

The uninsured population, whether covered for all or part of a year, is almost entirely under age 65. Nearly one-fifth of the non-aged population is uninsured for some or all of the year. Less than 1 percent of the aged, barely 200,000 persons, are uninsured during the year (Table 1). This is attributable primarily to Medicare which provides basic coverage for hospital and physician services to most older Americans. The success of Medicare in providing financial access to health care for the elderly is demonstrated by the extensive coverage of the elderly today in contrast to the dramatic lack of insurance prior to implementation of Medicare in 1966 (Davis 1982). Medicaid and private insurance help to fill the gap for those elderly persons ineligible for Medicare because they lack sufficient Social Security earnings contributions. The uninsured elderly are primarily individuals with incomes above the eligibility levels for welfare assistance and Medicaid.

Examination of the uninsured by age group reveals that young adults are the group most likely to be uninsured. As highlighted in Table 2, almost one-third of all persons aged 19 to 24 are

TABLE 1
Insurance Status during Year by Age and Race, 1977

Age and Race	Total	Always Uninsured	Uninsured Part of Year	Always Insured
	Number in millions			
Total, all persons	212.1	18.1	15.9	178.1
Persons under age 65	189.8	18.0	15.8	156.0
White	163.7	14.5	12.5	136.7
Black and Other	26.1	3.5	3.3	19.3
Persons age 65 and over	22.3	0.1	0.1	22.1
White	20.2	0.07	0.09	20.0
Black and Other	2.1	0.03	0.01	2.1
	Percentage			
All persons	100%	8.6%	7.5%	83.9%
Persons under age 65	100	9.5	8.3	82.2
White	100	8.9	7.6	83.5
Black and Other	100	13.3	12.7	74.0
Persons age 65 and over	100	0.4	0.5	99.1
White	100	0.3	0.5	99.2
Black and Other	100	1.0	0.8	98.2

Source: Data from the U.S. Department of Health and Human Services, National Center for Health Services Research, National Medical Care Expenditure Survey.

uninsured during the course of a year. Roughly 16 percent of this age group are without coverage all year, and an additional 14 percent lack coverage at least part of the year. This rate is nearly double that of other age groups. A variety of factors undoubtedly contribute to this situation. Young adults frequently lose coverage under their parents' policies at age 18. Many young adults may elect to forgo coverage when it is available, since coverage is costly and they assume themselves to be relatively healthy. High youth unemployment, as well as employment in marginal jobs without health benefits, make insurance difficult to obtain or afford for this group.

TABLE 2
Percent Uninsured during Year by Selected Population Characteristics, 1977

Population Characteristic	Percent Uninsured during Year	Percent Always Uninsured	Percent Uninsured Part of Year
All persons	16.1%	8.6%	7.5%
Age			
Under age 65	17.8	9.5	8.3
less than 6 years	19.6	8.3	11.3
6 to 18 years	16.1	8.6	7.5
19 to 24 years	30.3	16.0	14.3
25 to 54 years	16.1	8.7	7.4
55 to 64 years	12.6	8.2	4.4
Age 65 and over	0.9	0.4	0.5
Occupation			
Farm	22.3	15.9	6.4
Blue collar	19.8	11.3	8.5
Services	20.8	11.9	8.9
White collar	12.6	5.6	7.0
Region			
Northeast	10.7	5.4	5.3
North Central	12.5	5.7	6.8
South	20.5	11.6	8.9
West	20.8	11.7	9.1

Source: Wilensky and Walden (1981), and data from the U.S. Department of Health and Human Services, National Center for Health Services Research, National Medical Care Expenditure Survey.

Employment

Employment status and occupation are important factors in assessing the likelihood of being uninsured for all or part of a year. Most American workers receive their health care coverage through the workplace, but insurance coverage varies widely depending on the type of employer (Taylor and Lawson 1981). Employees of small firms are less likely to be insured than employees of large firms. For example, 45 percent of employees in firms of 25 or fewer employees do not have employer-provided health insurance compared with only 1 percent in firms with more than 1,000 employees. Yet, small firms employ over 20 percent of all workers. Unionized firms are six times more likely to have employee health insurance than are nonunionized firms.

Insurance status varies by type of employment (Table 2). Nearly one-quarter of all agricultural workers are uninsured during the year, with 16 percent uninsured for the entire year. As expected, white collar workers are the most likely to be insured, while blue collar and service workers fare only somewhat better than agricultural workers (Wilensky and Walden 1981). Among blue collar and service workers, insurance coverage is low in the construction industry, wholesale and retail trades, and service industries, and high in manufacturing. Of manufacturing employees, 96 percent have health insurance through their place of employment (Davis 1975).

Residence

These trends in coverage by employment are reflected in the regional picture of insurance status. In the heavily industrial and unionized Northeast and north central regions of the country, the percentage of uninsured during the year is half that of the South and the West. In these areas where agricultural interests are strong and unionization less extensive, over 20 percent of the population is uninsured during the course of a year. Of those living in the South and West, 11 percent are uninsured throughout the year compared with 5 percent in the Northeast and north central regions. Similarly, people in metropolitan areas are more likely to be insured than people living outside metropolitan areas (Wilensky and Walden 1981).

Income and Race

However, while nature of employment and unionization may explain some of the regional variations, a critical underlying factor in the analysis is the distribution in the population of poverty and minorities. Residents of the South comprise 32 percent of the total population under age 65. Yet 48 percent of the nation's minorities live in the South (Department of Health and Human Services 1982a). The higher concentration of poor and minority persons in the South in comparison with other parts of the country helps explain the high level of uninsured individuals.

Poverty and lack of insurance are strongly correlated. Of poor families with incomes below 125 percent of the poverty line, 27 percent are uninsured. The near-poor, with incomes between 125 and 200 percent of poverty, fare only slightly better, with 21 percent uninsured during the year. The poor are always more likely to be uninsured than the middle and upper income groups (Table 3) (Wilensky and Walden 1981).

The limited health insurance coverage for the poor and near-poor demonstrates the limits of coverage of the poor under Medicaid (Wilensky and Berk 1982). Many assume that Medicaid finances health care services for all of the poor. However, many poor persons are ineligible for Medicaid due to categorical requirements for program eligibility and variations in state eligibility policies. Two-parent families are generally ineligible for Medicaid and single adults are covered only if they are aged or disabled (Davis and Schoen 1978). Moreover, many states have established income eligibility cutoffs well below the poverty level. Many states have not adjusted income levels to account for inflation, resulting in a reduction in the number of individuals covered over the last few years (Rowland and Gaus 1983). As a result of the restrictions on Medicaid coverage, about 60 percent of the poor are not covered by Medicaid. Of the 35 million poor and near-poor in 1977, almost 5 million or about 15 percent had no insurance throughout 1977. Approximately 35 percent were on Medicaid for at least part of the year (Wilensky and Berk 1982). This situation can only be expected to worsen as the recession swells the numbers of poor and near-poor while cutbacks in social programs and Medicaid further erode the health coverage available to some of the poor.

TABLE 3
Percent Uninsured during Year by Ethnic/Racial Background and Income, 1977*

Ethnic/Racial Background	Percent Uninsured during Year	Percent Always Uninsured	Percent Uninsured Part of Year
White, all incomes	14.0	7.0	7.0
Poor	27.1	13.5	13.6
Other low income	21.0	10.9	10.1
Middle income	12.6	6.3	6.3
High income	8.8	4.2	4.6
Black, all incomes	23.2	9.7	13.5
Poor	32.2	10.6	21.6
Other low income	26.6	11.9	14.7
Middle income	17.4	8.6	8.8
High income	12.4	7.1	5.3
Hispanic, all incomes	24.3	12.8	11.5
Poor	29.6	9.5	20.1
Other low income	32.0	18.2	13.8
Middle income	17.7	12.4	5.3
High income	20.0	12.3	8.0

Source: Wilensky and Walden (1981).
*In 1977, the poverty level for a family of 4 was $8,000. Poor are defined as those whose family income was less than or equal to 125 percent of the 1977 poverty level. Other low income includes those whose income is 1.26 to 2 times the poverty level; middle income is 2.01 to 4 times the poverty level; and high income is 4.01 times the poverty level or more.

Thus, while the poor are obviously the least able to pay for care directly, they are the most likely to be without either Medicaid or private insurance. The poor are twice as likely to be uninsured as the middle class and three times as likely as those in upper income groups. Lack of insurance is inversely related to ability to bear the economic consequences of ill health.

Blacks, Hispanics, and other minorities are also more likely to be uninsured than whites regardless of their income; poor blacks are the most likely to be uninsured. As noted in Table 3, nearly one-third of poor blacks are uninsured during a year. If you are poor and a member of a minority group, your chances of being uninsured are four times as great as for a high income white.

Yet this relationship between race and income (Table 3) actually understates the situation because the aged are included in the population analyzed. The aged are overrepresented in the lower income groups, but, as noted in Table 1, almost all of the aged are insured. Thus, inclusion of the aged in Table 3 tends to overstate the insured status of the nonelderly poor.

Regional and racial differences in insurance coverage of the population under age 65 are enumerated in Table 4. When the aged are excluded from the analysis, the differentials become even more striking. Southerners are nearly 1½ times as likely to be uninsured as those from other parts of the country. But blacks in the South are 1½ times more likely to be uninsured as are whites from the South or nonsouthern blacks. Southern blacks are twice as likely to be uninsured as nonsouthern whites.

TABLE 4
Percent of Persons under Age 65
Uninsured during Year by Race and Residence, 1977

Race and Residence	Population (in millions)	Percent Uninsured during Year	Percent Always Uninsured	Percent Uninsured Part of Year
Total, all persons under 65	189.8	17.8%	9.5%	8.3%
South	60.5	22.4	12.7	9.7
White	47.9	20.4	11.8	8.6
Black and Other	12.6	30.0	16.2	13.8
Non-South	129.3	15.7	8.0	7.7
White	115.8	14.9	7.7	7.2
Black and Other	13.5	22.2	10.7	11.5
SMSA	132.6	16.3	8.2	8.1
White	111.3	14.9	7.6	7.3
Black and Other	21.3	23.2	11.1	12.1
Non-SMSA	57.2	21.4	12.5	8.9
White	52.5	19.9	11.6	8.3
Black and Other	4.7	38.2	23.3	14.9

Source: Data from the U.S. Department of Health and Human Services, National Center for Health Services Research, National Medical Care Expenditure Survey.

Similarly, when differences in insurance status are assessed from the perspective of metropolitan versus nonmetropolitan areas, blacks fare much worse than whites. Over 16 percent of nonelderly residents of Standard Metropolitan Statistical Areas (SMSAs) are uninsured compared with over 21 percent of those residing in non-SMSA areas. But, for minorities living outside SMSAs, almost 40 percent are uninsured—a rate twice that of whites residing in non-SMSA areas and 2½ times that of whites in SMSAs.

Thus, health insurance coverage in the U.S. is to some extent a matter of luck. Those fortunate enough to be employed by large, unionized, manufacturing firms are also likely to be fortunate enough to have good health insurance coverage. Those who are poor, those who live in the South or in rural areas, and those who are black or minority group members are more likely to bear the personal and economic effects of lack of insurance and the consequent financial barriers to health care.

Utilization of Health Services by the Uninsured

With the investment in primary care made by federal programs in the late 1960s and 1970s, significant progress in improving access to primary care for the poor and other disadvantaged groups was achieved. Virtually all of the numerous studies examining trends in access to health care conclude that differentials in utilization of physician services and preventive service by income have narrowed (Davis et al. 1981).

In the early 1960s the nonpoor visited physicians 23 percent more frequently than the poor even though the poor, then as now, were considerably sicker than the nonpoor. By the 1970s the poor visited physicians more frequently than the nonpoor, and more in accordance with their greater need for health care services. Blacks and other minorities also made substantial gains over this period. Utilization of services by rural residents also increased relative to urban residents (Davis and Schoen 1978).

However, use of preventive services by the poor, minorities, and rural residents continues to lag well behind use by those not facing similar barriers to health care. Some studies have also found that these differentials continue to exist for all disadvantaged groups even when adjusted for the greater health needs of the disadvantaged (Davis et al. 1981).

The major difficulty with past studies, however, is that they have not examined insurance coverage of subgroups of the poor to detect the cumulative impact of lack of financial and physical access to care. How do uninsured blacks in rural areas fare in obtaining ambulatory care services? Can nearly all disadvantaged persons get care from public hospitals or clinics, or do those facing multiple barriers to care simply do without?

Data and Methodology

New data from the 1977 National Medical Care Expenditure Survey (NMCES) shed some light on the cumulative effect of multiple barriers to care. Insured persons are those covered during the entire year; the uninsured are those uninsured for the entire year. Those insured for part of the year are excluded; presumably their utilization resembles that of the insured for the portion of the year in which they are insured and that of the uninsured for the portion of the year in which they are uninsured.

The NMCES sample was designed to produce statistically unbiased national estimates that are representative of the civilian noninstitutionalized population of the United States. Since the statistics presented here are based on a sample, they may differ somewhat from the figures that would have been obtained if a complete census had been taken. Tests of statistical significance are indicated in the tables included below (see Department of Health and Human Services 1982d, Technical Notes, for further detail on methodology). Particular caution should be taken in interpreting those data items for which the noted relative standard error is equal to or greater than 30 percent.

The statistics presented here show utilization differentials between insured and uninsured individuals under age 65. Analysis of age-specific differentials between the insured and uninsured showed patterns similar to the general pattern of the nonelderly population. The elderly were excluded from the analysis since the majority of the elderly population is insured.

Ambulatory Care

Most striking is the extent to which insurance coverage affects use of ambulatory care. Table 5 presents data on use of physicians' services from NMCES for the population under age 65; the insured average 3.7 visits to physicians during the year compared with 2.4 visits for the uninsured. That is, the insured receive 54 percent more ambulatory care from physicians than do the uninsured. However, the differential between the insured and uninsured for physician visits may understate the actual differential because variations in scope of coverage among the insured population are not accounted for. Some of the insured may only have insurance coverage for inpatient hospital care, not ambulatory care. Thus, although their utilization pattern is considered in the insured category, such individuals are actually uninsured for physician visits. Better data on ambulatory-

TABLE 5

**Physician Visits per Person under Age 65 per Year,
by Insurance Status, Residence, and Race, 1977**

Insurance Status, Residence, and Race	Uninsured	Insured	Ratio
Total	2.4	3.7	1.54*
South	2.1	3.5	1.67*
White	2.3	3.7	1.61*
Black and Other	1.5	2.8	1.87*
Non-South	2.6	3.8	1.46*
White	2.7	3.8	1.41*
Black and Other	1.9	3.5	1.84*
SMSA	2.4	3.8	1.58*
White	2.6	3.9	1.50*
Black and Other	1.7	3.2	1.88*
Non-SMSA	2.3	3.3	1.43*
White	2.4	3.4	1.42*
Black and Other	1.6	2.9	1.81

*indicates values for insured and uninsured are significantly different at the .05 level.
Source: Data from the U.S. Department of Health and Human Services, National Center for Health Services Research, National Medical Care Expenditure Survey.

care insurance coverage of the insured population therefore might indicate even greater differentials in use of ambulatory care.

Residence and race also affect utilization of ambulatory services. The lowest utilization of ambulatory care occurs for uninsured blacks and other minorities, including Hispanics. These persons use far less than more advantaged groups. For example, uninsured blacks and other minorities in the South make 1.5 physician visits per person annually, compared with 3.7 physician visits for insured whites in the South. That is, to be advantaged multiply leads to a utilization rate almost 2.5 times that of individuals who are disadvantaged multiply.

These data point to the importance of financial and physical barriers to access. It is not the case that the uninsured manage to obtain ambulatory care comparable in amount to that obtained by the insured by relying on public clinics, teaching hospital outpatient clinics, nonprofit health centers, or the charity of private physicians. Without insurance, many simply do without care.

The patterns of utilization for different groups provide some insight into the relative importance of financial, physical, and racial barriers to care. Financial access to care is clearly the most important factor affecting use. Insurance coverage reduces much but not all of the differential in use of ambulatory services. Insured blacks in the South, for example, average 2.8 physician visits annually, compared with 3.7 for insured whites in the South. That is, whites average about 30 percent more ambulatory care than blacks and other minorities even if both are insured. But this differential is substantially smaller than the 2½ times greater use of physicians between insured southern whites and uninsured southern blacks.

Location remains an important determinant of use of physician services. Lack of insurance coverage is more predominant in rural areas; however, even among the insured, urban residents are more likely to receive ambulatory care than are rural residents, whether white or black (see Table 5). Among insured groups, rural whites receive 3.4 physician visits annually compared with 3.9 visits for urban whites. Rural blacks and other minorities with insurance make 2.9 physician visits compared with 3.2 visits for their insured counterparts in urban areas. That is, a 10 to 15 percent differential in use between urban and rural areas occurs even when financial access to care is not a problem. It should be noted, however, that the quality of insurance for ambulatory care may not be as good in rural areas as in urban areas.

Racial differentials in utilization of ambulatory care are also ameliorated with insurance coverage. Insurance is particularly helpful in improving access to care for minorities. Insured minorities receive 80 to 90 percent more ambulatory care than do uninsured minorities, in both rural and urban areas. But even with insurance, strong racial differences persist.

Hospital Care

Despite the common perception that all disadvantaged persons can obtain hospital care from some charity facility, tremendous differentials in use of hospital care also exist by insurance status, residence, and race. The insured receive 90 percent more hospital care than do the uninsured (see Table 6). Differentials by insurance status are particularly marked in the South and in rural areas. In the South, insured persons receive three times as many days of hospital care annually as uninsured persons, regardless of race or ethnic background.

These hospital utilization differentials clearly demonstrate that the insured fare much better than the uninsured in obtaining health care services. Since those with insurance are likely to have basic coverage for hospitalization, the hospital utilization data provide a more accurate assessment of the role of insurance coverage in the use of health care services than do the ambulatory care differentials in the previous section.

These differentials remove any complacency about the accessibility of inpatient care. They reinforce similar findings by Wilensky and Berk (1982) who find that the insured poor use more hospital care than the uninsured poor. They find the biggest difference between those always uninsured and those on Medicaid all year. Those on Medicaid part of the year used fewer hospital services than those on Medicaid all year. The uninsured also used less hospital care than those privately insured. The analysis here extends these results to examine racial and regional differentials.

More disaggregated information is essential on the types of conditions for which the insured receive inpatient care and the

TABLE 6
Hospital Patient Days per 100 Persons under Age 65,
by Insurance Status, Residence, and Race, 1977

Insurance Status, Residence, and Race	Uninsured	Insured	Ratio
Total	47	90	1.91*
South	35	104	2.97*
White	33	100	3.03*
Black and Other	40†	119	2.98*
Non-South	56	84	1.50
White	51	81	1.59*
Black and Other	89†	114	1.28
SMSA	50	86	1.72*
White	44	83	1.89*
Black and Other	70†	106	1.51
Non-SMSA	42	99	2.36*
White	43	94	2.19*
Black and Other	39†	175	4.49*

*indicates values for insured and uninsured are significantly different at the .05 level.
†indicates relative standard error is equal to or greater than 30 percent.
Source: Data from the U.S. Department of Health and Human Services, National Center for Health Services Research, National Medical Care Expenditure Survey.

uninsured do not. Standards for appropriate utilization of hospital services are still the subject of wide debate. Some of the differential between the insured and uninsured seen here may be the result of overutilization of hospital services by the insured. However, this is unlikely to explain the entire differential.

Some of the greater utilization of hospital care by the insured may represent self-selection. Those who expect to be hospitalized may obtain such coverage. Hospitalization may itself result in Medicaid coverage of some of the poor and near-poor. However, this should affect primarily those who are insured part of the year and uninsured the remainder of the year. Such partially insured persons are excluded from this analysis. These explanations are unlikely to account for a three-fold differential in use.

Some of the results by region and race are surprising. It is interesting to note that outside the South uninsured blacks receive more hospital days per 100 persons than insured whites. Insured blacks have the highest use. This may reflect greater health problems among blacks, or the tendency of blacks to receive care in public hospitals which have longer stays. Another unexpected result is high hospitalization among insured blacks in nonmetropolitan areas. This is one of the smallest population groups in the study and results, in this case, may simply be statistically unreliable.

Barriers to access to hospital services for the uninsured need to be explored. To what extent do hospitals require preadmission deposits for the uninsured? What are the consequences of such policies on access to care? Which hospitals serve the uninsured and the insured? Do the differences between metropolitan and nonmetropolitan areas reflect the role of teaching hospitals and public hospitals in caring for the uninsured in the inner city? Do the uninsured have to travel sizeable distances to obtain services? What are the health problems of the insured and uninsured, for what conditions are the insured hospitalized but not the uninsured, and what are the health consequences of lack of hospital care for the uninsured? To what extent do any or all of these factors influence the use of hospital care by the uninsured? Further exploration is certainly warranted.

Health Status and Use of Services

Lower utilization of ambulatory and inpatient care by the uninsured is not a reflection of lower need for health care services. Instead, as measured by self-assessment of health status, the uninsured tend to be somewhat sicker than the insured. Fifteen percent of the uninsured under age 65 rate their health as fair or poor, compared with 11 percent of the insured. Blacks and other minorities in the South systematically rate their health the worst. Of insured blacks and other minorities in the South, 19 percent assess their health as fair or poor, compared with 9 percent of insured whites outside the South.

One possible explanation of the higher rate of poor or fair health among the uninsured is that the lack of insurance is itself related to health status. Those who rate their health as poor or fair are more likely to be unable to work because of illness than those who rate their health good or excellent. Since insurance coverage in the United States is related to employment, those who are unemployed due to poor health are also likely to be without insurance. Under an employment-based insurance system, the working population enjoys both good health and insurance coverage, while those too ill to work suffer both lack of employment and lack of insurance.

The sick who are uninsured use medical care services less than their insured counterparts. Utilization of ambulatory services, adjusted for health status, shows that the insured in poor health see a physician 70 percent more often than the uninsured in poor health. Physician visits per person under age 65 in fair or poor health average 6.9 among the insured, compared with 4.1 visits for the uninsured with similar health problems (Table 7).

TABLE 7
Physician Visits per Person under Age 65
in Fair or Poor Health per Year,
by Insurance Status, Residence, and Race, 1977

Insurance Status, Residence, and Race	Uninsured	Insured	Ratio
Total	4.1	6.9	1.68*
South	3.8	6.1	1.61*
White	4.4	6.4	1.45*
Black and Other	2.2†	5.0	2.27
Non-South	4.5	7.4	1.64*
White	4.6	7.6	1.65*
Black and Other	3.5†	6.5	1.86
SMSA	4.1	7.2	1.76*
White	4.7	7.6	1.62*
Black and Other	2.3†	5.9	2.57
Non-SMSA	4.2	6.3	1.50
White	4.3	6.4	1.49
Black and Other	3.2†	5.4	1.69

*indicates values for insured and uninsured are significantly different at the .05 level.
†indicates relative standard error is equal to or greater than 30 percent.
Source: Data from the U.S. Department of Health and Human Services, National Center for Health Services Research, National Medical Care Expenditure Survey.

Blacks and other minorities with fair or poor health who are insured receive twice as much care as their uninsured counterparts.

Among the uninsured in poor or fair health, the differentials in physician visits by race and residence are especially noteworthy. Uninsured whites have greater access to physician services than do uninsured minorities. A southern white in fair or poor health sees a physician twice as often as a southern minority person in fair or poor health. The same relationship exists for utilization of physician services in metropolitan areas. However, the utilization differential between whites and minorities narrows in areas outside the South and in nonmetropolitan areas.

The number of physician visits by the uninsured versus the insured in fair or poor health warrants further examination. It is expected that the individual in fair or poor health would require frequent physician visits for diagnosis and treatment of the condition. The average of five to seven visits annually by the insured would appear to provide a reasonable level of physician contact. But for uninsured minorities in the South in fair or poor health, the average number of visits is two per year. This rate would provide no more than an initial visit and one follow-up visit, which might be insufficient to treat serious or complex illnesses. Thus, lower rates of physician visits could impair adequate treatment and follow-up to promote a rapid recovery.

Dental Care

Dental care, unlike hospital care and most physician services, is not covered under most insurance plans. Therefore, differentials in dental visits between the insured and uninsured are not meaningful. However, the NMCES data do show a striking contrast between dental visits by whites and minorities.

Whites obtain dental care twice as often as minorities, averaging 1.5 visits per year compared to 0.7 visits for minorities. Nonsouthern whites had two times the number of visits as nonsouthern minorities and over three times the number of visits as southern minorities. Rural minorities appear to have the least access to dental services.

The significant differential between access to dental services for minorities and whites warrants further examination. The extent to which this differential reflects differences in health practices and attitudes toward dental care or differences in availability and accessibility to dental care should be explored.

Usual Source of Care

The NMCES data confirm other studies that have found that disadvantaged groups are less likely to have a usual source of ambulatory care and more likely to receive their care from a hospital outpatient department or a clinic than from a physician's office. Table 8, for example, enumerates that 84 percent of the insured have a physician's office as their usual source of care compared with 67 percent of the uninsured. About 50 percent of uninsured blacks and other minorities have a physician's office as their usual source of care. While this percentage is quite low in comparison with other groups, it does not fit the stereotype that all minorities in urban areas receive the bulk of their care from public facilities or hospital outpatient departments.

Uninsured residents of nonmetropolitan areas are more likely to have a physician as a usual source of care than are residents of a metropolitan area. In nonmetropolitan areas, 73 percent of the uninsured have a physician as a usual source of care in contrast to only 63 percent of the uninsured in metropolitan areas. However, nonmetropolitan residents are still likely to have fewer physician visits than their metropolitan counterparts (see Table 5). The nonmetropolitan uninsured get more of their care from physicians but receive less total care. These differences in utilization among the uninsured undoubtedly reflect differences between metropolitan and nonmetropolitan areas in the availability of alternatives to physician care. Residents of metropolitan areas are more likely to have access to clinic and outpatient hospital services that can substitute for care in physicians' offices.

The metropolitan and nonmetropolitan differential for physicians as a usual source of care is markedly reduced among the insured. As seen in Table 8, 86 percent of insured nonmetropolitan residents and 82 percent of insured metropolitan residents have a physician as a usual source of care. Insurance coverage significantly increases the proportion of minorities who have a physician's office as their usual source of care. Among the minority uninsured, 49 percent of those living in

TABLE 8
Percent of Persons under Age 65
Whose Usual Source of Care Is a Physician's Office,
by Insurance Status, Residence, and Race, 1977

Insurance Status, Residence, and Race	Uninsured	Insured	Ratio
Total	67	84	1.25*
South	66	81	1.22*
White	70	82	1.16*
Black and Other	53	76	1.41*
Non-South	68	85	1.25*
White	70	86	1.22*
Black and Other	45	69	1.53*
SMSA	63	82	1.31*
White	66	84	1.27*
Black and Other	49	71	1.43*
Non-SMSA	73	86	1.19*
White	76	87	1.15*
Black and Other	52	79	1.53*

*indicates values for insured and uninsured are significantly different at the .05 level.
Source: Data from the U.S. Department of Health and Human Services, National Center for Health Services Research, National Medical Care Expenditure Survey.

metropolitan areas and 52 percent of those in nonmetropolitan areas have a physician as a usual source of care. In contrast, for insured minorities, 71 percent in metropolitan areas and 79 percent outside of metropolitan areas have physicians as a usual source of care. This would suggest that Medicaid and private health insurance coverage enable a substantial number of minorities to obtain care in a physician's office.

Convenience of Care

When they are able to obtain care, the uninsured must travel longer distances than the insured to obtain it. As enumerated in Table 9, 25 percent of the uninsured travel 30 minutes or more to obtain care compared with 18 percent of the insured. Differentials in travel time between the insured and uninsured are somewhat more marked in rural areas than in urban areas, but travel time is a problem for uninsured persons everywhere. These data suggest not only that the uninsured receive less care, but also that when they do obtain care they do so by searching over a longer distance for providers willing to see them. The effort involved in such a search for care may discourage the use of preventive services, resulting in the uninsured only seeking care for serious illness or in crises. This would help explain the lower utilization levels of the uninsured.

When the uninsured arrive at a care provider, they generally have to wait longer for care to be delivered. Regardless of residence, the waiting time for insured blacks and other minorities is longer than the waiting time experienced by uninsured whites. Waiting times are longer in the South. Uninsured southern minority persons experience the longest waiting times. The

TABLE 9

**Percent of Persons under Age 65 Traveling
More Than 29 Minutes to Receive Medical Care,
by Insurance Status, Residence, and Race, 1977**

Insurance Status, Residence, and Race	Uninsured	Insured	Ratio
Total	25	18	1.39*
South	29	21	1.39*
White	30	20	1.48*
Black and Other	28	26	1.09
Non-South	21	16	1.29*
White	22	16	1.35*
Black and Other	17	21	.81
SMSA	22	17	1.27*
White	21	16	1.32*
Black and Other	24	24	1.00
Non-SMSA	29	20	1.46*
White	30	20	1.50*
Black and Other	23	19	1.24

*indicates values for insured and uninsured are significantly different at the .05 level.
Source: Data from the U.S. Department of Health and Human Services, National Center for Health Services Research, National Medical Care Expenditure Survey.

NMCES data show that they wait one-third longer than do insured southern whites (Department of Health and Human Services 1982a).

Policy Implications

The utilization differentials between the insured and uninsured underscore the importance of financial barriers to health care. Lack of insurance coverage is the major barrier. It markedly affects the amount of both ambulatory and inpatient care received. Without insurance coverage, many individuals obviously do without care. Those able to obtain care incur substantial travel and waiting times.

Lack of insurance coverage has three major consequences: it contributes to unnecessary pain, suffering, disability, and even death among the uninsured; it places a financial burden on those uninsured who struggle to pay burdensome medical bills; and it places a financial strain on hospitals, physicians, and other health care providers who attempt to provide care to the uninsured.

Research is limited on both the health of the uninsured and the health consequences of having no insurance. Extensive data on utilization patterns by the uninsured disaggregated by residence and race are presented for virtually the first time in this report. But a number of recent studies have shown that medical care utilization has a dramatic impact on health. A recent Urban Institute report by Hadley (1982) explores the relation between medical care utilization and mortality rates. It contains persuasive evidence that utilization of medical care services leads to a marked reduction in mortality rates. A recent study by Grossman and Goldman (1981) at the National Bureau of Economic Research has found that infant mortality rates have dropped significantly in communities served by federally funded community health centers. This growing body of evidence does provide considerable support to the importance of medical care utilization in assuring a healthy population—and at least indirectly provides a basis for concern that the lower medical care utilization of the uninsured contributes to unnecessary deaths and lowered health status.

Lack of insurance coverage also imposes serious financial burdens on those who try to make regular payments to retire enormous debts incurred in obtaining medical care. With the average cost of a hospital stay in the United States now in excess of $2,000, few individuals can afford to build payments for hospital care into their monthly living allowance (Department of Health and Human Services 1982b). Yet, since the uninsured are more likely to be poor, the economic consequences of lack of insurance fall heaviest on those least able to bear the burden.

In addition to its consequences for the uninsured, lack of insurance also takes its toll on the health care system. One result is that the financial stability of hospitals and ambulatory care providers willing to provide charity care for those unable to pay is jeopardized. Health care providers serving the uninsured—particularly inner city community and teaching hospitals, county and municipal clinics, and community health centers—absorb much of the cost of this as charity care or a bad debt. Yet this burden is not evenly distributed among hospitals and other providers. A recent study by the Urban Institute found that one-seventh of a national sample of hospitals studied provided over 40 percent of the free care (Brazda 1982).

Recent policy measures are likely to exacerbate this situation. The Omnibus Budget Reconciliation Act of 1981 reduced federal financial participation in Medicaid and curtailed eligibility under the Aid to Families with Dependent Children (AFDC) program. Actions by state governments in response to this legislation could swell the ranks of the uninsured poor by over 1 million people. Coupled with the highest rate of unemployment since the Great Depression and the loss of health insurance coverage frequently occurring with unemployment, the number of uninsured continues to rise. Undoubtedly the situation has worsened rather than improved since the NMCES study in 1977. Today, the access problems of the uninsured should be a pressing concern on the nation's health agenda.

For many of the uninsured, community health centers and migrant health centers have helped to fill the gap in access created by the lack of insurance. This was especially important for those ineligible for Medicaid. However, simultaneously with the cutbacks in Medicaid, major reductions were made in these service delivery programs. Overall funding was reduced by 25 percent in absolute dollars, which may lead to 1.1 million fewer people being served than the 6 million served in 1980. The National Health Service Corps, while not as seriously affected now, will be substantially reduced in future years since no new scholarships are being awarded with commitments for service in underserved areas (Davis 1981).

Financial strains on public hospitals and clinics supported by state and local governments are leading to further curtailment of services. Preadmission deposits, often sizeable in amount, impose serious barriers for many of the uninsured seeking hospital care. Teaching hospitals that have for years maintained an open-door policy are reevaluating the fiscal viability of continuing such a policy. In many areas, hospitals are beginning to transfer nonpaying patients to public facilities, further expanding the charity load of those facilities and reducing their ability to remain solvent (Brazda 1982).

Public hospitals, traditionally the care provider of last resort, are under new pressures to close or reduce services as local governments respond to shrinking revenues. Yet, shifting the responsibility of public hospitals to community hospitals will not solve the problem of caring for the uninsured. Recent hearings have documented the refusal of community hospitals to take uninsured patients, even in emergency situations. This has led to documented cases of deaths that could have been avoided with prompt medical attention (U.S. Congress. House. Committee on Energy and Commerce 1981).

Such disparities in access to care are unacceptable in a decent and humane society. Several actions are required to assure progress toward adequate access for all. Medicaid coverage should be expanded to provide basic insurance coverage for all low-income individuals. The Medicaid programs in southern states have tended to have very restrictive eligibility policies leaving many of the poor uncovered (Department of Health and Human Services 1982c). Expanded coverage of the poor through Medicaid would improve the scope of coverage in the South and could help to alleviate some of the extreme utilization differentials between the South and non-South. A minimum income standard set at some percentage of the poverty level would be an important first step. In 1979, 23 states, including most of the southern states, had income eligibility levels for Medicaid below 55 percent of the poverty level. Texas, Alabama, and Tennessee had the lowest standards in the nation—less than $2,000 for a family of four. Coupled with implementation of a minimum income standard, Medicaid coverage should be broadened to include children and ultimately adults in two-parent families. Such steps would help assure access to care for the nation's poorest families.

Yet, the near-poor and working poor without insurance cannot be forgotten. Today, under Medicaid, only 29 states cover the medically needy to provide health coverage for those with large medical expenses. In effect, this catastrophe coverage provides some measure of protection to working families and is undoubtedly the source of care for many of the "sometimes insured." Coverage for the medically needy is currently very limited in the South; implementation of coverage for the medically needy would be another step toward reducing the disparities between the South and the rest of the country. Expansion of this coverage option is an important component of a positive health care agenda.

Finally, the extensiveness of unemployment in today's economy underscores the need to refine the link between employment and health insurance coverage. "Out of work" ought not to translate to "without health care services." Often, health needs are greatest during periods of stress related to unemployment (Brenner 1973; Lee 1979). Health insurance coverage should be extended through employer plans for a period following unemployment, and guaranteed through public coverage until reemployment. Employers should also be encouraged to provide comprehensive coverage, including prevention and primary care services, to all workers and their families.

These measures would help to provide protection and improved access to care for the 34 million or more Americans now without health care insurance. However, as the metropolitan and nonmetropolitan differentials among the insured demonstrate, financing alone is not enough to correct access differentials. Resources development must be coupled with improved financing in underserved areas to assure that needed providers are available. Continued funding and expansion of the community and migrant health center programs to assure physical access to services for residents of high poverty, medically underserved communities is an essential adjunct to broadened financing for low-income populations. Other important ways to provide expanded insurance coverage without perpetuating the cost inefficiencies of the existing system include: reform of Medicaid, Medicare, and private health insurance plans to encourage ambulatory care in cost-effective primary care programs; and experimentation with capitation payments to individual primary care centers, networks of centers, hospitals, or other major primary care providers for providing ambulatory and inpatient services to Medicaid beneficiaries.

This agenda of improved financing and resource development represents a positive strategy that can be employed to reduce major inequities in American health care. Today, some will argue that this agenda is too ambitious and costly and would instead opt for a more targeted and incremental approach. For example, instead of expanding Medicaid coverage, advocates of the incremental approach would favor renewed support to public hospitals and financial aid to hospitals serving large numbers of uninsured to mitigate the worst problems. These approaches are piecemeal, however, and do not address the fundamental problems identified in this paper. Such targeted approaches focus on protecting institutions serving the uninsured rather than protecting the uninsured themselves. Thus, they provide for the continued existence of a source of care for the uninsured seeking care, but do not provide comprehensive coverage to the uninsured to encourage early and preventive services. The poor and uninsured who do without care either because they do not live near an "aided facility" or do not know they could obtain free care from a hospital with a financial distress loan would still suffer inequitable health care differentials.

This paper demonstrates that lack of insurance makes a difference in health care utilization. Studies such as the recent work by Hadley (1982) point out the positive impact of medical care on mortality. Society ultimately bears the burden for care of the uninsured. The choice is between paying up front and directly covering the uninsured or indirectly paying for their care through subsidies to fiscally troubled health facilities, higher insurance premiums, and increased hospital costs to cover the cost of charity care and pay for the ill health caused by neglect and inadequate preventive and primary care. Thus, the best and most pragmatic approach is to provide health insurance coverage to the uninsured and to use targeted approaches to improve resource distribution and to remove remaining differentials. The inequities in health care in the United States described here will deepen unless a positive agenda is pursued.

NOTES

Brazda, J., ed. 1982. Perspectives: Who Will Care for the Uninsured? (September 27) *Washington Report on Medicine and Health* 36 (38, Sept. 27): unpaged insert.

Brenner, H. 1973. *Mental Illness and the Economy*. Cambridge: Harvard University Press.

Davis, K. 1975. *National Health Insurance: Benefits, Costs, and Consequences*. Washington: Brookings Institution.

———. 1981. Reagan Administration Health Policy. (December). *Journal of Public Health Policy* 2(4):312–32.

———. 1982. Medicare Reconsidered. Paper presented at Duke University Medical Center Private Sector Conference on the Financial Support of Health Care of the Elderly and the Indigent, March 14–16.

Davis, K., and C. Schoen. 1978 *Health and the War on Poverty: A Ten Year Appraisal*. Washington: Brookings Institution.

Davis, K., M. Gold, and D. Makuc. 1981. Access to Health Care for the Poor: Does the Gap Remain? *Annual Review of Public Health* 2:159–82.

Department of Health and Human Services. 1982a. National Medical Care Expenditure Survey, 1977. Unpublished Statistics. Hyattsville, Md.: National Center for Health Services Research.

———. 1982b. *Health Care Financing Trends*, June. Baltimore: Health Care Financing Administration.

———. 1982c. *Medicare and Medicaid Data Book 1981*. Baltimore: Health Care Financing Administration.

———. 1982d. Usual Sources of Medical Care and Their Characteristics, Data Preview 12. Hyattsville, Md.: National Center for Health Services Research.

Grossman, M., and F. Goldman. 1981. The Responsiveness and Impacts of Public Health Policy: The Case of Community Health Centers. Paper presented at the 109th Annual Meeting of the American Public Health Association, Los Angeles, November.

Health Centers. Paper presented at the 109th Annual Meeting of the American Public Health Association, Los Angeles, November.

Hadley, J. 1982. *More Medical Care, Better Health?* Washington: Urban Institute.

Institute of Medicine. 1981. *Health Care in a Context of Civil Rights.* Washington: National Academy Press.

Kasper, J.A., D.C. Walden, and G.R. Wilensky. 1978. *Who Are the Uninsured?* National Medical Care Expenditures Survey Data Preview no. 1. Hyattsville, Md.: National Center for Health Services Research.

Lee, A.J. 1979. *Employment, Unemployment, and Health Insurance.* Cambridge, Mass.: Abt Books.

Rowland, D., and C. Gaus. 1983. Medicaid Eligibility and Benefits: Current Policies and Alternatives. In *New Approaches to the Medicaid Crisis,* ed. R. Blendon and T.W. Moloney. New York: Frost and Sullivan.

Taylor, A.K., and W.R. Lawson. 1981. Employer and Employee Expenditures for Private Health Insurance. National Medical Care Expenditures Survey Data Preview 7. Hyattsville, Md.: National Center for Health Services Research, June.

U.S. Congress. House. Committee on Energy and Commerce, U.S. House of Representatives. 1981. *Hearings on Medicaid Cutbacks on Infant Care.* Washington, 27 July.

Wilensky, G.R., and M.L. Berk. 1982. The Health Care of the Poor and the Role of Medicaid. *Health Affairs* 1(4):93–100.

Wilensky, G.R., and D.C. Walden. 1981. Minorities, Poverty, and the Uninsured. Paper presented at the 109th Meeting of the American Public Health Association, Los Angeles, November. Hyattsville Md.: National Center for Health Services Research.

Acknowledgments: This paper was prepared for the President's Commission for the Study of Ethical Problems in Medicine and Biomedical and Behavioral Research. We gratefully acknowledge the assistance of Susan Morgan and Kathryn Kelly of the commission staff, and reviewers for helpful comments. We also thank Gail Wilensky and Daniel C. Walden of the National Center for Health Services Research for supplying requested data and assisting in its interpretation, and Karen Pinkston and Mary Frances leMat of Social and Scientific Systems, Inc. for programming support.

The System
Behind the Chaos

Barbara and John Ehrenreich

THE American health crisis became official in 1969. President
Nixon announced it in a special message in July. Liberal academic observers of the health scene, from Harvard's John
Knowles to Einstein College of Medicine's Martin Cherkasky,
hastened to verify the existence of the crisis. Now the media is
rushing in with details and documentation. *Time, Fortune, Business Week,* CBS, and NBC are on the medical scene, and
finding it "chaotic," "archaic," and "unmanageable."

For the great majority of Americans, the "health care crisis"
is not a TV show or a presidential address; it is an on-going
crisis of survival. Every day three million Americans go out in
search of medical care. Some find it; others do not. Some are
helped by it; others are not. Another twenty million Americans
probably ought to enter the daily search for medical help, but
are not healthy enough, rich enough, or enterprising enough to
try. The obstacles are enormous. Health care is scarce and
expensive to begin with. It is dangerously fragmented, and
usually offered in an atmosphere of mystery and unaccountability. For many, it is obtained only at the price of humiliation,
dependence, or bodily insult. The stakes are high—health, life,
beauty, sanity—and getting higher all the time. But the odds of
winning are low and getting lower.

From *The American Health Empire: Power, Profits and Politics.* Copyright ©
1970 by Health Policy Advisory Center, Inc. Reprinted by permission of Random
House, Inc.

For the person in search of medical help, the illness or possibility of illness which prompted the search is quickly overshadowed by the difficulties of the medical experience itself:

Problem One: Finding a Place Where the Appropriate Care Is Offered at a Reasonable Price

For the poor and for many working-class people, this can be all but impossible. Not long ago it was commonly believed that sheer distance from doctors or hospitals was a problem only in rural areas. But today's resident of slums like Brooklyn's Bedford-Stuyvesant, or Chicago's south side, is as effectively removed from health services as his relatives who stayed behind in Mississippi. One region of Bedford-Stuyvesant contains only one practicing physician for a population of one hundred thousand. Milwaukee County Hospital, the sole source of medical care for tens of thousands of poor and working-class people, is sixteen miles outside the city, an hour and a half bus ride for many. A few years ago, a social science graduate student was able to carry out her thesis work on rural health problems in a densely populated Chicago slum.

After getting to the building or office where medical care is offered, the next problem which affects both poor and middle-class people is paying for the care. Except at a diminishing number of charitable facilities, health care is not free; it is a commodity which consumers purchase from providers at unregulated, steadily increasing prices. Insurance plans like Medicaid, Medicare, and Blue Cross help soften the blow for many, but many other people are too rich for Medicaid, too poor for Blue Cross, and too young for Medicare. A total of twenty-four million Americans have no health insurance of any variety. Even for those who are insured, costs remain a major problem: first there is the cost of the insurance itself, then there is the cost of all those services which are not covered by insurance. About 102 million Americans have no insurance coverage for visits to the doctor, as opposed to hospital stays. They spend about ten dollars just to see a doctor; more, if laboratory tests or specialists are needed. Otherwise, they wait for an illness to become serious enough to warrant hospitalization. Hardly anyone, of course, has insurance for such everyday needs as dental care or prenatal care.

Supposing that one can afford the cost of the care itself, there remains the problem of paying for the time spent getting it. Working people must plan on losing a full workday for a simple doctor's appointment, whether with a private physician or at a hospital clinic. First, there is a long wait to see the doctor. Middle-class people may enjoy comfortable chairs, magazines, and even coffee, while waiting in their doctor's anteroom, but they wait just the same. As busy private doctors try to squeeze more and more customers into their day, their patients are finding that upwards of an hour's wait is part of the price for a five- or ten-minute face-to-face encounter with a harried physician.

Not all kinds of care are as available, or unavailable, as others. In a city studded with major hospitals the person with multiple bullet wounds or a rare and fatal blood disease stands a far better chance of making a successful medical "connection" than the person with stomach pains, or the parents of a feverish child. Hospitals, at all times, and physicians, after 7:00 P.M. (if they can be located) are geared to handling the dramatic and exotic cases which excite professional interest. The more mundane, or less obviously catastrophic, case can wait—and wait. For psychiatric problems, which are probably the nation's single greatest source of disability, there are almost no outpatient facilities, much less sympathetic attention, when one finds them. Those of the mentally ill who venture forth in search of help are usually rewarded with imprisonment in a state institution, except for the few who are able to make the investment required for private psychiatric care. Even for the wealthy, borderline problems, like alcoholism and addiction, may as well be lived with—there are vanishingly few facilities of any kind to deal with them.

Problem Two: Finding One's Way Amidst the Many Available Types of Medical Care

Most of us know what buildings or other locations are possible sources of medical help. Many of us can even arrange to get to these buildings in a reasonable amount of time. But, having arrived at the right spot, the patient finds that his safari has just begun. He must now chop through the tangled morass of medical specialization. The only system to American health services, the patient discovers, is the system used in preparing the tables of contents of medical textbooks. Everything is arranged according to the various specialties and subspecialties doctors study, not according to the symptoms and problems which patients perceive.

The middle-class patient is relatively lucky. He has a private doctor who can serve as a kind of guide. After an initial examination, which may cost as little as five dollars or as much as fifty dollars, the patient's personal doctor sends him to visit a long list of his specialist colleagues—a hematologist, allergist, cardiologist, endocrinologist, and maybe a urologist. Each of these examines his organ of interest, collects twenty dollars and up, and passes the patient along to the next specialist in line. If the patient is lucky, his illness will be claimed by one of the specialists fairly early in the process. If he is not so lucky, none of them will claim it, or—worse yet—several of them will. Only the very wealthy patient can afford the expense of visiting and retaining two medical specialists.

The hospital clinic patient wanders about in the same jungle, but without a guide. The hospital may screen him for his ills and point him in the right direction, but, from then on, he's on his own. There's nobody to take overall responsibility for his illness. He can only hope that at some point in time and space, one of the many specialty clinics to which he has been sent (each at the cost of a day off from work) will coincide with his disease of the moment.

Just as exasperating as the fragmentation of medical care is the fragmentation of medical care financing. Seymour Thaler, a

New York state senator from Queens, likes to tell the story of one of his constituents who came to Thaler's office, pulled out his wallet, and emptied out a stack of cards. "Here's my Medicaid card, my Medicare card, my Blue Cross supplementary card, my workmen's compensation card, and my union retirement health plan card." "So what are you complaining about?" Thaler asked. "I've got a stomach ache," the old man answered, "so what do I do?"

A family makes matters even more complicated and confusing. Grandparents have Medicare, children have Medicaid, the parents may have one or several union hospitalization insurance plans. No one is covered for everything, and no mother is sure just who is covered for what. If three members of the family came down with the same illness, they would more than likely end up seeing three different doctors, paying for it in three (or more) different ways, and staying in separate hospitals. In 1968, a New York father of six quit his job and applied for welfare, claiming he couldn't work and see to his children's health care. One child, diagnosed as retarded, had to be taken to and from a special school each day. All required dental care, which was free at a Health Department clinic on Manhattan's lower east side. For dental surgery, however, they went to a clinic a bus ride away, at Bellevue. The youngest children went to a neighborhood pediatrician who accepted Medicaid patients. An older child, with a rare metabolic defect, required weekly visits to a private hospital clinic a half hour's trip uptown. The father himself, the victim of a chronic back problem, qualified for care at a union health center on the west side. For him, family health maintenance was a full-time job, not, as it is for most parents, just a busy sideline.

Doctors like to tell us that fragmentation is the price of quality. We should be happy to be seeing a specialist, twice as happy to be seeing two of them, and fully gratified to have everyone in the family seeing a special one of his own. In many difficult cases, specialization does pay off. But evidence is accumulating that care which is targeted at a particular organ often completely misses the mark. Take the case of the Cleveland woman who had both a neurological disease and a damaged kidney. Since the neurologist had no time to chat, and since she assumed that doctors know a good deal more than their patients, she never mentioned her kidney to her neurologist. Over a period of time, her urologist noted a steady deterioration of her kidney problem. Only after the kidney had been removed did the urologist discover that his colleague, the neurologist, had been prescribing a drug which is known to put an extra strain on the kidney.

The patient may have only one problem—as far as his doctors are concerned—and still succumb to medical fragmentation. Recently, an elderly man with a heart condition was discharged from a prestigious private medical center, assured he was good for another decade or two. Four weeks later he died of heart failure. Cause? Overexertion. He lived on the fifth floor of a walk-up apartment—a detail which was obviously out of the purview of his team of hospital physicians, for all the time and technology they had brought to bear on his heart. Until human physiology adapts itself to the fragmentation of modern medical practice, it is up to the patient himself to integrate his medical problems, and to integrate them with the rest of his life.

Problem Three: Figuring Out What They Are Doing to You

Many people are not satisfied to have found the correct doctor or clinic. They also want to know what is being done to their bodies, and why. For most, this is not just idle curiosity. If the patient has to pay all or some of the bill, he wants to know whether a cheaper treatment would be just as efficacious, or whether he should really be paying for something much fancier. The doctors' magazine *Medical Economics* tells the story of the family whose infant developed bronchopneumonia. The physician who visited the home judged from the furnishings that the family could not afford hospitalization. With little or no explanation, he prescribed an antibiotic and left. The baby died six hours later. The parents were enraged when they learned the diagnosis and realized that hospitalization might have helped. They wanted to know the risks, and make the decision themselves.

More commonly, the patients fear they will be overtreated, hence overbilled, for a medical problem. A twenty-five-year-old graduate student, a victim of hayfever, was told by an allergist at prestigious New York Hospital that his case would require several years of multiple, weekly, antiallergy injections. When he asked to know the probability that this treatment would actually cure his hayfever, the allergist told him, "I'm the doctor, not you, and if you don't want to trust my judgment you can find another doctor—or be sick forever for all I care!" Following this advice, the patient did, indeed, find a new doctor. And when the limitations of the treatment were explained to him, he decided the treatment was probably worth the trouble after all. The important thing is that *he* decided.

Some people, perhaps more trusting of doctors, never ask for an explanation until they have to in sheer self-defense. Residents of Manhattan's lower east side tell the story of the woman who was admitted to a ward at Bellevue for a stomach operation. The operation was scheduled for Thursday. On Wednesday a nurse told her she was to be operated on that day. The patient asked why the change. "Never mind," said the nurse, "give me your glasses." The patient could not see why she should give up her glasses, but finally handed them over at the nurse's insistence. Inside the operating room, the patient was surprised when she was not given general anesthesia. Although her English was poor, she noticed that the doctors were talking about eye cancer, and looking at her eyes. She sat up and said there was nothing wrong with her eyes—her stomach was the problem. She was pushed back on the operating table. With the strength of panic, she leapt up and ran into the hall. A security guard caught her, running sobbing down the hall in an operating gown. She was summarily placed in the psychiatric ward for a week's observation.

Even when confronted with what seems to be irrational therapy, most patients feel helpless to question or complain. A new folklore of medicine has emerged, rivaling that of the old witch doctors. Medical technology, from all that the patient has read in the newspapers, is as complex and mystifying as space technology. Physicians, from all he has seen on TV serials or heard thirdhand from other patients, are steely-nerved, omniscient, medical astronauts. The patient himself is usually sick-feeling, often undressed, a nameless observer in a process which he can never hope to understand. He has been schooled by all the news of medical "space shots"—heart transplants, renal dialysis, wonder drugs, nuclear therapy, etc.—to expect some small miracle in his own case—a magical new prescription drug or an operation. And miracles, by their very nature, are not explainable or understandable. Whether it's a "miracle detergent," a "miracle mouth wash," or a "miracle medical treatment," the customer can only pay the price and hope the product works.

Problem Four: Getting a Hearing If Things Don't Go Right

Everything about the American medical system seems calculated to maintain the childlike, dependent, and depersonalized condition of the patient. It is bad enough that modern medical technology has been infused by its practitioners with all the mystery and unaccountability of primitive shamanism. What is worse is that the patient is given absolutely no means of judging what care he should get or evaluating what he has gotten. As one Washington, D.C., taxi driver put it, "When I buy a used car, I know it might be a gyp. But I go over it, test it, try to figure out if it's O.K. for the price. Then take last year when I got started getting some stomach problem. The doctor says I need an operation. How do I know I need an operation? But what can I do—I have an operation. Later I get the bill—$1700—and Blue Cross left over $850 for me to pay. How should I know whether the operation should cost $50 or $1700? Now I think my stomach problem is coming back. Do I get my money back?"

Doctors and hospitals have turned patients into "consumers," but patients have none of the rights or protections which consumers of other goods and services expect. People in search of medical care cannot very easily do comparative shopping. When they're sick, they take help wherever they can get it. Besides, patients who switch doctors more than once are viewed by other doctors as possible neurotics. Health consumers know what they'd like—good health—but they have no way of knowing what this should entail in terms of services—a new diet, a prescription, or a thousand-dollar operation. Once they've received the service, the doctor, not their own perception, tells them whether it did any good. And if they suspect that the price was unduly high, the treatment unnecessarily complicated or drastic, there is no one to turn to—no Better Business Bureau or Department of Consumer Protection.

When something goes really wrong—a person is killed or maimed in the course of medical treatment—there is still no formal avenue of recourse for the patient or his survivors. Middle-class people, who know the ropes and have some money to spend, can embark on a long and costly malpractice suit, and win, at best, a cash compensation for the damage done. But this process, like everything else in a person's encounter with doctors and hospitals, is highly individualistic, and has no pay-off in terms of the general health and safety of the community. For the poor, there is usually no resource at all short of open resistance. A Manhattan man, infuriated by his wife's treatment in the emergency room of New York's Beth Israel Medical Center, beat up the intern on duty. Another man, whose child died inexplicably at a big city public hospital, solitarily pickets City Hall summer after summer.

Problem Five: Overcoming the Built-in Racism and Male Chauvinism of Doctors and Hospitals

In the ways that it irritates, exhausts, and occasionally injures patients, the American medical system is not egalitarian. Everything that is bad about American medicine is especially so for Americans who are not male or white. Blacks, and in some areas Native Americans or Hispanics, face unique problems of access to medical care, and not just because they are poor. Many hospitals in the south are still unofficially segregated, or at least highly selective. For instance, in towns outside of Orangeburg, South Carolina, blacks claim they are admitted to the hospital only on the recommendation of a (white) employer or other white "reference."

In the big cities of the north, health facilities are available on a more equal footing to blacks, browns, and poor whites. But for the nonwhite patient, the medical experience is more likely to be something he will not look forward to repeating. The first thing he notices about the large hospital—he is more likely to be at a hospital clinic than at a private doctor's office—is that the doctors are almost uniformly white; the nonskilled workers are almost entirely brown or black. Thus the nonwhite patient enters the hospital at the bottom end of its social scale, quite aside from any personal racial prejudices the staff may harbor. And, in medicine, these prejudices take a particularly insulting form. Black and Hispanic patients complain again and again of literally being "treated like animals" by everyone from the clerks to the M.D.'s. Since blacks are assumed to be less sensitive than white patients, they get less privacy. Since blacks are assumed to be more ignorant than whites, they get less by way of explanation of what is happening to them. And since they are assumed to be irresponsible and forgetful, they are more likely to be given a drastic, one-shot treatment, instead of a prolonged regimen of drugs, or a restricted diet.

Only a part of this medical racism is due to the racist attitudes of individual medical personnel. The rest is "institutional racism," a built-in feature of the way medicine is learned and practiced in the United States. As interns and residents, young doctors get their training by practicing on the hospital ward and clinic patients—generally nonwhite. Later they make their money by practicing for a paying clientele—generally white. White patients are "customers"; black patients are "teaching material." White patients pay for care with their money; black patients pay with their dignity and their comfort. Clinic patients at the hospital affiliated with Columbia University's medical school recently learned this distinction in a particularly painful way. They had complained that anesthesia was never available in the dental clinic. Finally, a leak from one of the dental interns showed that this was an official policy: the patient's pain is a good guide to the dentist-in-training—it teaches him not to drill too deep. Anesthesia would deaden the pain and dull the intern's learning experience.

Hospitals' institutional racism clearly serves the needs of the medical system, but it is also an instrument of the racist, repressive impulses of the society at large. Black community organizations in New York have charged hospitals with "genocidal" policies toward the black community. Harlem residents tell of medical atrocities—cases where patients have unwittingly given their lives or their organs in the cause of medical research. A more common charge is that, to public hospital doctors, "the birth control method of choice for black women is the hysterectomy." Even some doctors admit that hysterectomies are often performed with pretty slim justification in ghetto hospitals. (After all, they can't be expected to take a pill every day, can they? And one less black baby is one less baby on welfare, isn't it?) If deaths from sloppy abortions run highest in the ghetto, it is partly because black women are afraid to go to the hospital for an abortion or for treatment following a sloppy abortion, fearing that an involuntary sterilization—all for "medical" reasons—will be the likely result. Aside from their medical policies, ghetto hospitals have a reputation as racist because they serve as police strongholds in the community. In the emergency room, cops often outnumber doctors. They interrogate the wounded—often before the doctor does, and pick up any vagrants, police brutality victims, drunks, or addicts who have mistakenly come in for help. In fact, during the 1964 riots in New York, the police used Harlem Hospital as a launching pad for their pacification measures.

Women are the other major group of Americans singled out for special treatment by the medical system. Just as blacks face a medical hierarchy dominated by whites, women entering a hospital or doctor's office encounter a heirarchy headed by men, with women as nurses and aides playing subservient, hand-maid roles. And in the medical system, women face all the male supremacist attitudes and superstitions that characterize American society in general—they are the victims of sexism, as blacks are of racism. Women are assumed to be incapable of understanding complex technological explanations, so they are not given any. Women are assumed to be emotional and "difficult," so they are often classified as neurotic well before physical illness has been ruled out. (Note how many tranquilizer ads in medical journals depict women, rather than men, as likely customers.) And women are assumed to be vain, so they are the special prey of the paramedical dieting, cosmetics, and plastic surgery businesses.

Everyone who enters the medical system in search of care quickly finds himself transformed into an object, a mass of organs and pathology. Women have a special handicap—they start out as "objects." Physicians, despite their supposed objectivity and clinical impersonality, share all the sexual hangups of other American men. The sick person who enters the gynecology clinic is the same sex as the sexual "object" who sells cars in the magazine ads. What makes matters worse is that a high proportion of routine medical care for women centers on the most superstitious and fantasy-ridden aspect of female physiology—the reproductive system. Women of all classes almost uniformly hate or fear their gynecologists. The gynecologist plays a controlling role in that aspect of their lives society values most, the sexual aspect—and he knows it. Middle-class women find a man who is either patronizingly jolly, or cold and condescending. Poorer women, using clinics, are more likely to encounter outright brutality and sadism. Of course, black women have it worst of all. A shy teenager from a New York ghetto reports going to the clinic for her first prenatal check-up, and being used as teaching material for an entire class of young, male medical students learning to give pelvic examinations.

Doctors and hospitals treat pregnancy and childbirth, which are probably among the healthier things that women experience, as diseases—to be supervised by doctors and confined to hospitals. Women in other economically advanced countries, such as Holland, receive their prenatal care at home, from nurses, and, if all goes well, are delivered at home by trained midwives. (The Netherlands rank third lowest in infant mortality rate; the U.S. ranks fourteenth!) But for American women, pregnancy and childbirth are just another harrowing, expensive medical procedure. The doctor does it; the woman is essentially passive. Even in large cities, women often have to go from one obstetrician to another before they find one who approves of natural childbirth. Otherwise, childbirth is handled as if it were a surgical operation, even to the point of "scheduling" the event to suit the obstetrician's convenience through the use of possibly dangerous labor-inducing drugs.

Most people who have set out to look for medical care eventually have to conclude that there *is* no American medical system—at least there is no systematic way in America of getting medical help when you need it, without being financially ruined, humiliated, or injured in the process. What system there is—the three hundred thousand doctors, seven thousand hospitals and supporting insurance plans—was clearly not designed to deal with the sick. In fact the one thing you need most in order to qualify for care financially and to survive the process of obtaining it is *health*, plus, of course, a good deal of cunning and resourcefulness. The trouble is that it's almost impossible to stay healthy and strong enough to be able to tackle the medical system. Preventive health care (regular check-ups, chest X-rays, pap tests, etc.) is not a specialty or even an interest of the American medical system.

The price of this double bind—having to be healthy just to stay healthy—is not just consumer frustration and discomfort. The price is lives. The United States ranks fourteenth among the nations of the world in infant mortality, which means that approximately 33,000 American babies under one year old die unnecessarily every year. (Our infant mortality statistics are not, as often asserted, so high because they are "spoiled" by the death rates for blacks. The statistics for white America alone compare unfavorably to those for countries such as Sweden, the Netherlands, Norway, etc.) Mothers also stand a better chance of dying in the United States, where the maternal mortality rate ranks twelfth among the world's nations. The average American man lives five years less than the Swedish man, and his life expectancy is shorter than for males in seventeen other nations. Many American men never live out their already relatively short lifetime, since the chance of dying between ages forty and fifty is twice as high for an American as it is for a Scandinavian. What is perhaps most alarming about these statistics is that they are, in a relative sense, getting worse. The statistics improve a little each year, but at a rate far slower than that for other advanced countries. Gradually, the United States is slipping behind most of the European nations, and even some non-European nations, in its ability to keep its citizens alive.

These are the symptoms: unhealthy statistics, soaring costs and mounting consumer frustration over the quality and even the quantity of medical care. Practically everyone but the A.M.A.

agrees that something is drastically wrong. The roster of public figures actively concerned about the health care crisis is beginning to read like *Who's Who in America:* Labor leaders Walter Reuther of the Auto Workers and Harold Gibbons of the Teamsters, businessmen like General James Gavin of Arthur D. Little, Inc., politicians like New York's Mayor John Lindsay and Cleveland's Mayor Carl Stokes, doctors like Michael DeBakey of Baylor College of Medicine, and civil rights leaders like Mrs. Martin Luther King, Jr. and Whitney Young, Jr. With the help of eminent medical economists like Harvard's Rashi Fein and Princeton's Ann Somers, these liberal leaders have come up with a common diagnosis of the problem: the medical care system is in a state of near-chaos. There is no one to blame—medical care is simply adrift, with the winds rising in all directions. In the words of the official pamphlet of the Committee for National Health Insurance (a coalition of one hundred well-known liberals): "The fact is that we do not have a health care system at all. We have a 'nonsystem.' " According to this diagnosis, the health care industry is, in the words of the January, 1970, *Fortune* magazine, a "cottage industry." It is dominated by small, inefficient and uncoordinated enterprises (private doctors, small hospitals, and nursing homes), which add up to a fragmented and wasteful whole—a nonsystem.

Proponents of the nonsystem theory trace the problem to the fact that health care, as a commodity, does not obey the orderly, businesslike laws of economics. With a commodity like bacon, demand reflects people's desire to eat bacon and ability to pay for bacon. Since the supply gracefully adjusts itself to demand, things never get out of hand—there is a *system* of bacon production and sales. No such invisible hand of economic law operates in the health market. First, people buy medical care when they have to, not when they want to or can afford to. Then, when he does go to purchase care, the consumer is not the one who decides what and how much to buy—the doctor or hospital does. In other words, in the medical market place, it is the supplier who controls the demand. Finally, medical care suppliers have none of the usual economic incentives to lower their prices or rationalize their services. Most hospitals receive a large part of their income on a cost-plus basis from insurance organizations, and couldn't care less about cost or efficiency. Doctors do not compete on the basis of price. In fact, given the shortage of doctors (which is maintained by the doctors themselves through the A.M.A.'s prevention of medical school expansion), they don't have to compete at all.

Solutions offered by the liberal viewers of the medical nonsystem are all along the lines of putting the health industry on a more "rational," i.e., businesslike, basis. First the consumer should not have to fish in his pocket each time the need for care arises; he should have some sort of all-purpose medical credit card. With some form of National Health Insurance, all consumers, rich or poor, would have the same amount of medical credit, paid for by the government, by the consumer, or both through payroll taxes. Second, the delivery of health services must be made more efficient. Just as supermarkets are more efficient than corner groceries, and shopping centers are more efficient than isolated supermarkets, the medical system ought to be more efficient if it were bigger and more integrated at all levels. Doctors should be encouraged to come together into group practices, and group practices, hospitals and medical schools should be gradually knitted together into coordinated regional medical care systems. Since they are the centers of medical technology, the medical schools should be the centers and leaders of these regional systems—regulating quality in the "outposts," training professional and paraprofessional personnel, and planning to meet changing needs.

There is only one thing wrong with this analysis of the health care crisis: it's based on a false assumption. The medical reformers have assumed, understandably enough, that the function of the American health industry is to provide adequate health care to the American people. From this it is easy enough to conclude that there is no American health *system*. But this is like assuming that the function of the TV networks is to give comprehensive, penetrating, and meaningful information to the viewers—a premise which would quickly lead us to believe that the networks have fallen into wild disorganization and confusion. Like the mass media, the American medical industry has many items on its agenda other than service to the consumers. Analyzed in terms of all of its functions, the medical industry emerges as a coherent, highly organized system. One particular function—patient care—may be getting slighted, and there may be some problems in other areas as well, but it remains a *system*, and can only be analyzed as such.

The most obvious function of the American medical system, other than patient care, is profit-making. When it comes to making money, the health industry is an extraordinarily well organized and efficient machine. The most profitable small business around is the private practice of medicine, with aggregate profits running into the billions. The most profitable big business in America is the manufacture and sale of drugs. Rivaling the drug industry for Wall Street attention is the burgeoning hospital supply and equipment industry, with products ranging from chicken soup to catheters and heart-lung machines. The fledgling nursing home (for profit) industry was a speculator's dream in 1968 and 1969, and even the stolid insurance companies gross over ten billion dollars a year in health insurance premiums. In fact, the health business is so profitable that even the "nonprofit" hospitals make profits. All that "nonprofit" means is that the hospital's profit, i.e., the difference between its income and its expenditures, is not distributed to shareholders. These nonprofits are used to finance the expansion of medical empires—to buy real estate, stocks, plush new buildings, and expensively salaried professional employees. The medical system may not be doing too well at fighting disease, but, as any broker will testify, it's one of the healthiest businesses around.

Next in the medical system's list of priorities is research. Again, if this undertaking is measured in terms of its dividends for patient care, it comes out looking pretty unsystematic and disorganized. Although the vast federal appropriations for biomedical research are primarily motivated by the hope of improving health care, only a small fraction (much smaller than need be) of the work done in the name of medical research leaks out to the general public as improved medical care. But medical research has a *raison d'être* wholly independent of the delivery of health services, as an indispensable part of the nation's giant research and development enterprise. Since the Second World War, the United States has developed a vast machinery for R&D in all areas—physics, electronics, aerospace as well as biomedical sciences—financed largely by the government and carried out in universities and private industry. It has generated military and aerospace technology, and all the many little innovations which fuel the expansion of private industry.

For the purposes of this growing R&D effort, the medical system is important because it happens to be the place where R&D in general comes into contact with human material. Medical research is the link. The nation's major biomedical research institutes are affiliated to hospitals to a significant extent because they require human material to carry out their own, usually abstract, investigations. For instance, a sophisticated (and possible patentable) technique for investigating protein structure was recently developed through the use of the blood of several dozen victims of a rare and fatal bone marrow disease. Even the research carried out inside hospitals has implications for the entire R&D enterprise. Investigations of the pulmonary disorders of patients in Harlem Hospital may provide insights for designing space suits, or it may contribute to the technology of aerosol dissemination of nerve gas. Or, of course, it may simply lead to yet another investigation.

Human bodies are not all that the medical care system offers up to R&D. The sociological and psychological research carried out in hospitals and ghetto health centers may have pay-offs in the form of new counterinsurgency techniques for use at home and abroad. And who knows what sinister—or benignly academic —ends are met by the routine neurological and drug research carried out on the nation's millions of mental hospital inmates?

Finally, an important function of the medical care system is the reproduction of its key personnel—physicians. Here, again, there seems to be no system if patient care is the ultimate goal. The medical schools graduate each year just a few more doctors than are needed to replace the ones who retire, and far too few doctors to keep up with the growth of population. Of those who graduate, a growing proportion go straight into academic government, or industrial biomedical research, and never see a patient. The rest, according to some dissatisfied medical students, aren't trained to take care of patients anyway—having been educated chiefly in academic medicine (a mixture of basic sciences and "interesting" pathology). But all this is not as irrational as it seems. The limited size of medical school classes has been maintained through the diligent, and entirely systematic, efforts of the A.M.A. Too many—or even enough—doctors would mean lower profits for those already in practice. And the research orientation of medical education simply reflects the medical schools' own consuming preoccupation with research.

Profits, research, and teaching, then, are independent functions of the medical system, not just adjuncts to patient care. But they do not go on along separate tracks, removed from patient care. Patients are the indispensable ingredient of medical profit-making, research, and education. In order that the medical industry serve these functions, patient care must be twisted to meet the needs of these other "medical" enterprises.

Different groups of patients serve the ends of profit-making, research, and education in different ways. The rich, of course, do much to keep medical care profitable. They can afford luxury, so, for them, the medical system produces a luxury commodity—the most painstaking, supertechnological treatment possible; special cosmetic care to preserve youth, or to add or subtract fatty tissue; even sumptuous private hospital rooms with carpeting and a selection of wines at meals. The poor, on the other hand, serve chiefly to subsidize medical research and education—with their bodies. City and county hospitals and the wards and clinics of private hospitals provide free care for the poor, who, in turn, provide their bodies for young doctors to practice on and for researchers to experiment with. The lucky poor patient with a rare or interesting disease may qualify for someone's research project, and end up receiving the technically most advanced care. But most of the poor are no more interesting than they are profitable, and receive minimal, low-quality care from bored young interns.

The majority of Americans have enough money to buy their way out of being used for research, but not enough to buy luxury care. Medical care for the middle class is, like any other commodity, aimed at a mass market: the profits are based on volume, not on high quality. The rich man may have his steak dinners catered to him individually; the middle-class consumer waits for his hamburger in the check-out line at the A&P. Similarly, the middle-class patient waits in crowded waiting rooms, receives five minutes of brusque, impersonal attention from a doctor who is quicker to farm him out to a specialist than to take the time to treat him himself, and finally is charged all that the market will bear. Preventive care is out of the question: it is neither very profitable nor interesting to the modern, science-oriented M.D.

The crisis experienced by the poor and middle-class consumer of health care can be traced directly to the fact that patient care is not the only, or even the primary, aim of the medical care system. But what has turned the consumer's private nightmare into a great public debate about the health care crisis is that the other functions of the system are also in trouble. Profit-making, research, and education are all increasingly suffering from financial shortage on the one hand and institutional inadequacies on the other. The solutions offered by the growing chorus of medical reformers are, in large measure, aimed at salvaging profits, research, and education as much as they are aimed at improving patient care. They are simple survival measures, aimed at preserving and strengthening the medical system as it now operates.

No one, so far, has seen through the proposed reforms. Union and management groups, who have moved into the forefront of the medical reform movement, seem happy to go along with the prescription that the medical system is writing for itself. The alternative—to marshall all the force of public power to take medical care out of the arena of private enterprise and recreate it as a public system, a community service—is rarely mentioned, and never considered seriously. To do this would be to challenge some of the underlying tenets of the American free enterprise system. If physicians were to become community employees, if the drug companies were to be nationalized—then why not expropriate the oil and coal industries, or the automobile industry? There is an even more direct antipathy to nationalizing the health industry: a host of industries, including the aerospace industry, the electronic industry, the chemical industry, and the insurance industry, all have a direct stake in the profitability of the medical care system. (And a much larger sector of American industry stands to profit from the human technology spun off by the medical research enterprise.) Of course, the argument never takes this form. Both business and unions assert, in their public pronouncements, that only a private enterprise system is capable of managing medical services in an efficient, nonbureaucratic, and flexible manner. (The obvious extrapolation, that all medical services, including voluntary and city hospitals, would be in better shape if run as profit-making enterprises, is already being advanced by a few of the more visionary medical reformers.)

For all these reasons, business and unions (and, as a result, government) are not interested in restructuring the medical care system in ways contrary to those already put forth by the doctors, hospitals, and medical industry companies. Their only remaining choice is to go along with the reforms which have been proposed, in the hope that lower costs, and possibly even more effective care, will somehow fall out as by-products.

For the health care consumer, this is a slim hope. What he is up against now, what he will be up against even after the best-intentioned reform measures, is a system in which health care is itself only a by-product, secondary to the priorities of profits, research, and training. The danger is that, when all the current reforms are said and done, the system as a whole will be tighter, more efficient, and harder to crack, while health services, from the consumer's point of view, will be no less chaotic and inadequate. Health care will remain a commodity, to be purchased at great effort and expense, and not a right to be freely exercised.

But there are already the beginnings of a consumer rebellion against the reformer-managers of the medical care system. The demand is to turn the medical system upside down, putting human care on top, placing research and education at its service, and putting profit-making aside. Ultimately, the growing movement of health care consumers does not want to "consume" health care at all, on any terms. They want to take it—because they have to have it—even if this means creating a wholly new American health care system.

Health Maintenance Organizations and the Rationing of Medical Care

Harold S. Luft

HEALTH maintenance organizations (HMOs), with their capitation payments and contractual obligations to provide services, present a set of economic incentives that depart significantly from those of the conventional fee-for-service medical care system. It might be expected that these incentive differences will result in different approaches to the allocation of medical resources. Furthermore, these allocation or rationing mechanisms might have ethical implications because of the differential impact on various socioeconomic groups.

This paper will address a series of questions arising from the differences between prepaid and fee-for-service systems. The first section will examine the incentives under each system. In doing so, it will focus on incentives to the enrollee or patient, to the organization, and to providers within the system. This discussion will highlight the conflicting incentives inherent in various arrangements. The second section will examine how these incentives and conflicts may be dealt with in terms of the rationing or allocation of resources. The third section will expand the analysis to consider the probable effects of different systems with respect to various socioeconomic groups. This discussion will focus on both the microquestion of the impact of various mechanisms to allocate services among plan members, and the macroquestion of the effects of HMO enrollment and marketing decisions on who gets access to HMO options. To

From *Milbank Quarterly*, 1982, 60(2) Reprinted by permission of the *Milbank Quarterly*, Milbank Memorial Fund.

the extent possible, this discussion will include empirical evidence on the magnitude of such effects. The fourth section extends the discussion to speculate on the possible effects of an increasingly competitive environment for HMOs and other health care plans. Again, while this section will be based largely on conjecture, some evidence is available for analysis. The final section of the paper will consider the ethical implications of the issues already raised and will discuss some of the policy implications arising from them.

Economic Incentives in Various Medical Settings

Economic incentives and allocation mechanisms exist in all medical care delivery systems. Defining either optimally efficient or ethically just systems within the context of medical care realities is a task well beyond the scope of this paper. Instead, the focus here is on how various prepaid systems, of which HMOs are one notable example, *differ* from the conventional, primarily fee-for-service system. Subsequent discussions may then address the desirability of alternative systems.

Incentives in the Conventional Fee-for-Service Setting

The primary actors in the medical care system are: 1)consumers or, after they begin to receive medical care, patients; 2)insurance companies or other third parties; 3)physicians; and 4) hospitals. For most employed people and their families, health insurance is purchased through employer or union groups, often with a substantial employer contribution. The insurance plan or plans to be offered are selected by the employer or union and in most cases only one option is available to the employee. When ill, the patient selects a physician to diagnose the problem, provide treatment, and serve as an agent in arranging for the provision of services by hospitals and other physicians. All of these providers are typically paid on a fee-for-service or cost-reimbursement basis by the patient, the patient's insurer, or the government.

To the extent that insurance or other third-party payments such as Medicaid reduce the net price of services to the patient, more medical care will be demanded than if the patient paid the total bill (Newhouse et al., 1981). How much greater demand will be, or in economic terms the price elasticity of demand, is a much debated empirical question, but it is generally agreed that there is some increase, and that it is proportionately greater for discretionary and ambulatory services than for emergency and hospital services. Simultaneously, fee-for-service payments to the providers create a natural incentive to do more and respond to the increased demand.

Incentives in an HMO Setting

An HMO changes some of these linkages in ways that alter substantially the economic incentives. The patient no longer pays fee-for-service, except for an occasional small copayment of a dollar or two, so demand is likely to increase relative to conventional coverage. The HMO can also develop a set of financial linkages that tie together the physician, hospital, and insurer in a fashion quite unlike that of the conventional system. In contrast to the typical fee-for-service situation, the physicians and hospitals gain economically by doing less. This sets up a direct conflict with their patients whose comprehensive coverage leads them to demand even more than is usually the case.

In HMOs where the physicians practice as a group, two payment schemes are generally used: 1) salaries, with some type of bonuses if the group performs well; or 2) fee-for-service based payments modified to reflect the total pool of funds available. Salaries, of course, provide an incentive to exert oneself as little as possible unless there are other rewards for good performance. Fee-for-service payments tend to increase productivity—as measured by services per hour and hours worked per year—but increase the conflict between incentives to do more and the group incentives to do less (Held and Reinhardt, 1980).

In addition to the group model HMO, there is the individual

practice association (IPA) model which typically involves an HMO acting as a health plan which then contracts through an intermediary organization with independent office-based physicians to provide services. These physicians agree to accept payment by the HMO as payment in full and to allow a withholding of these fees to be placed at risk. The withheld fee is paid back only if the HMO meets its financial goals. Thus, while the individual physician can still earn more by performing more services, he or she can lose money if the physicians collectively provide or order too much or too expensive care.

The implications of these different economic incentives on the supply of services by the HMO and its providers are quite complex. When the physicians are essentially salaried and share in the financial success of the plan, they will collectively and individually probably try to reduce services. When physicians are essentially paid on a fee-for-service basis within a group or IPA type HMO, this incentive to do more will be only partially offset by the collective risk-sharing. This is especially true in IPAs in which the prepaid patients typically account for under 15 percent of the physicians' caseload.

Organizational Influences

While economic incentives are clearly different in HMOs, one must also consider a second dimension of difference—the organizational setting. The prepaid-group-practice type of HMO, which has been the economically most successful model, is characterized by both prepayment *and* the group-practice mode of delivery. Often, one of the attractions for physicians of large group practices is a more regularly scheduled life, with vacation time, educational leave, shorter hours, and on-call coverage. Such arrangements imply less doctor-patient continuity and typically a more bureaucratic organization (Luft, 1981; Mechanic, 1976). Prepaid groups, in particular, seem to have developed appointment and scheduling systems that reduce patient waiting time in the office but increase the time one must wait to obtain an appointment. Patients who drop in or request a visit the same day are typically seen in an urgent-care clinic, usually by a physician on rotation rather than their usual provider.

In the discussion that follows it will not be possible to examine all possible combinations of economic and organizational factors that may influence the provision of services. Instead, three models of practice will be discussed. The first is the conventional system of independently practicing fee-for-service providers with third-party insurance available for the patient. The second is the individual practice association or IPA model HMO involving primarily independent fee-for-service practitioners linked through a risk-sharing arrangement with an HMO. The third is the prepaid-group-practice or PGP model HMO composed of a large multispecialty-physician group practice which obtains most of its revenue from the HMO in the form of fixed capitation or salary payments plus some risk-sharing based on overall plan performance.

Methods of Allocating Services in HMOs

In classical market situations, goods and services are allocated through a price system. In medical care, various factors combine to cause substantial deviations from a market in which price is the only means of allocation. Information is scarce, both because of restrictions on advertising and, more importantly, because of the technical nature of the product, so consumers cannot make rational decisions (Arrow, 1963). Not only must the patient rely upon the physician to diagnose and provide services, but in many instances it is difficult to check on performance, so trust becomes an important factor. Medical services also require the presence of the patient and thus impose a time cost to obtain medical care and information about treatment alternatives.

Further complicating the analysis of the allocation of medical services is the fact that two levels of decisions are involved. The first decision is the type of insurance *cum* medical delivery system, that is, conventional insurance with independent fee-for-service providers or a prepaid system with a more limited choice of providers. (Of course, one also must consider *which* of the available providers one will choose within these two groupings.) The second level of decision concerns how much medical care will be consumed in treating a specific problem. Each type of decision reflects the preferences and behaviors of consumers/patients, on the one hand, and insurers/providers on the other. HMOs and insurers can attempt to influence the enrollment choices of consumers, and providers can influence or control the services delivered. Consumers often have strong preferences for practice setting (group vs. solo) and constrained vs. free choice of provider. Patients also have preferences, sometimes strongly held ones, as to the treatments they expect for specific illnesses. The following discussion will examine first the factors that influence treatment decisions and how these might vary among different practice settings; these might be termed "service allocation or rationing" issues. The focus will then widen to consider the allocation of consumers among systems; these might be termed "enrollment allocation or rationing" issues.

Decision Making in Three Types of Medical Treatment

When examining how medical care is allocated under various systems, it is useful to distinguish three major types of services: 1) patient initiated visits; 2) physician initiated or controlled visits; and 3) hospitalizations (Gertman, 1974). In a typical situation, a person recognizes certain problems or symptoms and decides that an examination by a physician is warranted. Obviously, whether a physician is actually seen will depend on the fee that must be paid, time costs, transportation and access costs, and whether the patient knows a potential provider. At the end of the examination, the physician may request a follow-up visit or may suggest a consultation with a specialist. (Of course, this is not entirely up to the physician; the patient may request such follow-up procedures for more reassurance and, likewise, the patient may refuse to follow through.) In some cases, the patient may continue to initiate follow-up visits by seeking out physicians. In general, the consumer has less control with respect to hospital services—admission can be gained only with the authorization of a physician, and once in the hospital, the physician essentially controls what services will and will not be provided.

A crucial point in this discussion is the idea that not only do physicians have a great deal of discretion in treatment and referral decisions, but that wide variation in practice patterns may be consistent with good quality care rendered in a careful and professional manner. Some physicians will have broad indications for surgery while others will impose stringent criteria for even suspected appendicitis. Some will make aggressive use of laboratory tests to rule out conditions while others will rely more upon the patient's history and physical examination. In most instances, large-scale trials have not been performed to identify the course of action leading to the best results. Wide variations in practice patterns often coexist in similar practice settings (e.g., among independent fee-for-service practitioners in the same state), with no noticeable difference in outcomes (Roos and Roos, 1981; Wennberg and Gittelsohn, 1973; Wennberg et al., 1980). This suggests that physicians in various HMOs and fee-for-service settings may consistently differ in their recommendations for treatment, yet still be within acceptable norms.

Likely Impact on Services in Different Settings

The likely impacts of the differences in price, accessibility, and practice styles on utilization of services in different settings are summarized in Table 1. While precise measurements of these effects are unavailable, in most instances each aspect can be identified as either increasing or decreasing utilization. One must note, however, that it is not always clear whether increased or decreased utilization is necessarily desirable. In general, increased access for patient-initiated visits is probably desirable, but one can even question that assumption. For instance, annual physical examinations for certain population groups are not cost-effective (Collen et al., 1973). Moreover, frequent testing of healthy people increases the likelihood of false-positive results and subsequent anxiety, invasive testing, and iatrogenesis.

The various factors listed in Table 1 influence utilization through different mechanisms. Some, like net price, travel time and costs, and waiting time, enter into the consumer's implicit calculation concerning whether the perceived problem is worth a visit. In general, because IPA-HMOs involve physicians primarily in fee-for-service office based practice, the only difference perceived by their HMO patients relative to their fee-for-service patients is more comprehensive coverage. The resulting lower net price will tend to increase utilization. Prepaid group-practice

(PGP) patients also face a lower (or zero) net money price, but other factors change simultaneously. They may not have a close relationship to a physician in the plan and thus may find it more difficult to take the initial steps to obtain treatment. PGPs are typically centralized so that for most patients a longer trip will be involved. The PGP also generally involves a different set of time costs—appointments must be scheduled further in advance, but once made, waiting time in the office is typically less (Mechanic, 1976; Richardson et al., 1977; Luft, 1981). Thus, while fees are not used by HMOs as a rationing device to influence demand, as is the case in the conventional system, there are other changes associated with the organization of group practice that make access both easier and more difficult. More importantly, as will be seen below, some of these influences on access may have different effects for people in different socioeconomic groups.

As one examines physician-initiated referral and follow-up visits and hospitalizations, differential physician behavior becomes more important relative to consumer factors. In part this is because conventional insurance policies provide better coverage for hospital services, tests, and procedures than for initial office visits, and because follow-up visits are more likely to be beyond the initial deductible. The greater physician influence also reflects the fact that when evaluating whether to make an initial visit, patients have only their own perceptions (as well as those of friends and family) concerning the need for a visit. For follow-ups, referrals, and hospitalizations, the physician's presentation of the severity of the problem will play a key role. Thus, differential clinical decision rules are a potentially major factor in the HMO's control over cost and utilization. This role is highlighted when one recognizes that in general, HMO enrollees are somewhat more likely than people in conventional plans to see a physician at least once a year, yet among utilizers, HMO enrollees have somewhat fewer office visits and substantially fewer hospitalizations (Luft, 1978).

Thus far, the discussion may have suggested that the capitation or risk-sharing incentives of the HMO lead HMO physicians to alter their practice patterns for their members. In fact, it is extremely unlikely that HMO physicians reflect upon the impact on their bonuses each time they consider a follow-up visit or an extra test. Instead, certain routine patterns are

TABLE 1

Probable Effects on Utilization of Services of Various Factors in Different Practice Settings

Type of Medical Care/ Rationing Factors	Conventional Fee-for-Service and Insurance		IPA-HMOs: Fee-for-Service Practitioners at Risk		PGP-HMOs	
Patient Initiated Visits						
Price to consumer	Initial and preventive visits often not covered	–	Comprehensive coverage of all visits	+	Comprehensive coverage of all visits	+
Knowledge of provider	Often a local physician with a longstanding relationship	+	Often a local physician with a longstanding relationship	+	Often a local physician with no prior contact with patient	–
Appointment lag	Typically short, urgent visits "squeezed in"	+	Typically short, urgent visits "squeezed in"	+	Typically long, urgent visits routed to separate clinic	–
Accessibility to provider	Decentralized, likely one close to patient	+	Decentralized, likely one close to patient	+	Centralized, generally further from patient	–
Waiting time in office	Variable, often long because patients "squeezed in"	–	Variable, often long because patients "squeezed in"	–	Typically short if appointment made in advance	+
Physician Initiated Visits						
Physician incentives	Follow-up increases revenue	+	Follow-up increases revenue more than risk sharing	+	Follow-up reduces net income; substitute call-backs	– +/–

Physician Initiated Referral

Physician incentives	Reciprocal referrals among different specialists encouraged by professional network, discouraged by prohibitions on fee splitting +	Referrals encouraged by professional network but discouraged by risk sharing +/-	Referral attractive to "dump" a problem patient, but collegial and financial costs if frequent +/-
Price to consumer	More likely covered than initial visit, still not complete +/-	Comprehensive coverage of all visits +/-	Comprehensive coverage of all visits +
Accessibility of provider	Typically at a different location -	Typically at a different location -	Centralized—"one stop care" -
Incentives to "return patient to primary care physician"	Depends on nature of referral network +	Depends on referral network, sometimes encouraged by HMO +	Typically encouraged by the system +/-
Hospitalization			
Price to patient	Often fairly comprehensive coverage but some copayments -	Comprehensive coverage pays in full +	Comprehensive coverage pays in full +
Incentives for physician	Hourly income higher in hospital +	Hourly income higher, but risk sharing tends to counter +	No additional income, costs are borne by plan +/-

+ = tends to increase utilization
- = tends to decrease utilization
+/- = mixed effects

probably developed that tend to be consistent with their economic incentives. Inconsistent patterns may be reexamined and slowly adjusted to reduce conflict with system incentives.

As before, the situation in IPA and PGP HMOs differs markedly. While the research has yet to be done, it seems unlikely that many physicians will use different decision rules for their fee-for-service and prepaid patients. The available evidence supports the notion that current levels of risk sharing and patient loads in IPAs (10–20 percent withheld fees and under 15 percent of the patients) have little impact on performance (Meier and Tillotson, 1978). Instead, IPAs exercise controls through hospital-based utilization review and through educational efforts to change general practice patterns by showing that certain less costly techniques are equally effective.

PGP physicians typically see only HMO patients, so the altering of practice styles may be easier because a "two-class" system is not necessary. Some HMOs develop extensive data bases on the use of tests by physicians and feed back this information. Merely seeing that he or she has an ordering pattern very different from the rest of the group is often sufficient incentive for a clinician to rethink decision rules. In other cases, active physician-education programs have been undertaken by the HMO (Thompson, 1979). Another, perhaps crucial factor is self-selection by physicians. PGPs are often perceived by outside physicians as imposing restrictions on the practices of their clinicians and this is likely to deter even initial investigation by physicians who value highly the unconstrained ability to aggressively use any treatment. (Interestingly, PGP physicians often mention as one of the advantages of prepaid practice the ability to select treatments without having to worry about the financial cost to the patient [Cook, 1971].) Similarly, physicians who value a wait-and-see approach may be attracted by the HMO setting, which does not penalize them financially for not ordering batteries of tests. In this way prepaid and fee-for-service settings may attract physicians with previously developed practice styles consistent with their subsequent economic incentives.

Allocation of Consumers Among Systems

Thus far, the focus has been on the provision of services within an HMO or other medical care setting. However, it is important to also take a broader view and examine the question of who is allowed into the setting. HMOs, like other insurers, receive most of their members through employee groups. Generally only a small number of people are allowed to enroll as individual (nongroup) contracts and their premiums are typically higher. (In fact, the record of HMOs on this issue is generally better than that of most commercial insurers. The HMO Act of 1973 requires federally qualified HMOs to provide an open enrollment season and allow individual subscribers to enroll at community rates. Conventional insurers are under no such obligation.)

If an HMO wishes to select a certain type of enrollee—healthy, white, female, upper income, or whatever—two strategies may be used. The first involves careful selection of the employee groups to whom the HMO option will be offered. For instance, firms with primarily white collar workers might be placed high on the marketing list while other firms might be ranked lower. (The mandating provisions of the HMO Act allow a federally qualified HMO to require certain employers to offer the HMO as an option. There is no parallel requirement of an HMO to offer enrollment to any employer requesting coverage.) In general, it is difficult to document instances in which firms were not approached because their employees were thought to be too risky—numerous explanations for marketing patterns can be described. However, there are some examples of behavior toward firms already in the HMO that support the notion of these techniques. In one case, an HMO in Minneapolis-St. Paul dropped its contract with a large local employer because maternity use within the group was too high (Matlock, 1980). In another case, an HMO that phased in mental health benefits offered them first to working class groups least likely to use them while delaying coverage of university groups anticipated to be higher users.

The second strategy for selection would be to attract certain types of people *within* the employee group. Various tactics can be used to influence enrollment. Premiums are often weighted so that family coverage is proportionately less expensive than individual coverage, thus attracting families with children who tend to cost less per capita than single persons or two-person families. (This strategy is also used by conventional insurers.) HMOs have traditionally offered more comprehensive coverage of maternity care, again attracting young, relatively healthy families. (Note that not all selection strategies are socially undesirable.) In other instances, the same factors that influence the use of services by members also influence who becomes a member. The single most important determinant of whether someone will choose a prepaid group practice when given the option is whether that decision will break a strong existing tie to a physician; people with strong ties do not join, whereas those without such ties are much more likely to join prepaid groups (Berki and Ashcraft, 1980). One explanation for the absence of a strong physician-patient relationship is low utilization of services. By chance or design, the PGP structure both attracts people without strong physician bonds and does not foster their development—and both features may lead to lower use of services (Scitovsky et al., 1979).

Another approach is in the careful location of facilities. While enrollment may be offered to any employee within a relatively wide region, if the clinics are only convenient to certain population subgroups, then enrollment is likely to reflect those locational factors. Similarly, access might be differentially altered for certain types of patients. For instance, appointment scheduling might be made easy and flexible for pediatrics and difficult for adult or geriatric medicine. The dual-choice option in the HMO is, in part, designed so that dissatisfied enrollees can leave the plan, removing both the source of complaint and the pressure on the organization to change (Hirschman, 1970; Phelan et al., 1970).

Because the typical IPA-model HMO utilizes the practices of a large number of independent practitioners, it has less control than the PGP over certain features of its delivery system, but it has more control over others. In particular, IPAs occasionally drop physicians from their roster because of excessive utilization. The situation may not have to get to the point of formal severance. Repeated review and questioning of a physician's treatment patterns is probably sufficient to cause withdrawal.

While some of the factors that have been discussed are rather subtle, they need only to result in relatively small differences among certain people to have a major cost impact from the perspective of the HMO. In general, a small fraction of the plan's enrollees account for the majority of its costs. Most people are fairly healthy and use ambulatory care and occasional hospital services. Clearly, it is in the plan's interests if certain features, whether by design or accident, tend to keep out those people who are frequent users of costly services. Note that not only does the plan benefit, but the relatively low-cost people who do enroll receive comprehensive coverage and usually excellent service at lower average cost, at least in part because they do not have to share the costs of their fellows. Conventional insurers have the same incentives to select healthy enrollees.

This leads to a consideration of the environment in which HMOs exist. The notion of risk-spreading through community rating whereby everyone in an area pays the same premium has been almost universally replaced by experience rating whereby firms with young, healthy employees pay lower premiums while those with older and more costly employees have higher premiums. In spite of this, HMOs were traditionally community rated long before the HMO Act required them to do so. Only recently, in the Omnibus Budget Reconciliation Act of 1981, P.L. 97-35, has the law been changed to allow HMOs to take into account differences in enrollment mix. How they will use the increased flexibility will depend in part on future changes in the competitive environment.

Socioeconomic Differences in the Effects of Alternative Allocation Systems

The major feature of the HMO system from the consumer's perspective is that prices in the form of coinsurance and deductibles are absent. This suggests immediately that income and ability to pay will not influence utilization, so the distribution of care may be expected to be more equitable. (In this case, equitable is taken to mean that services are allocated according to need rather than effective demand.) However, the previous section identified other variables that may influence utilization and these may have differential effects by income group, race, sex, residence, or other factors.

To economists, the most familiar device used by HMOs to constrain patient demand is time. Waiting time in an office is "dead," unproductive time. Many economists value time at the individual's wage rate so that an hour for someone earning $10 per hour is worth four times that of someone earning $2.50 per hour. Other economists would argue that wage rates alone are not appropriate measures of the value of time to an individual. At a minimum, wage rates must be compared to total income. Furthermore, a highly paid professional typically has more sick leave, flexibility in hours, and discretion than a dishwasher paid the minimum wage. For the dishwasher, a long appointment wait may mean peremptory firing, not just an inconvenience. In any case, it is difficult to determine the relative time costs in HMOs. Travel time is generally increased in PGPs, but waiting time in the office is reduced. Furthermore, patients with appointments probably experience less variability in waiting time in PGPs. While it is difficult to know whether the shorter office waits benefit more the higher or lower income groups, they may make less difference to the retired who are probably not pressed for time, and there are numerous anecdotes of the waiting room as a social hall.

The long appointment lag in PGPs has a different type of effect. It has little impact on people who have postponable, schedulable problems with a low anxiety component. Middle-class professionals are likely to fall into this category. The poor, parents of small children, and those elderly persons with recurrent urgent or acute problems may not be served as well by such a system. However, most PGPs offer 24-hour emergency coverage and urgent drop-in visits at the clinic, so services are available, albeit with longer waits and usually an unfamiliar provider. The PGP does have a substantial advantage over the typical emergency room in that the patient's medical record is usually available.

Physical access to PGP HMOs may have a differential effect on various subgroups. The centralized location means that the poor and others without automobiles may find access more difficult. However, the presence of consultants, laboratory, X-ray, and pharmacy at the same site may be a special convenience to such people. Like institutions, large PGPs are also more likely to enhance access for certain subgroups, such as non–English-speaking minorities and the disabled. For instance, Kaiser offers a special teletypewriter (TTY) telephone line for hearing-impaired persons, a convenience not offered by many independent physicians.

The large, bureaucratic structure of some PGPs may create barriers for the less educated. There is often a "system" that one must learn how to "work," rather than the helpful receptionist in an independent practitioner's office. On the other hand, the conventional system often offers no assistance in getting from one provider to another. The HMO also eliminates the need for complicated claim forms which often increase substantially the cost to the poor and uneducated because they do not claim the benefits due them.

Prepaid group practices are by their nature closer to some people than others. This may lead to much higher travel costs for residents of some neighborhoods. In most instances, because HMOs concentrate on enrolling employed populations, this implies reduced accessibility for people in lower-class areas. However, some HMOs have targeted their services to Medicaid recipients and thus are inaccessible to the middle and upper class.

HMOs can selectively try to enroll certain population subgroups. Clearly, they have incentives to avoid those groups with higher-than-average costs and utilization unless their premiums are commensurately higher. (Note that, in part, this incentive is caused by the HMO's community rating while other insurers rate by experience. An experience-rating HMO might even find high-risk people especially desirable because of the larger potential savings it could offer relative to the conventional system.)

Enrollment Choices by HMOs and the Poor

The most important factors in HMO selection with respect to the aged and the poor are policies set by the federal and state governments. Current Medicare provisions do not make it attractive for HMOs to enroll the elderly, nor are Medicare beneficiaries given any incentives to enroll in HMOs (Luft et al., 1980). The Medicaid program allows states to contract with

HMOs to provide care for the poor. In some states this has resulted in rather large programs, but in many areas Medicaid enrollment is minimal even though HMOs are available.

The poor, almost by definition, enter HMOs under circumstances different than those of the middle class who have a dual-choice option through their employers or unions. In general, the conventional health-insurance alternative for employees provides fairly comprehensive coverage with some copayments and deductibles. Moreover, the middle-class family can generally use their conventional health insurance at a wide range of medical care providers. For those who join, the HMO is the better of several fairly good options.

Poor enrollees in HMOs have generally entered through either of two routes—a demonstration project or a Medicaid contract. In a demonstration project or experiment, a government or private agency offers to pay the premiums for those people who enroll in the HMO. In a few instances, the family is given a choice of plans, but in almost all of these instances special monitoring programs and evaluations are included. (Such efforts are likely to influence, as well as measure, performance.) These demonstration projects often include special features such as outreach coordinators and transportation programs not normally provided by the HMO (Freeborn et al., 1980; Coltin et al., 1978; Richardson et al., 1977). In some cases the experiment provided comprehensive coverage as long as the family stayed enrolled, but disenrollment would imply a loss of benefits. It is also the case that most demonstration projects for which data are available were undertaken by mature HMOs with large stable enrollments of employed populations. Many of the HMOs supported substantial research staffs and most undertook the demonstration at least in part out of perceived social responsibility. All of these factors render such situations somewhat atypical and may alter the actual or perceived performance of the plan relative to a simple competitive market model.

In several states HMO enrollment has been made available as an option to Medicaid beneficiaries. Although on the surface such arrangements appear analogous to the multiple-choice options available to employees, there are also some important differences. One is that conventional Medicaid programs generally do not include copayments or a premium paid by the enrollee, nor is the HMO able to offer additional benefits to the enrollee should it realize savings. Thus, the Medicaid recipient is not attracted to the HMO by its better financial coverage, lower cost, or improved benefits, as is the case for middle-and working-class enrollees. Instead, the reason many Medicaid beneficiaries take an HMO option is that few fee-for-service physicians in their area are willing to accept Medicaid patients. Rather than being attracted by a better system, the HMO may offer the only viable system and thus be under less pressure to perform well. In addition to the enrollees' incentives, it is important to examine the motives of the HMO in negotiating a Medicaid contract. In most instances, this process is long and difficult, and the capitation rates offered by the state are often unattractive relative to premiums paid by employee groups. Thus, some plans that choose to attract Medicaid beneficiaries may do so because of their own precarious position in the market. This is certainly not always the case, however, and some well-known and highly successful HMOs have tried to enroll the poor out of a sense of community.

Service Allocation Differences for Different Socioeconomic Groups

One problem in searching for differential consequences by socioeconomic group is choosing the appropriate comparison population. One can argue that the poor have more health problems than the nonpoor, so the poor in an HMO should be compared to the poor in the traditional system. Alternatively, one might reason that the fee-for-service system is not now meeting the needs of the poor. Thus the experience of the poor in an HMO should be compared to that of the middle class in the same organization. Studies of both types are available.

Most of the findings concerning utilization of comparable groups of the poor in HMOs and fee-for-service settings are discussed in Luft, 1981 (see also Vignola and Strumpf, 1980). The major studies are those of Gaus, Cooper, and Hirschman (1976) on ten HMOs; Fuller and Patera (1976) on Group Health Association in Washington, D.C.; Richardson et al. (1977) on the Seattle Model Cities Project; Johnson and Azevedo (1979) on Kaiser-Portland; and Salkever, German, Shapiro, Horky, and Skinner (1976) on East Baltimore Health Plan. For ambulatory care, the results are mixed; in half, there are more visits by the poor in HMOs, and in half, the results are reversed. These average findings are misleading because it is much more frequently the case that the poor in HMOs have at least one visit more than the poor seeing fee-for-service physicians. This suggests that access is easier for the poor in HMOs than for those in the conventional systems, even with Medicaid coverage.

For hospitalization, the results are remarkably consistent—lower admission rates for HMO enrollees in all cases. The prevailing opinion is that this generally is not due to an inability of patients to gain admission. In fact, somewhat lower utilization is probably good because of the presumed excessive hospitalization in conventional settings. While exceedingly low utilization rates may not be good practice, more detailed studies are necessary in order for us to determine if this is the case.

The second type of comparison involves the poor and nonpoor in the same organization. The question is: Does enrollment of the poor in the same plan with the middle class, and with the same financial coverage, eliminate the general underservice of the poor found in the conventional system? In general, ambulatory utilization rates of the poor in mature HMOs approximates that of the middle class.

However, some differences appear in the *types* of utilization by different socioeconomic groups. The poor are more likely than the middle-class enrollees to walk in or use the hospital emergency room instead of a regularly scheduled appointment. The former results in fragmented care, but may better fit the life circumstances of the poor. Further adding to the fragmentation was the fact that when appointments were made, the poor had a higher no-show rate (Hurtado et al., 1973; Richardson et al., 1977; Group Health Cooperative of Puget Sound, 1970; Shragg et al., 1973). It is difficult to identify the cause of these utilization patterns, but it appears that to some degree the style of service provided by the HMOS does not match that desired by the poor enrollees. Of course, the life circumstances of the poor may lead them to favor drop-in visits, emergency room use, and cancelled appointments in all settings, not just in HMOs.

These studies examined the behavior of special subgroups of the poor who were introduced to an ongoing HMO as part of a demonstration project. Such an arrangement requires adjustments by both the HMO staff and the new enrollees. An alternative research design examines whether different utilization patterns occur by socioeconomic group within the regularly enrolled populating. While this approach is limited to employed people with an HMO option (and thus omits the very poor), it provides better measures of long-run equilibrium. Furthermore, if differences appear, they are likely to be larger if coverage is extended to the very poor.

Much of this work has been done by the Kaiser Portland Research Center. Freeborn, Pope, Davis, and Mullooly (1977) summarize their results concerning outpatient utilization with respect to socioeconomic status. Health status measures appear to be the dominant factors, and once they are held constant, education, income, and socioeconomic class have little effect on utilization. The one exception is preventive service, which is not related to health status but, for women, is positively related to education and income. These studies also exhibit differences in the patterns of ambulatory use that are related to socioeconomic status—the middle class is more likely to use the telephone for reporting symptoms and is less likely to use walk-in clinics (Pope et al., 1971; Weiss and Greenlick, 1970; Nolan et al., 1967).

Hetherington, Hopkins, and Roemer (1975) argue that in PGPs people with more education and higher incomes can more easily "work the system." While it is true that higher-income enrollees in Kaiser and Ross-Loos have more visits per year than lower-income enrollees, their own data show that this is also the case in the conventional plans. More importantly, low income PGP enrollees were much less likely to go without a physician visit, suggesting that the lower out-of-pocket cost in the PGPs more than compensates for any bureaucratic deterrent.

Taken together, these studies in large, mature PGPs suggest some important differences in utilization patterns among regularly enrolled HMO members. While overall use of ambulatory services does not differ very much, especially when factors such as age, sex, and health status are held constant, the types of services vary. The middle class is much more likely to use the telephone to report symptoms. Walk-in visits and appointments, both of which are held during normal working hours, also appear easier for the middle class. While the unemployed may have a low time cost, the working poor probably have less flexible schedules than the middle class. Thus the poor are more likely to use the emergency room, and they are more likely to miss appointments without cancelling them.

The California Prepaid Health Plan Program Under Medicaid

The previous discussion provides substantial evidence that many HMOs have adequately served the poor and that their systems to constrain costs have not had noticeably adverse impacts. Yet, the history of HMOs and the poor contains one chapter with a different tone—reports of fraud, abuse, poor quality, and inaccessible services by some prepaid health plans serving Medicaid beneficiaries in California. To gain a better understanding of how HMO-type services can lead to undesirable outcomes, it is useful to examine the California experience.

In 1970 California began a policy of encouraging the development of HMOs to serve its Medicaid population. These organizations, called prepaid health plans (PHPs), were supposed to save the state money by reducing unnecessary utilization and administrative costs of claims reimbursement. The then governor, Ronald Reagan, also attempted to control utilization of fee-for-service providers by limiting office visits and requiring prior authorization for hospital admissions. (See, e.g., Goldberg, 1975; California Department of Health, 1975; Chavkin and Treseder, 1977.) This strategy was also designed to make HMO enrollment more attractive to the Medicaid population, because no such external restrictions on utilization would be imposed on HMO enrollees. Implicit constraints were imposed because the HMO capitation rates were pegged to the average fee-for-service costs. Most observers agree that the initial program was poorly designed with problems arising from marketing abuses, excessive administrative costs and profits, and poor quality of care (Goldberg, 1975; D'Onofrio and Mullen, 1977; Moore and Breslow, 1972; California State Legislative Analyst, 1975; U.S. Senate Committee on Government Operations, Permanent Subcommittee on Investigations, 1975, 1978).

The principal charges concerning marketing stemmed from PHP use of door-to-door salespeople to enroll Medicaid eligibles. These people often posed as physicians or Medicaid officials and rarely explained fully the options available to consumers. Promises often far exceeded reality. Salespeople attempted to enroll only healthy individuals and told people with ongoing problems to stay in the fee-for-service system. These marketing abuses were at least partially attributable to the intense competition for enrollees among plans, which, in turn, was fostered by the ground rules laid down by the state (U.S. General Accounting Office, 1974). A PHP would sign a contract allowing it to receive a fixed monthly capitation fee of no more than 90 percent of the average fee-for-service cost of similar enrollees. No funds were available for start up or fixed costs, so it was imperative that the PHP enroll members as quickly as possible. Furthermore, in an effort to encourage competition and promote choice for Medicaid eligibles, the state took a laissez-faire attitude and authorized many plans to operate in the same service areas. While creating a situation in which there was a rush to enroll people, the state refused to release the names of Medicaid eligibles, so the PHPs had to use door-to-door salespeople paid on commission. There was also little control over PHP attempts to enroll only the healthy and to keep dissatisfied members from disenrolling. The situation was almost perfectly designed to lead to an aggressive attempt to enroll healthy members.

There was almost no concern for even minimal quality audits in the early years of the PHP program, and only after June 1973 were medical professionals assigned by the state to audit PHPs (California State Legislative Analyst, 1975). A detailed investigation in 1974 of five PHPs in operation prior to December 1972 showed substantial variability in quality, with some significantly better than fee-for-service Medi-Cal (the California Medicaid program) and some significantly worse. Plans with a high proportion of non–Medi-Cal enrollees scored consistently better (Louis and McCord, 1974).

These differences in quality which appear related to the proportion of non–Medi-Cal enrollees are consistent with the notion that plans tend to provide comparable services for all enrollees and that the competitive environment has a major influence on the overall level of service. Large, mature HMOs have had to compete with conventional insurers and providers for the employed population. In contrast, some of the PHPs were established to serve only Medi-Cal prepaid enrollees while others were large fee-for-service Medi-Cal practices prior to converting to prepayment. In many areas, the poor have few alternatives—in 1972 less than 20 percent of Medi-Cal eligibles in Orange County saw "mainstream" providers (Auger and Goldberg, 1974).

This review suggests that in the past competition for employed populations has led to a high quality of care and service by HMOs. (These mature HMOs were also established by individuals committed primarily to the development of innovations in medical care rather than profitability, an issue to be discussed below.) But, competition per se is not necessarily good; the intense competition among PHPs for Medi-Cal enrollees encouraged their marketing abuses. Thus, future policy strategies should examine the nature and level of competition most likely to lead to socially desirable results.

Potential Effects
Under Increased Competition

It is important to remember that the preceding discussion of HMO incentives and performance relates to a specific market environment and historical context. Most mature HMOs (i.e., those developed before the 1970s, which account for the bulk of total enrollment and most of the research studies) were started in an environment actively hostile to prepayment. The founders of these plans were often visionaries with strong beliefs concerning the superiority of prepayment and group practice (MacColl, 1966; Rothenberg et al., 1949; Williams, 1971). They often enlisted community support in their struggles with organized medicine and sought to provide a better service at reasonable cost. Few of these HMOs were operated on a for-profit basis and those aspects that were technically for profit, e.g., the physician groups, rarely seemed to act as if profit were a major goal. The market environment has also been relatively noncompetitive. Often only one HMO existed in an area. Although

HMOs competed with conventional insurers for enrollees, tax subsidies for health insurance benefits and employer ignorance or unconcern made the market orderly and quiet. Current proposals to increase competition in the medical care market suggest that it may be inappropriate to extrapolate from the past.

Changes in the Competitive Environment

Several changes are proposed or in process to substantially increase competition. Various bills have been introduced to alter the tax laws to increase employee sensitivity to the cost of health insurance (Iglehart, 1981). Current law allows all employer contributions to be tax deductible for the employer and tax free to the employee. Many employers contribute more for more expensive plans. The proposed changes would place a cap on the employer contribution, require equal contributions, or give tax-free rebates to people choosing less expensive plans. Some employers provide "cafeteria style" benefit packages whereby employees receive a lump sum in fringe benefits to allocate among various health, life insurance, pension, vacation, and other options. The proposed changes in the tax law would increase the desirability of such cafeteria plans.

Employers have also become more aware of the cost of health insurance contributions and that this fringe benefit is a largely uncontrollable cost. Some employers have begun to alter their health insurance packages to increase cost control. One very popular approach is self-insurance and administrative-services-only arrangements in which the employer bears the risk and the carrier merely handles claims processing. The employer can then develop a substantial data base on cost and utilization and can exercise substantial control over reimbursement levels and payment flexibility.

New delivery systems and insurance arrangements are also beginning to enter the market. The older generation of PGPs and IPAs has been joined by new HMOs with a frankly entrepreneurial orientation. Some are local organizations, often controlled by a few physicians, while others are owned and operated by large statewide or national insurers. In some instances it has been alleged that these new plans have a very short (two- to three-year) time horizon on profitability, rather than the long-run perspective focusing on service delivery attributed to the older plans. (For example, the innovative United Healthcare plan sponsored by Safeco has been closed [Moore et al., 1980].) The currently high interest rates make imperative the rapid payback of start-up capital. New firms have entered the administrative services market with an emphasis on fast, inexpensive processing and a get-tough attitude toward providers. Such firms will sometimes offer a fixed fee, perhaps well below the physician's usual charge, and if that is not accepted, threaten interminable negotiations. Other plans are establishing "preferred provider organizations" in which selected cost-conscious providers are identified. If the enrollee goes to one of these providers, charges are covered in full, while for other providers standard copayments are required.

Simultaneously, the provider market is becoming increasingly competitive. Falling hospitalization rates are leading to increasing bed surpluses so hospitals are more willing to grant concessions (Kralewski and Countryman, 1982). For-profit hospital chains are expanding and sometimes concentrate on handling only certain types of cases. In some instances HMOs are owned by these for-profit chains. The supply of physicians is also increasing rapidly relative to the population, and in some parts of the nation it is becoming difficult for physicians to start an independent practice and meet income expectations and debts incurred during training. This is leading to an increased willingness and sometimes eagerness by new, young physicians to accept a position with one of the new HMOs or other plans.

Possible Effects of Increased Competition

As competition increases, consumers and employers become more cost-conscious, and providers become more squeezed, various tactics may be used to ration resources inside and out of HMOs. Plans will probably attempt to control costs much more tightly than is currently the case. This may lead to the firing or dropping from provider lists of those physicians who appear to overutilize services (Physicians Health Plan, 1980). Both approaches have been used in selected plans. The question, of course, is whether the cuts are aimed only at the true "abuser" such as the physician who gives a vitamin B-12 shot to every patient. In a cost-cutting environment a plan may fail to distinguish the abusing physicians from those who have a sicker patient load. In either case, the patients of those physicians will lose a provider and the ones who will be most affected are the frequent users with chronic high-cost problems. Similar approaches are not difficult to imagine. For instance, plans generally cover all but "experimental" services. By not updating the coverage list frequently, patients desiring such new and usually expensive procedures will be encouraged to switch insurers (Rybin, 1981). Alternatively, the indications for a service or its delivery method may be structured to shift certain users out of the plan. Many HMOs provide fairly comprehensive coverage of outpatient mental health care—often 20 or more visits per year, usually in a group therapy setting. While this may be sufficient for most acute problems, it may not be very attractive to patients who wish long-term insight-oriented individual therapy. Such people will switch to conventional insurers with outpatient mental health benefits. Plans could attract well-trained board-certified physicians yet make sure that, while the primary-care physicians are well liked by the enrollees, most of the specialists are foreigners with limited command of conversational English. Such a strategy would, if associated with low premiums, attract the young and healthy, and repel the old and sick.

Even more subtle tactics could be used by IPAs or insurers through manipulation of reimbursements. The allowable fees for certain types of expensive specialists could be held down, either as a matter of policy or by updating usual, customary, and reasonable fee screens less frequently for low-volume specialties (Showstack et al., 1979). Such an approach would increasingly shift costs to the patient and might even lead to a change of plan. A crucial factor in such approaches is that a small number of enrollees account for a large fraction of the costs (Roos and Shapiro, 1981; Eggers, 1981; McCall and Wai, 1981). Small changes that may affect only high users can have a major cost impact with little apparent effect on enrollment. Moreover, changes in administrative procedures or providers affecting this small segment are difficult or impossible to monitor from the outside.

Competitive strategies are even more likely to occur in marketing. Some of the procompetitive bills would eliminate minimum basic benefit packages. If such minimums are dropped,

HMOs and insurers could compete for low-cost enrollees by offering benefits attractive to the healthy, like eyeglasses, while limiting coverage for services required by high-cost enrollees. Plans are likely to target their enrollment toward the healthier groups, and within groups toward healthier and less expensive individuals.

Employers may also structure their benefit packages to reduce their own costs. For instance, it is reported that one Washington, D.C.–based firm has designed its health-benefits option so employees married to federal workers will choose coverage under their spouse's plan, thus reducing costs to the firm. (While such anecdotal evidence is difficult to generalize, it is indicative of the types of behavior already observed which are likely to become more common. The examples are drawn from interviews during which anonymity was assured) In another situation, a firm with a self-insured plan and a community-rated HMO option had personnel staff counsel people with health problems to join the HMO—and thus lower the firm's costs. Some employers with administrative-services-only contracts have their carriers identify high-utilizing employees for special counseling. It is only a small additional step to pressure such employees to quit. Preemployment physical exams can be used to screen out not only people unable to perform their jobs, but those who may have costly medical expenses.

These are just a few of the possible ways by which increased competition may lead to a situation in which the young and healthy receive good low-cost coverage and the old and sick face expensive inadequate coverage—just the opposite of the risk-pooling implicit in socially desirable insurance. Many more tactics are likely to be developed as competitive pressures increase. While the old and sick are more likely to be poor, other factors will also increase the burden of such a competitive strategy for poor and female workers. Unions are likely to resist the fragmentation envisioned in this scenario and employers of upper-income workers are also less likely to adopt penny-pinching strategies. For instance, one electronics firm was said to avoid aggressive intermediaries because it did not want to offend its engineers with a hard line on claims. Low-income and nonunion workers have much smaller employer contributions and are likely to be especially sensitive to the self-selection inducements of a competitive strategy (Taylor and Lawson, 1981).

If Medicare and Medicaid are brought into the competitive strategy, similar outcomes are possible. The experience with the "Medigap" policies suggests that many of the elderly are not informed consumers of health insurance; the poor are apt to be even more vulnerable. Depending upon the value of the "voucher" offered by the government, the Medicare and Medicaid beneficiaries could be very attractive markets. On average, their medical expenditures (and implicit premiums) are high, but again, a small fraction accounts for a very large fraction of the expenditures (Roos and Shapiro, 1981). Furthermore, in contrast to employed groups, high expenditures among Medicare and Medicaid beneficiaries are probably more likely to be associated with chronic conditions than sudden trauma so the importance of preexisting physician ties is even stronger. It may also be easier to attract people with certain chronic, but low-cost conditions while discouraging others. For instance, a plan may emphasize a program for the blind, who are relatively low-cost patients, while making access difficult to cardiologists. The relative absence of informed agents, such as union negotiators, may make such strategies particularly easy if there is no government monitoring of the process.

Ethical and Policy Implications of Rationing of Medical Care in HMOs

The previous sections have pointed out that the systems of controlling utilization or rationing in HMOs are rather different than they might appear at first glance. While fees are not used to influence consumer demand, the burden is placed only partially on time prices. The seemingly endless queues reported in England are not evident in most HMOs. Instead, there is a different tradeoff between waiting time and appointment delay in PGPs and, while physical accessibility is more difficult in some ways, it is easier in others. Rationing tends to occur in much more subtle ways. Controls over services provided take place through an environment that encourages the medical staff to be more conservative in its use of medical resources. Hard and fast rules on when a patient should be admitted have not been uncovered. Instead, although clinicians make decisions on a case-by-case basis, the overall pattern of decisions is more conservative. This may be the result of changing the practice patterns of physicians or of attracting those physicians who already have conservative practice patterns. Perhaps a more important type of rationing occurs through the process by which consumers enroll in HMOs. A complex mixture of decisions by government, insurers, HMOs, employers, unions, and the individuals themselves results in HMO options being unavailable to some, expensive to others, and attractive to a relatively small proportion of the nation.

The effects of these rationing devices on various subgroups of the population are similarly complex. By and large, the poor and other disadvantaged groups enrolled in HMOs probably have better access to services than would be the case for them in the conventional system. Similarly, the differences in utilization among socioeconomic groups in HMOs are far smaller than in conventional settings. This is not to say that all differences are erased or that utilization of services is strictly in proportion to need. However, many of the remaining differences seem attributable to difficulties faced by the poor in all settings, rather than to specific hurdles imposed by the HMOs. Somewhat broader differential effects can be seen in those who have the option of joining HMOs. However, this rationing through the availability of enrollment options is to a substantial degree a reflection of market forces and government policies.

Ethical Issues in Approaches Used by HMOs to Constrain Utilization

Two major ethical issues arise when considering the methods used by HMOs to allocate medical services: 1) whether the economic incentives present in an HMO create unethical behavior by their physicians; and 2) whether the allocation system appropriately reflects medical need. Unethical physician behavior may arise from the loss of the physician as an impartial and trusted agent for the patient. This important issue lies at the heart of traditional opposition to the corporate practice of medicine. Abstracting from the rhetoric of such discussions, one can say that the appropriate level of treatment within the current market environment is that level of treatment which the fully informed patient would choose after weighing its risks and benefits, as well as its financial costs (Pauly, 1979). (To simplify matters, we will assume the patient's insurance coverage is equivalent under both systems. Various redistributive schemes would add complexity to the discussion but not alter its major conclusion.) A physician acting as a perfect agent for this patient would reach a similar conclusion. A physician who is also a provider of care to this patient may no longer be a perfect agent and may be swayed by the economic incentives inherent in the payment scheme. If paid fee-for-service, he or she will have an incentive to offer more services, while if paid on a salary or capitation basis, there is an incentive to offer fewer services. The question is whether it is better to err on the high or low side of the correct amount. Too many services increase not only cost but risk.

Unfortunately, it is rarely the case that the patient's problem is diagnosed with such certainty and that a course of treatment is so clear that the "correct" amount is known. Instead, there is generally some uncertainty about the true nature of the disease and often there are several courses of treatment with no clear objective evidence as to which is best for the particular patient (Wennberg et al., 1980). The patient does not have the expertise to really evaluate the potential choices, and I suspect that few physicians are able to deal explicitly with the uncertainty. In fact, even consciously recognizing the relative "softness" of the decision may be such a burden that many physicians develop a "standard approach" to dealing with particular problems. Some may choose a very aggressive testing and treatment approach while others may choose to "wait and see" with minimal intervention. Yet both approaches may yield similar outcomes, especially since our measures of outcome are rather insensitive. The similarity in results will reinforce each practitioner in his or her chosen approach. Wide variations in practice styles have been observed among independent fee-for-service practitioners, as well as within apparently similar physicians in both fee-for-service and prepaid group practices (Wennberg and Gittelsohn, 1973; Schroeder et al., 1973; Roos and Roos, 1981).

While there may be a wide distribution across physicians in how they might treat a particular problem, fee-for-service physicians are more likely to be concentrated at the high service end and prepaid physicians at the low service end. This may reflect the role of incentives in altering their clinical decision-making. Alternatively, it may reflect a process of selection. Physicians who order fewer tests and procedures and hospitalize less frequently—perhaps because that is the way they were trained—will find it difficult to earn as much in a fee-for-service environment as will more aggressive physicians. Similarly, physicians with an aggressive approach will find a prepaid environment less rewarding than fee-for-service (McClure, 1982). Yet each type may be practicing within the generally accepted range of clinical behavior.

There are very few studies of different practice patterns in fee-for-service and prepaid settings that examine what is or would be done for identical patients. Overall measures of the use of services are confounded by patient copayments, differences in case mix, and other factors. One very recent study queried board-certified cardiologists on how they would treat a series of patients described in brief case histories (Hlatky et al., 1981). As might be expected, the independent fee-for-service physicians on average were much more likely than the prepaid group-practice cardiologists to recommend invasive testing and cardiac bypass surgery. However, the recommendations of the HMO physicians were similar to those of university-based cardiologists. In general, recommendations were comparable across practice settings for patients with the most severe manifestations, and major discrepancies occurred for patients with only one or two blocked arteries, a situation in which there is no clear consensus on appropriate treatment in the research literature (McIntosh, 1981; Kouchoukos, 1982). Furthermore, some fee-for-service cardiologists were *more* conservative than the PGP cardiologists, supporting the notion that while the average recommendation may differ significantly, the PGP physicians are within a range acceptable to fee-for-service providers. In general, current studies of the quality of care in HMOs indicate standards at least as high as those in the fee-for-service community (Cunningham and Williamson, 1980; Luft, 1981).

The second ethical issue is whether the systems used by HMOs to ration their services result in an allocation that reflects medical need. HMOs seem to perform well in allocating care *among their enrollees* largely according to need, rather than ability to pay. In this respect, their performance is superior to the conventional system in which copayments often serve as greater deterrents for those with lower incomes.

From a broader perspective, however, one may ask whether *access to health plans* should be independent of ability to pay. There are two problems raised by this question. The first relates to the inability of the poor to pay for health insurance premiums. This problem can, in theory, be solved by giving the poor and low-income workers a voucher scaled to their income and family size that can be used to purchase basic health insurance. If they wish a more expensive plan they will have to pay the extra cost out-of-pocket, just as would be the case for the middle class. Everyone would be placed on an equal footing and access to good basic coverage would be available to all. Such an approach is outlined in Alain Enthoven's "Consumer Choice Health Plan" (1980) and is incorporated in the "Project Health" system in Multnomah County, Oregon (Lewis, 1979; Multnomah County, Oregon, Project Health Division, 1977). The "Project Health" system provided not only a basic voucher, but provided subsidies so that low-income enrollees did not have to pay the full marginal cost of more expensive plans.

The second problem in assuring equal access to health plans arises from the higher cost of covering sick people and the resulting incentives for plans to avoid or push out such enrollees. As indicated earlier, increasing competition is likely to increase the attempts by plans—both HMOs and conventional insurers—to enroll only the healthy. This suggests that people with high needs for medical care will have to purchase coverage at substantial out-of-pocket cost or else they will be forced out of the system. The proposed scenario is analogous to the change in insurance during the 1950s and 1960s which led to the virtual replacement of community rating by experience rating. An area would start out with a uniform rate for all persons. Insurers would identify firms with younger-than-average employees and offer a lower rate. As low-cost firms dropped out of the pool, the premium for those remaining would increase and the process accelerate. The result was a wide variation in rates charged to different firms with some gaining and others losing. Increased competition in the 1980s is likely to result in conventional insurers and HMOs trying to attract low-cost *individuals* within firms, leaving the older or sicker persons to high-cost plans. Furthermore, as the California PHP example and other early indications suggest, the competitive techniques that may be used are not always aboveboard.

Implications for Health Policy

The crucial policy issue that derives from this discussion is how can a competitive system be designed to allow for diversity and encourage innovation and efficiency without getting caught by an analogue to Gresham's law in which cheap plans attract the healthy and exclude the sick. Unfortunately, it is far easier to raise concerns and identify problems than it is to propose solutions, but a few suggestions will be offered to promote discussion.

The basic approach in these suggestions is to reduce the benefits to those plans that select healthy enrollees and increase the penalties they would pay for pursuing such strategies. The first step would be to require a rather broad basic-benefit package for all plans so that people with specific health problems would not be deterred by benefit exclusions. Plans would be encouraged to compete primarily on the basis of price rather than coverage options. This will also make it easier for consumers to evaluate alternatives (Luft, 1982).

The major difficulty with any competitive approach is that the effective premiums for the sick must be above those for the healthy; otherwise plans will develop strategies to avoid enrolling people whose expected costs exceed the premium. If it is possible to identify with reasonable accuracy those people at risk for high expenses, they can be categorized and charged a higher premium. This would entail a system analogous to, but much more complicated than, the point system used by carriers to adjust insurance premiums for drivers with poor accident or traffic violation records. A social decision might be made that most health problems are not the individual's responsibility, so government vouchers or employer contributions would be adjusted to reflect the individual's risk category. While a rather complex system might result, the philosophical precedent is already implicit in the current willingness to pay high premiums for Medicare coverage of the elderly, persons with kidney failure, and the permanently disabled.

The actuarial feasibility of designing risk-adjusted premiums and vouchers is quite another problem. Making the premium a smooth function of several factors such as age, sex, family medical history, and the like might avoid many of the problems associated with the yes/no decisions on disability eligibility. Such a system would make the sick and healthy equally desirable to plans because each brings a premium commensurate with expected costs. Very careful screening by plans might still produce some selection, but most of the benefit to plans of such approaches would be lost. The vouchers could be set at some constant fraction of the risk-adjusted premiums if price sensitivity were desired. Furthermore, the plan's actual premium might be above or below the voucher level depending on the plan's efficiency.

Enthoven (1980) includes a more restricted version of this notion in his discussion of actuarial risk categories. My major difference with him is in emphasis. I think we agree that without such adjustments competition will result primarily in a rush for healthy enrollees. However, I am much more skeptical than Enthoven about the technical feasibility of devising a sufficiently sensitive categorizing scheme, but this is a research question which has not to my knowledge even been explored in a preliminary fashion. The government's willingness to maintain its contribution levels for the most costly categories is a crucial political question that must also be addressed. This becomes particularly important if high-cost patients tend to enroll in certain plans (e.g., those utilizing tertiary-care hospitals) and the plan's high costs are attributed to inefficiency rather than to patients with more complicated problems.

The rewards a plan can reap by pushing out its high-cost enrollees can also be reduced. It may be possible to develop monitoring systems whereby people who change plans report on the problems they experienced and whether they felt pushed out. For instance, the California Public Employees Retirement System, which provides multiple-choice options for state employees, sends a questionnaire to all enrollees switching plans. Because such a system must be sensitive enough to identify important but infrequent complaints, it may be necessary to pool the data from many employee groups to obtain a sufficient sample. Such a system might be analogous to that used to evaluate automobile failures nationwide.

The incentives to keep nonusers while disenrolling users might be blunted by allowing enrollees to build up credits over several years for below-average use. If they switch to another plan, say after incurring an illness, some of those credits would be transferred and drawn down by the new plan. If the previous plan induced them to stay, it could use some of the credits to offset the patient's higher expenses. Although such an approach may be criticized as contrary to general insurance principles, it is designed to counter strong market incentives that may destroy the basic foundation of risk-spreading insurance.

It should be clear that these are only preliminary ideas presented to encourage discussion. They rest upon the belief that HMOs currently provide an important alternative to the conventional system, but that potential changes in the market environment may result in rather objectionable behavior by HMOs and other health plans. Whether it will be possible to design the appropriate policies to encourage desirable, and discourage undesirable, performance rests on improving our knowledge of how the medical care system works and on creating the correct incentives.

NOTES

Arrow, K.J. 1963. Uncertainty and the Welfare Economics of Medical Care. *American Economic Review* 53(5):941–973.

Auger, R., and Goldberg, V. 1974. Prepaid Health Plans and Moral Hazard. *Public Policy* 22:353–393.

Berki, S.E., and Ashcraft, M.L.F. 1980. HMO Enrollment: Who Joins and Why: A Review of the Literature. *Milbank Memorial Fund Quarterly/Health and Society* 58(4):588–632.

California Department of Health. 1975. Prepaid Health Plans: The California Experience. In U.S. Senate, Committee on Government Operations, Permanent Subcommittee on Investigations, *Prepaid Health Plans*, Hearings, March 13–14, 1975, 94th Congress, 1st Session. Washington, D.C.: U.S. Government Printing Office.

California State Legislative Analyst. 1975. A Review of the Regulation of Prepaid Health Plans by the California Department of Health, Sacramento, November 15, 1973. In U.S. Senate, Committee on Government Operations, Permanent Subcommittee on Investigations, *Prepaid Health Plans*, March 13–14, 1975, 94th Congress, 1st Session. Washington, D.C.: U.S. Government Printing Office.

Chavkin, D.F., and Treseder, A. 1977. California's Prepaid Health Plan Program: Can the Patient Be Saved? *Hastings Law Journal* 28 (January):685–760.

Collen, M.F., Dales, L.G., Friedman, G.D., Flagle, C.D., Feldman, R., and Siegelaub, A.B. 1973. Multiphasic Checkup Evaluation Study. 4. Preliminary Cost Benefit Analysis for Middle-Aged Men. *Preventive Medicine* 2(2): 236–246.

Coltin, K., Neisuler, R., and Lurie, R.S. 1978. Utilization of Preventive Services by Poor, Near-Poor, and Non-Poor Members of an HMO. Presented at 106th Annual Meeting of the American Public Health Association, October 16. (Unpublished.)

Cook, W.H. 1971. Profile of the Permanente Physician. In Somers, A.R., ed., *The Kaiser-Permanente Medical Care Program: A Symposium*. New York: Commonwealth Fund.

Cunningham, F.C., and Williamson, J.W. 1980. How Does the Quality of Health Care in HMOs Compare to That in Other Settings—An Analytic Literature Review: 1958 to 1979. *Group Health Journal* 1(1):4–25.

D'Onofrio, C. N., and Mullen, P.D. 1977. Consumer Problems with Prepaid Health Plans in California. *Public Health Reports* 92(2):121–134.

Eggers, P. 1981. Pre-Enrollment Reimbursement Patterns of Medicare Beneficiaries Enrolled in "At Risk" HMOs. Health Care Financing Administration, Office of Research Demonstration and Statistics. (Unpublished draft.)

Enthoven, A. 1980. *Health Plan: The Only Practical Solution to the Soaring Cost of Medical Care*. Reading, Mass.: Addison-Wesley.

Freeborn, D.K., Pope, C.R., Davis, M.A., and Mullooly, J. P. 1977. Health Status, Socioeconomic Status, and Utilization of Outpatient Services for Members of a Prepaid Group Practice. *Medical Care* 15(2):115–128.

———, Greenlick, M.R., Mullooly, J.P., and Burnham, V. 1980. *The Kaiser-Permanente Neighborhood Health Center Project: Ambulatory Care Utilization Patterns*. Health Services Research Center, Research Report Series, Report No. 5. Portland, Oreg.: Kaiser-Permanente Medical Care Program.

Fuller, N., and Patera, M. 1976. *Report on a Study of Medicaid Utilization of Services in a Prepaid Group Practice Health Plan*. Washington, D.C.: U.S. Department of Health, Education, and Welfare, Public Health Service, Bureau of Medical Services.

Gaus, C., Cooper, B.S., and Hirschman, C.G. 1976. Contrasts in HMO and Fee-For-Service Performance. *Social Security Bulletin* 39(5):3–14.

Gertman, P.M. 1974. Physicians as Guiders of Health Services Use. In Mushkin, S.J., ed., *Consumer Incentives for Health Care*. New York: Prodist.

Goldberg, V.P. 1975. Some Emerging Problems of Prepaid Health Plans in the Medi-Cal System. *Policy Analysis* 1(1):55–68.

Group Health Cooperative of Puget Sound. 1970. Non-Appearance of Appointed Enrollees for Care among Public Assistance Enrollees for Comprehensive Prepaid Medical Care. *GHC Research Note* No. 9, summarized in Vignola and Strumpf, 1980.

Held, P.J., and Reinhardt, U. 1980. Prepaid Medical Practice: A Summary of Findings from a Recent Survey of Group Practices in the United States—A Comparison of Fee-for-Service and Prepaid Groups. *Group Health Journal* 1 (Summer):415.

Hetherington, R.W., Hopkins, C.E., and Roemer, M.I. 1975. *Health Insurance Plans: Promise and Performance*. New York: Wiley-Interscience.

Hirschman, A.O. 1970. *Exit, Voice, and Loyalty: Responses to Decline in Firms, Organizations and States*. Cambridge, Mass.: Harvard University Press.

Hlatky, M., Botvinick, E., and Brundage, B. 1981. A Controlled Comparison of Cardiac Diagnostic Test Use in a Health Maintenance Organization. Presented at Annual Meeting of Robert Wood Johnson Clinical Scholars, San Antonio, Texas, November 11–14. (Unpublished.)

Hurtado, A.V., Greenlick, M.R., and Colombo, T.J. 1973. Determinants of Medical Care Utilization: Failure to Keep Appointments. *Medical Care* 10(3):189–198.

Iglehart, J.K. 1981. Drawing the Lines for the Debate on Competition. *New England Journal of Medicine* 305(5):291–296.

Johnson, R.E., and Azevedo, D.J. 1979. Comparing the Medical Utilization and Expenditures of Low Income Health Plan Enrollees with Medicaid Recipients and with Low Income Enrollees Having Medicaid Eligibility. *Medical Care* 17(9):953–966.

Kouchoukos, N.T. 1982. *An Overview Paper—a Surgeon's Perspective on Coronary Artery Bypass Surgery*. Washington, D.C.: National Center for Health Care Technology.

Kralewski, J.E., and Countryman, D.D. 1982. The Interaction of Community Hospitals with HMOs: A Case Study of the Minneapolis/St. Paul Metropolitan Area. *Health Care Financing Review*.

Lewis, R. 1979. Oregon County Buying Prepaid Care for the Needy. *American Medical News* (July 17):1,14,15.

Louis, D.Z., and McCord, J.J. 1974. *Evaluation of California Prepaid Health Plans: Executive Summary*. Santa Barbara: General Research Corp.

Luft, H.S. 1978. How Do Health Maintenance Organizations Achieve Their "Savings"?: Rhetoric and Evidence. *New England Journal of Medicine* 298 (June 15):1336–1343.

———. 1981. *Health Maintenance Organizations: Dimensions of Performance*. New York: Wiley-Interscience.

———. 1982. On the Potential Failure of Good Ideas: An Interview with the Originator of "Murphy's Law." *Journal of Health Politics, Policy and Law*.

———, Feder, J., Holahan, J., and Lennox, D.K. 1980. Health Maintenance Organizations. In Feder, J., Holahan, J., and Marmor, T., eds., *National Health Insurance: Conflicting Goals and Policy Choices*. Washington, D.C.: Urban Institute.

MacColl, W.A. 1966. *Group Practice and Prepayment of Medical Care*. Washington, D.C.: Public Affairs Press.

McCall, N., and Wai, H.S. 1981. *An Analysis of the Use of Medicare Services by the Continuously Enrolled Aged*. Menlo Park, Calif.: SRI International.

McClure, W. 1982. Toward Development and Application of a Qualitative Theory of Hospital Utilization. *Inquiry, The Journal of Health Care Organization, Provision and Financing,* Vol. XIX, No. 2, 117–135, Summer 1982.

Matlock, M.A. 1980. Birth Rate Begets HMO Cancellation. *Business Insurance* (December 22):1,31.

McIntosh, H.D. 1981. *Overview of Aortocoronary Bypass Grafting for the Treatment of Coronary Artery Disease: An Inter-*

nist's Perspective. Washington, D.C.: National Center for Health Care Technology.

Mechanic, D. 1976. *The Growth of Bureaucratic Medicine.* New York: Wiley-Interscience.

Meier, G.B., and Tillotson, J. 1978. *Physician Reimbursement and Hospital Use in HMOs.* Excelsior, Minn.: InterStudy.

Moore, S.H., Martin, D.P., Richardson, W.C., and Reidel, D.C. 1980. Cost Containment through Risk-Sharing by Primary Care Physicians: A History of the Development of United Healthcare. *Health Care Financing Review* 1(4):1–14.

Moore, T.G., Jr., and Breslow, L. 1972. California Medical Group Evaluation Report. California Council for Health Plan Alternatives, December 6. In U.S. Senate, Committee on Government Operations, Permanent Subcommittee on Investigations, *Prepaid Health Plans,* Hearings, March 12–14, 1975, 94th Congress, 1st Session. Washington, D.C.: U.S. Government Printing Office.

Multnomah County Oregon, Project Health Division. 1977. *National Health Insurance through State/Regional/Local Government and Private Sector Health Care Brokerage.* Portland, Oreg.: Department of Human Services.

Newhouse, J.P., Manning, W.G., Morris, C.N., Orr, L.L., Duan, N., Keeler, E.B., Leibowitz, A., Marquis, K.H. Marquis, M.S., Phelps, C.E., and Brook, R.H. 1981. Some Interim Results from a Controlled Trial of Cost Sharing in Health Insurance. *New England Journal of Medicine* 305(25):1501–1507.

Nolan, R.L., Schwartz, J.L., and Simonian, K. 1967. Social Class Differences in Utilization of Pediatric Services in a Prepaid Direct Service Medical Care Program. *American Journal of Public Health* 57(1):34–47.

Pauly, M.V. 1979. What is Unnecessary Surgery? *Milbank Memorial Fund Quarterly/Health and Society* 57(1):95–117.

Phelan, J., Erickson, R., and Fleming, S. 1970. Group Practice Prepayment: An Approach to Delivering Organized Health Services. Part II. *Law and Contemporary Problems* 35(4):796–816.

Physicians Health Plan. 1980. *The Physicians Health Plan of Minnesota: A Case Study of Utilization Controls in an IPA.* DHHS Publication No. (PHS) 80-50128. Washington, D.C.: US. Government Printing Office.

Pope, C.R., Yoshioka, S., and Greenlick, M.R. 1971. Determinants of Medical Care Utilization: The Use of Telephone for Reporting Symptoms. *Journal of Health and Social Behavior* 12 (June): 155–162.

Richardson, W.C., Boscha, M.V., Diehr, P.K., Drucker, W.L., Efird, R.A., Green, K.E., LoGerfo, J.P., McCaffree, K.M., Richardson, W.C., Shortell, S.M., Weaver, B.L., and Williams, S.J. 1977. *The Seattle Prepaid Health Care Project: Comparison of Health Services Delivery.* PB 267488-SET. Springfield, Va.: National Technical Information Service.

Roos, N.P., and Roos, L.L. 1981. High and Low Surgical Rates: Risk Study Factors for Area Residents. *American Journal of Public Health* 71(6):591–600.

Roos, N.P., and Shapiro, E. 1981. The Manitoba Longitudinal Study on Aging: Preliminary Findings on Health Care Utilization by the Elderly. *Medical Care* 19(6):644–657.

Rothenberg, R.E., Pickard, K., and Rothenberg, J.E. 1949. *Group Medicine and Health Insurance in Action.* New York: Crown.

Rybin, V. 1981. Cry for Help: Can HMOs Afford to Listen to Their Patients? *St. Paul Sunday Pioneer Press* (November 15).

Salkever, D.S., German, P.S., Shapiro, S., Horky, R., and Skinner, E.A. 1976. Episodes of Illness and Access to Care in the Inner City: A Comparison of HMO and non-HMO Populations. *Health Services Research* (Fall):252–270.

Schroeder, S.A., Kenders, K., Coopers, J.K., and Piemme, T.E. 1973. Use of Laboratory Tests and Pharmaceuticals: Variation among Physicians and Effects of Cost Audit on Subsequent Use. *Journal of the American Medical Association* 225(8):969–973.

Scitovsky, A.A., Benham, L., and McCall, N. 1979. Use of Physician Services under Two Prepaid Plans. *Medical Care* 17(5):441–460.

Showstack, J.A., Blumberg, B.D., Schwartz, J., and Schroeder, S.A. 1979. Fee-for-Service Physician Payment: Analysis of Current Methods and Their Development. *Inquiry* 16(3): 230–246.

Shragg, H., Fagenbaum, M.E., Kovner, J.W., Caro, H.M., and Bunting, E.D. 1973. Low Income Families in a Large Scale Prepaid Group Practice. *Inquiry* 10(2):52–60.

Taylor, A.K., and Lawson, W.R., Jr. 1981. Employer and Employee Expenditures for Private Health Insurance. *NCHSR National Health Care Expenditures Study Data Preview 7.* DHHS Publication No. (PHS) 81-3297. Washington, D.C.: U.S. Government Printing Office.

Thompson, R.S. 1979. Approaches to Prevention in an HMO Setting. *Journal of Family Practice* 9(1):71–82.

U.S. General Accounting Office. 1974. *Better Controls Needed for Health Maintenance Organizations under Medicaid in California.* Washington, D.C.: General Accounting Office. September 10.

U.S. Senate. Committee on Governmental Affairs, Permanent Sub-committee on Investigations. 1978. *Prepaid Health Plans and Health Maintenance Organizations,* 95th Congress, 2nd Session, Report 95-749. Washington, D.C.: U.S. Government Printing Office.

U.S. Senate. Committee on Government Operations, Permanent Subcommittee on Investigations. 1975. *Prepaid Health Plans,* Hearings, March 13–14, 1975, 94th Congress, 1st Session. Washington, D.C.: U.S. Government Printing Office.

Vignola, M.L., and Strumpf, G.B. 1980. *Medicaid Beneficiaries in Health Maintenance Organizations: Utilization, Cost, Quality, Legal Requirements—An Annotated Bibliography.* DHHS Publication No. 10012. Washington, D.C.: American Public Welfare Association and U.S. Health Care Financing Administration.

Weiss, J.E., and Greenlick, M.R. 1970. Determinants of Medical Care Utilization: The Effects of Social Class and Distance on Contacts with the Medical Care System. *Medical Care* 8(6):456–462.

Wennberg, J.E., and Gittelsohn, A. 1973. Small Area Variations in Health Care Delivery. *Science* 182(4117):1102–1108.

Wennberg, J.E., Bunker, J.P., and Barnes, B. 1980. The Need for Assessing the Outcome of Common Medical Practices. In Breslow, L., Fielding. J.E., and Lave, L.B., *Annual Review of Public Health,* Vol. I. Palo Alto: Annual Reviews, Inc.

Williams, G. 1971. *Kaiser-Permanente Health Plan: Why It Works.* Oakland, Ca.: Henry J. Kaiser Foundation.

Acknowledgments: This paper was prepared for the President's Commission for the Study of Ethical Problems in Medicine and Biomedical and Behavioral Research. I am grateful for comments by Mary Ann Baily, Barbara Cooper, Lauren LeRoy, Susan Maerki, Lawrence Stern, Joan Trauner, and anonymous reviewers.

SECTION II

SOCIAL ETHICS AND MEDICAL SCARCITY

The New Ethical Demand in the Crisis of Primary Care Medicine.

Nancy F. McKenzie, Ph.D.

Introduction

The corporatization of medicine in the twentieth century, culminating in the proliferation of HMOs and corporate medical entities, has left a large segment of American citizens without primary care. Though not by design, the encouragement of high-profit, technological medicine has resulted in a kind of "franchise–middle-class–medicine" mentality that has grave consequences for urban health needs. In our cities, as groups age, become physically or mentally dysfunctional, or otherwise marginalized, they become medically indigent. In 1989, 37 million Americans were without any form of public or private health insurance. Those that were on public entitlement programs could purchase only those medical goods that were offered and defined within the payment schedule of such programs.[1] This means that if their suffering or prospect of suffering was not defined as a medical necessity, they could not receive medical care.

The changes in health care delivery in the United States in the last fifty years, both in access and distribution and in the kinds of care offered, have brought a new set of ethical dilemmas for the health care provider. These dilemmas don't fit nicely into either the ethical framework of absolute duties constituting the Hippocratic ethos or the instrumental duties constituting for-profit medicine. The emerging dilemmas are more about being a patient advocate in a structural sense. They are about the responsibilities the provider has to bring about the social change necessary to allow him or her to dispense basic clinical care. These ethical difficulties require the caretaker to confront what has been true all along: Ethical issues cannot rest merely upon the demands of the dyadic relationship.

The last fifty years have been witness to vast technological changes in medical intervention, as well as the economic reorganization of health care delivery. The advancement in biological, clinical, and genetic research wedded to this economic reorganization is only now seen to have far-reaching effects. The effects are paradoxical, both conceptually and practically. The first—advancement in medical technology—has changed the way in which we think about the limits to "natural" or "biological" life and has *opened up* great possibilities for medical intervention. The other—the economic reorganization of American health care from a predominantly private physician care system to one controlled by centrally organized, corporately owned hospitals[2] —has *restricted* our conception of health care, its availability, and its distribution. In the past twenty years what is "natural" has been seen to have fewer and fewer limits and what is "man made"—the social distribution of medical care goods—has been viewed as immutable and not open to refinement. These views are now changing. The views that medical progress is technical progress and that the medical marketplace should be immune to public control are now being called into question.

The current crisis in primary health care is one that calls for the restructuring of the health care system: a restructuring that can only take place with the input and participation of health care providers themselves.

I. Frameworks of Medical Ethics

Traditional medical ethics has had two basic frameworks within which the medical professional has been able to articulate issues of health care. One kind of ethics is client-centered and driven by the nonutilitarian value of patient beneficence and patient autonomy.[3] Much of medical or biomedical ethics arose from fears that medical progress would impact upon the individual. In the late 1960s many also worried that the technologies of abortion, amniocentesis, resuscitation, and genetic research would bring with them disregard for traditional values: family, children, the *naturalness* of the processes of being born and dying. Additionally, due to the increased authority of the physician, "bioethics" took on the burden of discussions about increasing threats to patient autonomy brought about by a new and more augmented professional expert.

In the late 1960s, client-centered ethics began to address issues of access to health care. The debate was not very extensive and essentially resulted in the position that health care is not organized and should not be organized to the ends of equal access. What ethical questions pertaining to access that remained were restricted to issues of the distribution of finite resources. The need to reorganize health care delivery to more adequately meet medical needs was ignored; the question of distribution became the secondary question of scarcity: Who shall live when not all can live?[4]

However, even this debate was short-lived, and this was for two reasons: 1) It quickly became clear that, with the exception of questions of medical viability, no truly reasonable criteria could be found to refuse treatment to patients without disrupting the essential democratic spirit of American life. Criteria for *who* deserved *what kind* of medical treatment and *who did not* amounted to a kind of access elitism, the consequences of which were, for the nonelite, death. The only fair system for the social allocation of health care goods was a "lottery" or random selection. Physicians were not required to play God, and medical review committees were not required to allocate medical benefits according to any criteria other than "first come, first served," although there were other nonsocial criteria to be utilized.[5] 2) More importantly, however, the issue of health care distribution left the arena of ethics altogether as the American health care system became, for the most part, a corporate enterprise. What had been an ethical issue became an issue of cost containment. Scarcity, much like today but with considerably less severe consequences, still dictated limitations on treatment but discussions were internalized within the frameworks of health finances and fiscal planning. The fact that some people received no care, or were "rationed" out of adequate care, was disguised through health financing. The distribution of health care ultimately lost its meaning as an ethical question. Respect for scarcity became the duty of each physician working in a for-profit institution.[6] The ends of cost/benefit competed openly with patient beneficence as a professional goal.

II. Medical Ethos and Institutional Demand

Two ethical models, client-centered and cost-benefit ethics, have essentially exhausted the dialogue of medical ethics until the present.[7] The current crisis in primary health care requires us to reevaluate our "ethical reach" in the conduct of health care delivery. The emerging issues are ones that pertain directly to the organization of medical care, its limits, its caretaking advantages, or the lack of them. These are issues of account-ability by physicians as advocates of health care change. They are issues of access to health care goods in a shrinking medical economy. Most critically, they are issues of health care technol-ogy versus primary health care and they demand an expanded view of ethical action.

Much of the recent literature in medical ethics reflects the fact that client-centered goals and institutional goals come into conflict, resulting in severe working conditions for the health care provider.[8] The collision became visible as more and more American physicians worked under the requirements of DRG policy or, increasingly, in HMOs. As Veatch points out:

> Asking physicians to be cost-conscious, however, would be asking them to abandon their central commitment to their patients. In effect they would be asked to remove the Hippocratic Oath from their waiting room walls and replace it with a sign that reads, "Warning all Ye who enter here. I will generally work for your rights and welfare, but if benefits to you are marginal and costs great, I will abandon you in order to protect society."[9]

Veatch's view reflects the best face of the conflict. Many caretakers know that the cost containment they marshal their energies under in prospective payment institutions is one dictated purely by the corporate requirements of profitability. This realization has greatly exacerbated the confrontation between the caretaker's wish to practice medicine and the requirements that they do so within corporate financial profiles. Graphically illustrating the conflicting agendas of for-profit medicine and the ensuing pressures upon the present health caretaker is the AIDS epidemic. By the 1990s some major cities in America will be allocating 20 percent of their hospital beds and health resources to people with AIDS—people who, under the current and emerging system of medicine, have no way of paying for those resources. While AIDS paradoxically shows us the impossibility of a technological fix for human suffering, it reminds us, for this very reason, how specific and limited our expectations are with respect to medical care and its possibilities. AIDS stands out as the daunting exception in our otherwise seamless assurance of the last hundred years that health can be negotiated through medical technology.

Ethics in general is not limited to the relationship individuals have to each other; it also includes those relationships as they are conditioned by the history, organization, and policy of institutions. Hence, when we speak of "bioethics" or "ethics in medicine," we are addressing the quality of the relationships between persons made possible by the principled decisions of those medical professionals themselves, *as well as what the system of health care, as both an economic and a social institution, makes possible, or impossible, for its agents.* With prospective payment medicine, for example, the institution becomes the obstacle to care. As Luft points out with HMOs:

> Two major ethical issues arise when considering the methods used by HMOs to allocate medical services: 1) whether the economic incentives present in an HMO create unethical behavior by their physicians: and 2) whether the allocation system appropriately reflects medical need.[10]

Ethical discussion obviously includes an examination of the *quality of the institutions* themselves. As Luft indicates, health care is not only limited by purely professional duties to the patient and the obligations of a corporate or for-profit institution. Medical action is intimately tied to questions of service and advocacy as they are helped or hindered by medical institutions. The new ethical dilemmas are those that address the *structure* of health care within which the medical professional practices.

Providing the American caregiver with increasing difficulty is not merely the collision of a nonutilitarian and a utilitarian view of *their own* actions. More difficult, is *conceptualizing* a health care system with such a paradox; where very little primary care takes place in the areas of greatest need. If one practices medicine in the traditional Hippocratic sense of caring for patients, there is either *too little* to do—because the technical skills of machine-use dictate and intrude on care or are completely adequate to care needs—or there is *too much* to do— because one's patient, using the emergency room for all medical complaints, presents with myriad health care needs unamendable or unresponsive to purely technical intervention.[11]

The demands of the AIDS epidemic alone[12] disclose that our primary health care system, traditionally a system of care for chronic illness, is disintegrating. We simply do not have the infrastructure for a massive number of chronically and terminally ill individuals. Neither do we have treatments for the chronic conditions being disclosed by the American media coverage of AIDS: a heretofore invisible population of the indigent poor; the elderly; the drug-dependent population; the young and very young children of single, unemployed parents; the forcibly deinstitutionalized; and the homeless. What these populations have in common is not merely their poverty and objectification as groups but rather their lack of access to preventive health care and health monitoring by stable and reliable health care personnel. For the poor, medical care is rationed to such an extent that they are almost completely without services.

Health care delivery in America has been centralized in the university hospital. The rationale for this organization, called the Flexner Revolution, was the requirement of teaching and developing technical knowledge. This revolution in medical education changed what was formerly a physician apprenticeship within community health care settings into a method for the imparting of technical know-how, now a quite complex system of technologically refined health care training. Physicians today receive six years of schooling during which the research and development of electronic techniques is coupled with their training as technicians to use them. Such a focus on technologically adept physicians and the institutions to house them has not only resulted in the neglect of basic health care needs, it has functioned to discourage a wide range of health care needs from becoming visible *as* health care needs. Those needs are principally public health needs, which were once served by the general practitioner in neighborhood clinics and are now emerging in urban emergency rooms. They are essentially the needs of primary care: trauma care, preventive strategies, nutrition, prenatal and postnatal regimens, stress control care, psychiatric medicine, and rehabilitative strategies. It is the lack of this basic system of health care delivery that has brought about the collapse of primary care in urban settings. There are too many patients who present with multiple severe problems and are more difficult to treat due to their mistrust of the medical system and their lack of extrahospital resources.

The emerging collapse has been a very subtle disappearing act. The lack of health care delivery for the poor over the last decade has resulted in the redefinition of their plight as a social issue. What were medical or public health problems are now recast as social conditions. This is entirely obvious in the drug-dependent populations for whom the collateral effects of drug dependency, homelessness, physical and mental abuse, and malnutrition are seen as various forms of social degeneracy.

The disappearance of primary care in America operates on two fronts. It is not due only to an increasing scarcity of hospital or clinic access for indigent patients. It is due to a social redefinition of chronic disease as individual social action—the demedicalization of basic health needs and health vulnerabilities. The redefinition of smoking as a form of voluntarism makes the point for the middle-class person just as intravenous drug use does so for the veteran of urban streets. Yet both know that addiction is a medical problem. More funding from public agencies will not solve the national health problem. As one state health commissioner put it:

> The hospital-occupancy crisis will not be solved by more beds. Unless there is a concomitant expansion of other services, we will simply perpetuate a system in which expensive hospital-based technological interven-

tions are substituted for more appropriate primary care services. (David Axelrod, New York State Health Commissioner, *New York Times,* December 4, 1988)

The AIDS epidemic is now showing us the limit of our national system. In the most urgent situations, state and city agencies must step in and offer public assistance when a medical category is lacking or when private insurance or for-profit medicine is no longer operative as in, again, drug dependency or our soaring infant mortality rate. This "stepping in" is occurring increasingly across America, as growing numbers of people find themselves medically homeless. Such a piecemeal approach cannot go on indefinitely.

III. Medical Demand and Ethical Action

The crisis in American health care delivery can be ignored but at great social and moral cost. Confronting the issues of the severe inadequacies of the system with intellectual honesty will be no easy task. The ethical analysis will have to include not only questions of justice in health care access and distribution but an expanded sense of patient beneficence.[13]

One lesson we can learn from Kant, the philosopher of autonomy, is that the respecting of autonomy is the respecting of institutions that further it. This is the meaning of the Categorical Imperative and its required universalization. The respect for the independence and self-determination of persons that is at the heart of patient beneficence includes the responsibility for instituting principles that allow such respect to have a context. Respect for persons is respect for the furtherance of their autonomy. It is a futural concept. Beyond a purely Rousseauian world of nature, this furtherance can only mean the making of institutions that allow autonomy to be empowered and enriched. Ultimately, this must be true for both patient and caretaker. But, caretakers are the agents of this responsibility. The evolved crisis in health care shows us that caretakers must begin to acknowledge that they are as responsible for the quality of the institutions of which they are agents as for their patient-centered action. To split off the dyadic relation to patients as the only province of ethical conduct is to miss the set of external relations that sometimes makes the dyadic relation so problematic. Since the origin of the applied ethics movement, ethical problems have been understood to be internal to the practice of medicine and entirely distinct from the social problems emerging out of its changing social and economic organization. This narrow view of ethical action has led, in part, to the current crisis in primary health care. It can no longer be maintained. It is clear that much of what is happening in medical care today is "external" and that unless caretakers participate in the debate about *who* and *how* and *what* medical care serves, they will find themselves in increasing ethical triage.

Conclusion

A new social reorganization of medicine and an ensuing debate about social change within medicine are now beginning to occur because the economics of health care and the growing numbers of indigent patients dictate that it must.[14] What we will encounter in the next twenty years of ethical debate in medicine will largely be a debate about universal access to health care. This debate must include a reflection on primary health care needs, and this can most effectively be done by caretakers in concert with communities. The health provider, frustrated by an inability to treat a broad and urgent set of medical needs, will have to work in a permanent state of demoralization or begin to formulate a structural solution. As in the late 1950s and 1960s, physicians will enter the debate or have a solution to medical scarcity foisted upon them by public agencies.[15]

The awareness needed to bring about a reformed medical system is already occurring. There is an increased acknowledgment of the hidden and, now, not so hidden needs in America for chronic care delivery. This is already a quest for a redefinition of health provision beyond that artificially instituted under prospective payment plans. AIDS has shown us the dubious roles hospitalization plays in community medical care and the pragmatic and fiscal advantages of home and clinic care. Emergent is the realization of the wastefulness, cost inefficiency, and conflicts of interest at the heart of the hospital/industrial complex. This awareness, coupled with a slow-down in the growth of for-profit medicine,[16] will bring about state health plans, much like that developed recently in Massachusetts.[17] But financing national health care is only the beginning. The debate will have to include a redefinition of health care goods.

America has flirted with setting up a wholly privatized and corporate health care system. It seems, however, that short of the dream's realization, the nation found itself with a two-class system of medical care and one with egregious consequences. There is now broad acknowledgment that the two-class system cannot be maintained. Perhaps Ginzberg is right that the response is almost a moral one:

> [This] underscores the fact that the American people never came close to giving up their voluntary community hospitals and private medical practitioners for an investor-dominated, professional management structure whose goal has been the maximization of profit. Such a transformation would have required even more than short-term illusion on Wall Street and a pro-competition ideology run amok.[18]

It looks like America may, in fact, miss developing a wholly for-profit health care system in the next twenty years. However, for at least one third of the American population this "near miss" comes too late. The lack of preventive care, natality care, health education, rehabilitation therapies, and basic diagnostic care will furnish America with severe health needs well into the next century. The alarming rise in infectious diseases of another era—syphilis and tuberculosis, as well as a soaring rate of infant mortality—indicates quite forcefully how late it is with a "pro-competition ideology run amok."[19] The medically marginalized will fill hospital beds in great numbers for the next few decades.

As the stepchild in distribution of health care, the poor, however, may not be the only victims of this century's collision course with medical cost/benefit. The quality of the entire system of health care, one which should be designed to maintain the integrity of the human organism as well as the human spirit, may have degenerated to such an extent that the human body is merely the sum of its replaceable or usable parts while the medical spirit is one of fragmentation and passivity.

The next century will tell how close we came to the collapse of American medical viability and how far away we truly are from an adequate institutional definition of health. The health care provider is now well aware of the lack of a true health agenda in American medicine. The AIDS epidemic, as well as the candid admittance that our urban health care systems are inadequate, even dangerous to public health, has moved us a long way toward ending the class denial at the heart of health care delivery. Diagnosing the problem as two-class medicine under severe scarcity conditions is half a solution. The other half resides in the caretakers, their imagination, courage, and willingness to discard a system designed to satisfy mostly researchers' intellectual curiosity at the expense of the poor.

NOTES

1. For instance, Medicaid will not pay for such preventive strategies as pap smears.
2. *The Social Transformation of Medicine*, Paul Starr, Basic Books, 1982.
3. "DRGs and the Ethical Reallocation of Resources," Robert Veatch, *Hastings Center Report*, Vol. 16, No. 3, June 1986, p. 33.
4. "Who Shall Live When Not All Can Live," James Childress, in *Ethical Issues in Medicine*, MIT Press, p. 620–626.
5. Triage in the emergency rooms, medical viability, etc. *op. cit.*, Childress.
6. "DRGs: The Counterrevolution in Financing Health Care," Danielle A. Dolenc and Charles J. Dougherty, *Hastings Center Report*, Vol. 15, No. 3, June 1985.
7. In order to see the tension between the two models, it is necessary to provide a description of the ends of medical action that each entails. The context of medicine today is a highly complex one that requires to be understood on at least two traditional levels: One level is the ethos of medicine— our understanding of medicine as an institution or social practice of care, as human action organized by a particular

purpose or end which, put quite simply, is the alleviation of suffering. This description of medicine has endured as a rationale since Hippocrates. The ethos of care is not a simple one or one without conflicting duties. Traditionally, healing has been constituted by these conflicts whether between immediate clinical concerns tied to increasing the autonomy of the patient and the necessity for paternalism; or between current care and the progress of medicine. Most of "medical ethics" has been organized around these patient-centered conflicts. Topics such as truth telling; issues of advocacy in care-giving related to the cessation of suffering and life prolongation; issues of progress in research as well as issues brought about by dramatic technological advancements that change the very nature of birth, disease, and dying. All have served in the last millennia to complicate an apparently otherwise clear set of professional mandates to heal the patient and to serve the future of medicine.

The second level on which to understand medicine considerably changes the traditional picture and is a level now so highly developed as to be an open competitor with the rationale of the alleviation of suffering. This level of analysis is necessitated by the fact that in America medicine is an industry—a system of goods designed, developed, marketed, and sold as products for the alleviation of suffering. The for-profit agenda of medical care, unacknowledged by Americans for the past fifty years, adds a paradoxical quality to the system of care outlined by Hippocrates and adopted by every medical school graduate. This agenda has recently been made visible by the emergence of corporate medicine, which now funds and administers what has come to be called "corporated health care systems." This economic organization has a great influence upon ethical action for it affects the way and ends to which health care is developed, distributed and paid for. Nothing reflects this economic re-organization more clearly than the national change in choice of health care providers. According to the *Milbank Quarterly*:

> During the first half of the 1980's the number of individuals enrolled in capitated health care systems such as health maintenance organizations (HMOs) prepaid group practices (PGPs), and competitive medical plans (CMPs) has grown at an average annual rate approaching 20 percent. This rapid rate of growth is projected

by some analysts to continue until at least the year 2000, when an estimated 63 percent of the population may be enrolled in HMOs (Salomon Brothers 1985).

A for-profit (or "corporated") health care system is one in which the exigencies of profit, scarcity, and efficiency are taken explicitly as ends or goals of the institution and hence serve as limits to the action upon the agents who practice within it.

8. "How Do Health Maintenance Organizations Achieve Their "Savings?": Rhetoric and Evidence, H.S. Luft, *New England Journal of Medicine,* 298 (June 15): 1336–1343.

9. *Op. cit.,* Veatch [p. 38].

10. "Health Maintenance Organizations and the Rationing of Medical Care," Harold Luft, *Milbank Memorial Fund Quarterly,* Health and Society, Vol. 60, No. 2, 1982, p. 295.

11. Many of the over 35 million Americans that use emergency rooms as primary care facilities present with multiple ailments, often requiring interdisciplinary treatment. The waiting time in the public hospital emergency rooms in New York City can figure into days.

12. Not to mention many other alarming rates of infectious diseases such as syphilis, tuberculosis, and pelvic inflammatory disease in women.

13. Patient beneficence usually refers to the province of obligation a caretaker has to an existent patient. However, if those in most need of health care have the least access to health care, the result is ethical paradox. As a conclusion to the paper, I contend that the paradox is not one to be addressed by the obligations of health care justice but, rather, by an extension to patient welfare—an obligation that falls to health care providers. I go on to expand patient beneficence, as many do, to include patient autonomy and its external relations. This final point, made very early by Alisdair MacIntyre, was one that applied ethicists refused to acknowledge.

14. "For-Profit Medicine," Eli Ginzberg, *New England Journal of Medicine*, Vol. 319, No. 16, September 22, 1988, pp. 757–761:

The strongest of the for-profit chains continues to have considerable financial strength, experienced managerial personnel, and entrepreneurial know-how that enable them to move quickly from unattractive situa-

tions into more promising markets. . . . If their success is to continue, they will have to move beyond
health care to a new area of the economy. (p. 760)

15. Cf. the way in which Blue Cross/Blue Shield was used to
stave off national health care and the ways in which the
American Medical Association was allowed to develop
Medicare and Medicaid as alternatives to national health
care. "The Evolution of the Right to Health Concept in the
United States," Chapman and Talmadge, *Pharos*, Vol. 34,
1971, pp. 30–51.
16. *Op. cit.*, Ginzberg.
17. "Prices of Equitable Access: The New Massachusetts Health
Insurance Law," Alan Sager, *Hastings Center Report*, Vol.
16, No. 3, June 1986.
18. *Op. cit.*, Ginzberg.

Acknowledgments: Many thanks to Edna McCown and Jennifer Church, both of
whom read and commented substantially on earlier versions of this paper.

The Evolution of the Right to Health Concept in the United States

Carleton B. Chapman
and John M. Talmadge

Introduction

"Medicine is at the crossroads," incoming president Milford O. Rouse warned the American Medical Association in 1967. He went on to say:

> We are faced with the concept of *health care as a right rather than a privilege* .... We face proposals and possibilities of increased government control . . . , emphasis on a nonprofit approach to medicine, increasing coercion . . . , and emphasis on the academic and institutional environment.[1] (Italics ours.)

In striking contrast, the AMA's House of Delegates passed a resolution two years later (17 July 1969) that said in part: "It is the basic *right* of every citizen to have available to him adequate health care."[2] (Italics ours.)

Dr. Rouse was stating a point of view which was clearly in keeping with policy of the AMA as it was officially laid down nearly half a century ago. But the House of Delegates' action in 1969 represented a modification of official policy that may,

From *Pharos*, Vol. 34, 1971, pp. 30–51. Reprinted by permission of Alpha Omega Alpha, Honor Medical Society.

depending on the actual meaning the Delegates assigned to the resolution, prove to be a profound one.

In linking the word *right* to the word *health*, Dr. Rouse and the House of Delegates were employing a convention that has gradually received wide acceptance in the United States. *Right to health* appears, in modified form, in the Congressional Record (Annals of Congress) as early as 1796 and reappears, largely by inference, at many points during the nineteenth and early twentieth centuries. It came into full flower in Franklin Roosevelt's Economic Bill of Rights (1944) and has been employed by various groups, in and out of government, with increasing frequency ever since.

The meaning assigned to the phrase in 1796 was a very limited one but, even at that early date, it implied a guarantee of protection from certain health hazards to all citizens, regardless of economic or social status. In this sense, it diverged from the ancient view that health care should be provided by government—as a charity, not as a right—only to the indigent. The question of what level of government should concern itself with the right to health entered the debate from the first. And although the question, like the concept, has evolved down the years, it has not been fully resolved even in our own time.

For well over a century, the meaning of right to health had to do with the health of the millions, not of the individual. In the 1870s, leaders of organized medicine specifically excluded curative medicine—treatment of the individual—from their definition of the phrase, leaving preventive medicine, as applied to whole communities and populations, to government. There was no quarrel between government and the then relatively young American Medical Association at the time.

Right to health began to assume a much more comprehensive meaning shortly after the turn of the century and the AMA at first went along. But then came reaction.

Since World War One, and especially since the New Deal, the federal government has intermittently broadened its definition of right to health while the AMA has clung to a conservative view of the matter. But there can be no doubt that when Roosevelt used the phrase ("the right to adequate medical care and the opportunity to achieve and enjoy good health"), he was equating it with the most fundamental social and political rights, guaranteed to every citizen. And while the American electorate has never directly expressed its view of the matter, the broadened definition has almost certainly carried the day. Very few elected officials would, at present, be so rash as to declare publicly for the definition of the eighteen seventies. Right to health in today's usage refers to the health of the individual as well as to that of the millions; to curative as well as to preventive medicine.

Virtually by common agreement, the right to health question is about to become a national political issue of major proportions. Linked as it is with the recognition of a national health crisis, no federal administration, conservative or liberal, can evade the moment of truth that is at hand. Neither can the AMA.

The legislation that actually results will unquestionably be massively influenced by many precedents, some of which are already visible in existing laws but many of which have been largely forgotten.

The paper that follows attempts to display most of those precedents, more or less chronologically, and to put them into some sort of context. It is necessarily a wide-ranging chronicle since it involves some of the most fundamental of American political developments and much of the policy-making activity of the AMA. It ends with the dilemmas faced both by the Nixon Administration, and by the present leadership of the AMA.

Parts of the story have been told before but never in continuous form. The AMA's progressive era has been depicted but its origins and effects seem to have been somewhat slighted. So has the very slow process by which the federal government—all three branches—has laid the groundwork for comprehensive federal health legislation, yet to be achieved. In sum, the present account is part, but only a part, of the background needed by medical and lay observers to comprehend the shape of the battlelines now being formed.

Government and Health, 1796 to 1846

When the United States began life as a nation, most of the states already had in force a considerable body of health legislation. Several of the original colonies had acknowledged the obligation of the community to care for the indigent sick; Rhode Island did so as early as 1662 and Connecticut in 1673.[3] Where the total population was concerned—rich or poor—the only health measures passed by the colonies had to do with quarantine. Massachusetts passed a quarantine law (against yellow fever) in 1647 and repealed it two years later when the threat had passed.[4] New York City enacted a quarantine ordinance in 1755 specifying Bedloe's Island as the quarantine site. The Carolinas and Georgia passed similar laws, also in the mid-eighteenth century.[5]

The menace of summer epidemics of yellow fever plagued the new nation as much as it had the colonies. But the Constitution made no mention of health and Congress found no authority to act in the field of health until it was forced to do so by a crisis precipitated by a new yellow fever epidemic. Virtually by default, it turned to the Commerce Clause (Article I, Section 8),* the inference being that if state quarantine laws interfered with interstate and foreign commerce, federal authority was superior to that of the states. But the right to promulgate quarantine laws belonged to the states.

The precedent was a far-reaching one. For decades it had the effect of denying authority to the federal government in health matters, even those relating to quarantine. It was the continuing threat of yellow fever that finally broke the impasse.

Early Federal Health Laws

On 11 September 1793 the *Gazette of the United States* reported on one of its inner pages that "Yesterday, the President of the United States left town [Philadelphia], on a visit to

---

*"To regulate Commerce with foreign Nations, and among the several States, and with the Indian Tribes."

Mount Vernon."[6] For good reason, the *Gazette* did not tell the whole story. The President was actually fleeing a stricken city as almost his entire cabinet had done earlier. Yellow fever, which had appeared in Philadelphia in July, had paralyzed the city and a week after it reported the President's departure, the *Gazette* itself suspended publication until 11 December. The epidemic, which was at its height when Washington headed south, took 4044 lives before it was brought to a halt by cold weather. The President attempted to keep vital government business going from Mount Vernon, but for practical purposes the new nation had no government until the epidemic had run its course. Sensing the great danger in such a hiatus, Washington wrote to the Attorney General and other cabinet members from Mount Vernon to ascertain whether or not he possessed the power to convene Congress elsewhere if epidemics threatened.[7] Since opinions on the matter differed, he asked Congress early in 1794 for the authority to call meetings outside the Capital, if "... the prevalence of contagious sickness, or the existence of other circumstances [would] . . . be hazardous to the lives and health of the members. . . ."[8] An Act to this effect was approved on 3 April 1794.[9] On the surface, Congress appears by its action to have been concerned primarily with its own right to health rather than with that of the citizens of the new nation. But the move was a pragmatic one, initiated by an anxious chief executive and designed to keep the nation's government intact at a critical moment. Beyond this, it had no political or philosophic implications.

The severity of the epidemics of 1793 and 1794, and the paralysis they produced in the new nation's commercial life, were not soon to be forgotten. Congress might move its meetings to locations that were not threatened but the country's great seaports were fixed and the populace itself was less mobile than the Congress. Since nothing was known about the nature or mode of transmission of yellow fever except that it was introduced by ships coming from other countries, the resort was to control by quarantine. The inference of proponents of a national quarantine law was that the national government could administer quarantine action more effectively than the individual states. In the spring of 1796, a quarantine bill was introduced by Representative S. Smith of Maryland, requiring federal revenue officers to assist ". . . in the execution of the health laws of the states . . . in such manner as may . . . appear necessary."[10] But very significantly, the proposal gave the President the power to prescribe the conditions of quarantine, a feature that stimulated lively and fundamental debate in Congress. The debate, which went on for two days, centered primarily on questions relating to state and federal authority, a singularly sensitive issue at the time. The limits and extent of federal authority in general were very much in question, and Hamilton's federalist views were strongly contested by the opponents of strong central government headed up by Jefferson.

In the House debate on the quarantine proposal, seventeen representatives from ten states took part. The principle of national, as opposed to state, quarantine was fought most strongly by representatives from Pennsylvania, New York, and Massachusetts, all of which had their own quarantine laws. Southern representatives favored the proposal on the ground that epidemics affect the whole country and ". . . not only embarrass the commerce but injure the revenues of the United States." Representatives from Connecticut and Rhode Island (which had no quarantine laws) agreed.

Only one Representative seems to have been concerned as much with the health issue as with the question of state versus federal authority. He was William Lyman, of Massachusetts.* Although opposed to giving quarantine authority to the national government Lyman, a staunch Jeffersonian and antifederalist, acknowledged that government at some level may assume an obligation to protect its citizens from epidemic disease. *"The right to the preservation of health,"* said Lyman, *"is inalienable."*[12] (Italics ours.)

This was the first mention of the right to health in Congress and the meaning inferred by Lyman was a limited one. But the question of protecting the public's health was overwhelmed by the battle over the authority of the states versus that of the Congress, and the antifederalists carried the day. The quarantine measure was voted into law shorn of its provisions that were designed to give the federal government more than a permissive role in the matter of quarantine.[13] Within a few

---

*Lyman, born at Northampton in 1755, served in the House from 1793 to 1797. He belonged to the most radical wing of the Jeffersonian Party and was later rewarded by Jefferson with a Consulship in London. He died in England in 1811 and is interred at Gloucester Cathedral.[11]

years both New York and Phildelphia, whose Representatives had opposed the first national quarantine proposal, asked Congress for a strong national quarantine law but no action was taken owing to the fact that "Congress now had a precedent to worship."[14] It was, with regard to quarantine, a precedent that would remain largely intact for nearly a century.

Three years later (1799) the Fifth Congress revised the quarantine law of 1796, strengthening the hand of federal authority to a very small degree.[15] By that time, however, all moves to strengthen the central government had come under suspicion as the federalist era neared its end. The oppressive Aliens and Sedition Laws of the previous year[16, 17] had raised the specter of oligarchy and tyranny; and Thomas Jefferson (along with Madison) had, in cold fury, responded by secretly authoring the Kentucky Resolution (later adopted also by Virginia) with its extreme emphasis on States' Rights. Partly as a result, basic quarantine authority came to be even more firmly fixed in the hands of the states, a position that was subsequently upheld by Chief Justice John Marshall.

The occasion was the famous *Gibbons vs Ogden* decision which was precipitated when New York State awarded a steamboat monopoly on its navigable streams to Robert Fulton and Robert Livingston. The issue was one of interstate commerce but the question of quarantine authority was brought into the argument by analogy. In his decision, Marshall denied that quarantine (inspection) laws derive from the right to regulate commerce:

> That inspection laws may have a remote and considerable influence on commerce will not be denied; but that a power to regulate commerce is the source from which the right to pass them is derived, cannot be admitted. . . . They form a portion of that immense mass of legislation, which embraces everything within the territory of a State, not surrendered to the general government. . . . Inspection laws, quarantine laws, health laws of every description . . . are component parts of this mass. No direct general power over these objects is granted to Congress; and consequently they remain subject to State legislation. If the legislative power of the Union can reach them, it must be for national purposes.[18]

Although somewhat ambiguous, Marshall's opinion stood virtually unchallenged for decades. It recognized an obligation at the level of state government to protect the health of the public but made it clear that where quarantine laws ". . . might interfere with . . . the laws of the United States made for the regulation of Commerce . . . , the Congress may control the State laws. . . ." The decision went a long way toward consolidating federal control on interstate and foreign commerce but it clearly confirmed the precedent of the 1796 quarantine law in that it assigned basic quarantine authority to the states.

But an earlier Congress had already acknowledged a degree of federal obligation in protecting the nation's health. In an action which has been surprisingly neglected by historians, Congress had, in 1813, rejected the view that health matters belong solely in the hands of the states and acknowledged some degree of obligation at the federal level to guarantee the citizen's right to health. The law was one that required the federal government to guarantee the efficacy of cowpox vaccine and to distribute it, free of charge, to anyone requesting it. Cowpox vaccination had been introduced into the United States by Benjamin Waterhouse, Professor of the Theory and Practice of Physick at Harvard, in 1800. Waterhouse sought the patronage of Thomas Jefferson by sending him a copy of his pamphlet on the subject later the same year and Jefferson responded, expressing great interest, in a letter written on Christmas Day.[19] Once Jefferson's interest was aroused, he pursued the problem of obtaining a potent and safe vaccine with characteristic thoroughness and was instrumental, in the first decade of the nineteenth century, in making effective vaccine available to the country's major population centers.

State government had entered the effort three years earlier when the Commonwealth of Massachusetts required "towns, districts, and plantations," to choose three or more suitable persons to superintend inoculation of Massachusetts residents.[20] But the problem of obtaining an effective vaccine was (and sometimes still is) a difficult one. Partly at Jefferson's urging, the Twelfth Congress passed a law (27 February 1813) requiring the President to appoint an agent" . . . to preserve the genuine vaccine matter, and to furnish the same [free of charge] to *any citizen* of the United States."[21] (Italics ours.) It was, in effect, a reversal of Jefferson's antifederalist stand and suggests that, where health was concerned, he was willing to modify his customary views.

The vaccination law, in principle, went a good deal further than earlier quarantine legislation and came close to demonstrating a positive across-the-board concern for the health of all American citizens up to and including the supply of the necessary biologic agent at federal expense. The law was apparently enacted with little or no opposition and remained in force for nine years. It might have remained permanently on the books had not a federal vaccine agent sent a batch of smallpox (instead of cowpox) vaccine to North Carolina with dire results. As a result, the House set up a Select Committee to inquire into the matter and the conclusion was that the 1813 law should be repealed. The Committee doubted ". . . that Congress can, in any instance, devise a system which will not be more liable to abuses in its operation, and less subject to a prompt and salutary control, than such as may be adopted by local authorities.[22] Congress repealed the law of 1813 on 4 May 1822,[23] the honorable members having obviously been moved more by the outcry from North Carolina than by their concern for constitutional principles. But unlike quarantine legislation, a relatively passive exercise of police power, the 1813 act had reached out to the individual citizen by offering him guaranteed vaccine if he applied for it. In this sense, it was a precedent of considerable importance. And although the vaccination law was finally repealed on the ground that it constituted federal intrusion on the states' prerogatives, it was never actually challenged on that ground.

Subsequent decades saw a decline in federal interest in health legislation except for measures that were concerned with special groups including the military and various wards of the government. The quarantine system continued virtually unchanged except for a minor procedural alteration enacted in 1832 (for one year only).[24] The system was not, judging from the record, effective against yellow fever, which continued to afflict the nation's seaport areas, often in epidemic proportions, almost every year.[25]

But the health of the nation was, by existing standards, undoubtedly good. As its territory expanded (it doubled between 1790 and 1840), and as the center of population shifted from just east of Baltimore (in 1790) to the vicinity of Clarksburg, West Virginia (1840), food supply and distribution improved rapidly.[26] Except in a few large cities, overcrowding was no problem. Under the circumstances government, both federal and state, felt little need to consider health legislation.

Organized Medicine and Government, 1846 to 1910

The medical profession to this time, having no national organization, found itself at a disadvantage where health matters of national significance were concerned. The impetus for a national medical organization came from the New York State Medical Society, which organized a convention of delegates from medical societies and schools primarily to discuss means of improving medical education. The convention met in New York in 1846 and laid the groundwork for the formal founding of the American Medical Association the next year in Philadelphia.[27] The founding resolution listed the Association's purposes as ". . . cultivating and advancing medical knowledge . . . , elevating the standard of medical education, . . . , promoting the usefulness, honour, and interests of the Medical Profession . . . [etc.]."[28,29] Speaking at the Association's first annual meeting, held in Baltimore in 1848, its first president introduced another theme. The profession, said Nathaniel Chapman of Philadelphia, had fallen to a low state and should, through the Association, cleanse itself. But, he added, "we do not want, nor will condescend to accept of any extraneous assistance."[30] Chapman's emphasis on the profession's territorial rights struck a responsive chord; the emphasis remains to this day, although the boundaries of the profession's exclusive territory have been repeatedly redefined.

The new organization devoted its attention at first to medical ethics, education, and scientific matters; but, in its first year, it urged Congress to pass a law concerning adultered drugs and medicines.[31] Congress quickly obliged.[32] In 1849, however, the Association set up numerous committees (Hygiene and Sanitation, Vital Statistics, and others), and also sought to protect the public, within the limits of its power, from quacks and nostrums. Its concern for the public good became apparent very early through these and other actions; but it as yet lacked the strength and status to influence legislation very effectively. As late as 1901, the AMA had, in the words of its president for that year (Charles Reed) ". . . exerted relatively little influence on legislation, either state or national . . ." during its first fifty years.[33]

In the first decade of its life, the new association seems to have attracted relatively little attention in the press. The *New York Times* first mentioned it on 6 May 1858 and next day, poked fun at it ("a little business and a large row") because of a ruckus at its annual meeting over the seating of a delegate.[34,35] The *Times* continued thereafter to report its meetings more or less favorably but on 9 June 1882 a *Times* editorial writer delivered a blast against the Association. The occasion was the ejection of the New York State Medical Society for not conforming to the AMA's ban on consulting with homeopaths. The AMA, said the *Times*, had in this action ". . . displayed . . . an amount of bigotry and stupidity which is to the last degree discreditable to them. . . ."[36] The *Times* was also critical of the poor quality of the papers read at AMA meetings (only 20 percent worthwhile) but, in general, press comment was either noncommittal or favorable.

The Association quite early recognized the need for a federal department of health and for federal legislation in support of adequate vital statistics. In the seventies and eighties, it was pressing at the state level for adequate licensure laws and, in the last quarter of the century, for the establishment of state boards of health. In this noble endeavor, the Association was, in effect, stressing the obligation, as well as the power, of local and state government to guarantee the implied right of all citizens to protection from public health hazards. But the policy was still thoroughly in accord with Congressman Lyman's eighteenth-century concept of the right to health.

The first suggestion that the Association should be better informed about federal actions in health affairs came in 1867 when one of the founders, Dr. Nathan Smith Davis, moved that the annual meeting be held on alternate years in Washington.[37] The motion passed and the 1870 session was held in the capital; but meetings on alternate years proved to be impracticable. A section on State Medicine and Hygiene was created in 1872 and a definition of state medicine was composed for the first time. It ran: ". . . State Medicine consists in the application of medical knowledge and skill to the benefit of communities, which is obviously a very different thing from their application to the benefit of individuals in private or curative medicine."[38] A similar view was put forward in 1878 by the Association's incoming president, Dr. T. G. Richardson of New Orleans, who told the members that public hygiene was the ". . . prevention or arrest of all diseases which are not in their nature strictly limited to the individual . . . but which have a tendency to spread throughout . . . communities and which cannot otherwise be controlled. . . ."[39]

These semi-official definitions may be taken as the beginning of conflict between the AMA and government; but at the time they were put forward, the AMA was actually ahead of the national government in its attitude toward the right to health. Yet in defining public and private health as they did, the Association's leaders were drawing a very fine line, one which was even then rapidly becoming blurred.

At the state level, Massachusetts had (in 1850) taken a significant action when it set up a Sanitary Commission to inquire into conditions affecting the public's health in the Bay State. The result was a memorable report written largely by Lemuel Shattuck, a statistician.[40] In the report, Shattuck firmly points to the need for control of the public's health by "public authority and public administration." He thought the state should protect the citizen ". . . from injury from any influences connected with his locality, his dwelling house, his occupation, or those of his associates or neighbors; or from any other social causes." His emphasis was obviously on the prevention of disease rather than on curative medicine (". . . measures for prevention will affect infinitely more, than remedies for the cure of disease."). But there is an unmistakable implication in his comments that the individual citizen has the *right* to be protected by government from identifiable health hazards.

Shattuck's recommendations led to the establishment of the Massachusetts Board of Health (1869) but apparently had little immediate effect on federal legislation. Congress did, however, move a year later to give the Marine Hospital Service coherent structure. To that time, the Service had been concerned solely with the health of merchant seamen and was badly organized even for that limited purpose. It now began to take shape as a health unit of more general purpose. The Act of 29 June 1870 put the Service under the Treasury Department and authorized the appointment of a Supervising Surgeon at $2,000 a year.[41] Viewed at the time as a necessary but routine administrative action, it was to assume much greater significance after the turn of the century.

The National Board of Health

Eighteen seventy-eight was a major turning point in federal attitudes toward the government's obligation to protect the health of the nation and, once again, it was a massive epidemic of yellow fever that produced the change. An epidemic of the disease had been reported in Rio de Janeiro in April[42] and by mid-summer had reached New Orleans. By late August the city was paralyzed and the disease had made its appearance in cities well upriver from New Orleans. Credence was given in retrospect to an earlier prediction by a black voodoo sorcerer that a plague would strike New Orleans in the summer of 1878 and that it would not begin to subside until the daily death toll equalled the degrees of the thermometer.[43] He turned out to be approximately, if not exactly, correct. By December, the epidemic had taken an estimated total of 30,000 lives in the Mississippi Valley and, well before it had run its course, the country was in an uproar. While the disease was still localized in the New Orleans area, Congress passed an inoffensive quarantine measure requiring U.S. Consuls at foreign posts to report epidemics of contagious disease to the Marine Hospital Service on a regular basis. The new law also authorized the Service to make new rules and regulations on quarantine as appropriate provided that ". . . such rules and regulations shall not conflict with or impair any sanitary or quarantine laws or regulations of any State or municipal authority. . . ."[44]

The action was much too weak to influence the catastrophe that was so soon to break and events during the epidemic showed with abundant clarity that local quarantine laws were inadequate in time of crisis.[25] The epidemic ran its natural course largely uninfluenced by quarantine measures, local or federal.

The subsidence of the epidemic in November 1878 brought with it vigorous debate concerning the best means of excluding the disease from the United States. The American Public Health Association, meeting in Richmond, Va., called for effective quarantine measures and assigned responsibility for it to the "General Government."[45] The AMA had earlier passed several resolutions to the same effect.[46] In December 1878, both houses of Congress set up special committees to investigate ways and means of controlling epidemics of all types of contagious disease and the Senate's Select Committee, reporting on 7 February 1879, made a number of recommendations mostly aimed at centralization of quarantine authority; one proposal was the creation of a National Board of Health.[47]

There ensued several weeks of contest and conflict within the federal government,[48] the net effect of which was the hasty passage of a law on 3 March setting up a National Board which was charged, among other things, with ". . . *obtaining information* upon all matters affecting the public health. . . ."[49]

The Board was organized on 2 April and included in its membership some of the most able medical men in the country; John Shaw Billings, Henry I. Bowditch, and Samuel Bemiss were among them. The Board was reluctant to accept responsibility for administering national quarantine laws until it had the benefit of epidemiologic research on yellow fever, but despite this, Congress gave it rather vaguely defined authority over quarantine in a law passed on 2 June.[50] It was hotly debated in the House.[51] Representative Jonas H. McGowan of Michigan (who had introduced the Bill setting up the National Board) derived federal authority over quarantine squarely from the Commerce clause of the constitution, a view that was contested by many other members. Representative Van H. Manning of Mississippi sought to settle the conflict by resort to semantics: He noted that the word commerce meant much more than exchange of merchandise and must include other types of interstate and international relations as well. Most southerners, however, opposed the proposal on the grounds of states' rights and Representative Omar D. Conger of Michigan finally lost patience: "Show me a Southern States-rights democrat on this floor . . . and I will show you the man whose conscience has been relieved from all obligations as a States-rights man if he has a harbor to build within his district, or a river to deepen and improve."[51]

But the bill, which was to run for four years, passed despite the foes of centralization. The nation thus, in time of crisis, acquired its first national health authority, which, although badly designed and in difficulty from the start, was the closest Congress has ever come to sanctioning a Ministry of Health. The Board was charged with redesigning and implementing the nation's quarantine system, and ostensibly, it had the legal authority to do so. But in Billings' words, "the only power possessed by the National Board lay . . . in the character and reputation of its members and the probability that their advice would be received with respect by local organizations."[52] Its authority to initiate a research program was, however, much clearer. It was authorized to spend $500,000 as grants-in-aid for the purpose and it allocated a portion of the sum to nonfederal scientists working in private laboratories.

It was, in fact, the federal government's first move to support biomedical research *pro bono publico*, and as it turned out, the Board's sponsorship of extramural research was its most successful activity.* It funded a large number of epidemiologic and laboratory studies, some of them quite sophisticated for the time, during the four years of its existence.[48] Among its grantees were Ira Remsen of Johns Hopkins, P. C. Chandler of Columbia, James Low of Cornell, and George Sternberg of the U.S. Army.

The Board's chief problems arose in connection with the charge to design and implement a new national quarantine system. The effort to do so quickly brought it into conflict with the state health authorities (especially in Louisiana), officials of the Marine Hospital Service, and the Treasury Department. Probably its most implacable enemy was the Marine Hospital Service which saw itself being displaced by the National Board. The Board was commended for its sponsorship of research by the National Academy of Science, but by 1882 its demise was a foregone conclusion.[53] It ceased to meet in 1884 when the law that created it expired.

---

*The practice of awarding research grants to private individuals working in nonfederal institutions was reinstated briefly during World War I. In 1937 it was incorporated in the National Cancer Act and, from 1948 onward, formed a major feature of the vastly expanded activities of the National Institutes of Health.

The National Board episode was an important but unsuccessful step toward consolidation of quarantine authority in federal hands. Probably a good deal more important was its demonstration to Congress of the value of research in the public interest. But the consensus in later years was that it was well ahead of its time and too hastily conceived to be viable.

Objections to a national quarantine authority were, however, unmistakably subsiding and an effective national quarantine law, giving appropriate authority to the Marine Hospital Service, was finally passed in 1893.[54] A Supreme Court decision handed down six years earlier had virtually invited the action. The Court at that time had said:

> But it may be conceded that whenever Congress shall undertake to provide for the commercial cities of the United States a general system of quarantine, or shall confide the execution . . . of such a system to a national board of health . . . all state laws on the subject will be abrogated, at least so far as the two are inconsistent.[55]

It was, in Faulkner's words, the beginning of the decline of *laissez-faire,* a process which he dates to the Interstate Commerce Act of 1887.[56] But, in fact, the process may be viewed as having begun much earlier when Congress made its first timid moves to establish national authority over quarantine, attempting unsuccessfully to separate the right to protection from epidemic disease from the right to free enterprise in economic affairs.

In later years, the U.S. Public Health Service, successor to the Marine Hospital Service, became the federal government's health arm, but in health matters other than quarantine, it was forced by weak federal legislation to carry on its work more by diplomacy and tact than by legal authority. The precedent of the 1796 quarantine law, backed up by the Supreme Court decision of 1824, still applied in many respects at the turn of the century.

The American Medical Association had, unofficially but effectively, gone further. It had distinguished between the public's health and private health; government at all levels could only be concerned with the public's health—the health of the millions—and not with private health—the health of the individual. The distinction also involved another line of cleavage: preventive versus curative medicine. Preventive medicine was public; curative medicine was private with few exceptions.

The turn of the century saw the passing, for the most part, of huge epidemics of infectious disease. A federal health research arm was reestablished in 1887 with the founding of the Hygienic Laboratory within the Marine Hospital Service, and funds for a building were appropriated in 1901.[57] On 14 August 1912 an act of Congress completed the conversion of the Marine Hospital Service to the U.S. Public Health Service and specified that the Service should ". . . *study and investigate* the diseases of man and conditions influencing the propagation and spread thereof. . . ."[58] (Italics ours.) As in the case of the National Board Act of 1879, the research provision of the action taken in 1912 was clearly a pragmatic one in the minds of federal legislators: research was one means—and a politically inert one at that—by which the national government could guarantee the citizen's right to protection from disease.

Reform and Reorganization

The Age of Reform, by Hofstader's definition,[59] ran from 1890 to 1920, his reference being primarily to reform in economic affairs. It brought federal action limiting *laissez-faire* and monopolistic practices in business, the individual income tax, and other legislation, all of which had the effect of strengthening the central government. But federal action in the health field was unimpressive. There was continued agitation for a National Department of Health, which came to naught despite the recommendations of several presidents and the continuing support of the AMA. The Pure Food and Drugs law[60] was finally passed in 1906 owing, in considerable measure, to active support by the AMA. The Association continued the battle when the 1906 law proved to be inadequate and was instrumental in inducing Congress to pass the Sherley Amendment in 1912.[61]

But for some time prior to the turn of the century, AMA leaders had realized that the structure of the organization was too loose and clumsy to permit it to act effectively in the formation of policy. Under its old general assembly system, it was difficult to reach convincing agreement, especially on controversial matters, and concerted political action was well-nigh impossible. A few years after its founding it had disclaimed unofficial statements of AMA views,[62] but it lacked an efficient mechanism for creating or proclaiming official policy. In 1901, a new system was adopted which vested policy-making authority in an all-powerful House of Delegates whose members were chosen by the governing bodies of constituent state medical societies, instead of by direct popular vote.[63] In adopting the procedure, the AMA may well have been following the constitutional precedent of placing the selection of U.S. Senators in the hands of state legislatures, a practice that was abolished in 1913 when the seventeenth amendment was ratified. And by this means, the AMA converted itself into a less representative but much more cohesive and politically effective organization. Under the old system, said an editorial at the time, ". . . prolonged discussion almost always meant defeat or postponement."[64] Under the new, power could be channeled and concentrated for specific purposes. The Association retains the House of Delegates' structure today. Delegates are, not unnaturally, chosen from the relatively small group of physicians, usually conservative, who have shown a sustained and active interest in medical politics.

The power structure in the AMA came, in succeeding decades, to be misunderstood within and without the Association. In practice, editorials in the *Journal of the AMA* and statements by its officers are usually in line with official policy, but no policy is binding unless it has been approved by the House of Delegates. At times, editorials and widely publicized comments by AMA officers seem to have been used as straws in the wind, like many so-called leaks within the federal government, that can be disowned if the response is unfavorable. But the one thing the Association cannot disown is an action of the House of Delegates. Even the Board of Trustees, where policy is concerned, is subordinate; it is chosen by—and responsible to—the House of Delegates.

By 1910 the Association had sought to increase its influence on health legislation by the creation of special committees, bureaus, and councils to deal with the topic. Beginning much earlier, it had undertaken to improve and standardize medical education. Probably its most effective move in this direction

was the creation of a permanent Council on Medical Education
(1904). The Council laid the ground work and set the stage for
a joint effort with the Carnegie Foundation, beginning in 1908.
The result was the Flexner Report of 1910; but the basic work,
without which the Flexner Report would have had little or no
effect, was done by the AMA's Council.

With so much good work to its credit, the Association acquired an unchallengable reputation in the minds of laymen and
legislators alike. It seldom came under public attack, except
from dissident health groups; and in the public eye, more
prominently than the federal government, it was the primary
protector of the public's health.

Health Insurance and the
Genesis of Conflict, 1908–1932

On the national scene, economic reform and federal legislation designed to check monopolistic practices, along with demands for better conditions for the worker, were becoming
daily news items. Emerging labor unions very early turned their
attention to industrial safety and to compensation insurance,
and in this climate, European social and health insurance schemes
began to come under national scrutiny.

Except for active interest in the prevention of industrial accidents, the AMA at first showed little interest in such matters.
But between 1902 and 1914, eighteen states passed workmen's
compensation laws. In 1908, the Russell Sage Foundation financed a study of European social and health insurance systems
and the resulting report, published in 1910,[65] aroused the
interest of a great many liberal groups in this country. The
Journal of the AMA, at the time, published no original comments on health insurance, but from 1905 on it abstracted
many articles from foreign journals on the topic.

It was the passage of the National Health Insurance Act in
Britain toward the end of 1911* that stimulated the *Journal*'s

*It went into force on 1 July 1912.

first editorial on health insurance. The editorial said, in part:
". . . this law marks the beginning of the end of the old system
of the individual practice of medicine, and of the old relationship between patient and physician. . . ."[66]

The developments in Britain were reported sketchily in the
American press but the medical profession received detailed
coverage in the *Journal of the AMA* beginning in early 1911.*
The British Medical Association (BMA) had, by mid-1911,
begun a campaign that was sometimes in total opposition, sometimes in favor of modifications that seemed to be designed
basically to protect the physician's income and autonomy. Ultimately, the controversy split British physicians into two camps,
both in effect opposed to the national health insurance bill as it
had been introduced. A threat by the BMA to refuse service
under the new law could not, in the end, be enforced, and after
obtaining certain concessions from the government, the BMA
reluctantly went along. The final result was damage to public
confidence in the BMA itself, and a legislative compromise
providing inadequate coverage to wage-earners and excluding
their families altogether.

In the United States, the right to health concept was unquestionably coming to be defined more broadly. One of the most
vocal proponents of the concept was the American Section of
the International Association for Labor Legislation, organized
in 1906, which espoused the health insurance cause about 1910.†
In 1911 Louis Brandeis echoed the views of the country's
Progressives‡ when he told the Conference on Charities and
Corrections that a comprehensive system of workingman's insurance was an "incentive to justice," and that government
should not permit the existence of conditions that made large
classes of citizens financially dependent. If it does, he continued, it should ". . . assume the burden incident to its own
shortcoming."[67] The next year, the same organization called for
insurance against accident, sickness, old age, and unemploy-

---

*In the form of *London Letters*, written by a correspondent. The first to deal with
the British health insurance proposal appeared on 3 June 1911. There were about
30 of them over the next eighteen months.
†The American Association held its first meeting in Madison, Wisconsin 30–31
December 1907 and was disbanded in 1942.
‡Members of a political movement which was later to become Theodore Roosevelt's "Bull Moose" third party.

ment. And in the same year, Teddy Roosevelt's Progressive Party pledged itself to work increasingly for a ". . . system of social insurance [including health insurance] adapted to American use."[68]

Undoubtedly influenced by Brandeis, Woodrow Wilson lent impetus to the agitation for social legislation in his first inaugural address. Anticipating presidential health messages of the sixties, Wilson said:

> There can be no equality of opportunity if men and women and children be not shielded in their lives, in their very vitality, from the consequences of great industrial and social processes which they cannot alter, control, or singly cope with. . . . The first duty of law is to keep sound the society it serves. Sanitary laws, pure food laws, and laws determining conditions of labor which individuals are powerless to determine for themselves are intimate parts of the very business of justice and legal efficiency. *We have not . . . studied and perfected the means safeguarding the health of the nation, the health of its men and women and its children, as well as their rights in the struggle for existence.*[69] (Italics ours.)

Wilson seems, in all probability, to have had in mind a considerable expansion of the right to health concept and not to have been bound in his outlook by the rigid distinction between the public's health and private health. But his administration, so soon to be preoccupied by other matters, never followed the health issue up.

Health Insurance Viewed with Interest

The AMA seems to have taken no official notice of Wilson's reference to health, but in 1914 the *Journal* published an article favorable to health insurance by Dr. James P. Warbasse of Brooklyn, a surgeon and medical sociologist. Warbasse condemned commercialization in medicine and emphasized the need for preventive health care. "The socialization of medicine is coming," Warbasse declared, "and medical practice withholds itself from the field of science as long as it continues [to be] a competitive business."[70] And less than six months later, the *Journal* carried an authoritative article on compulsory health insurance by Isaac Max Rubinow, M.D., then the nation's leading authority on the subject, urging American physicians to react constructively to the matter (as British physicians had conspicuously failed to do in 1911).[71]

Two years earlier, the American Association for Labor Legislation had set up a Committee on Social Insurance (December, 1912) which included Rubinow in its membership. Within a few months two other physicians were added to the committee, one of whom was Dr. Alexander Lambert of New York.[72]

Rubinow and Lambert were later to join forces in temporarily converting the AMA to a position which, on balance, favored compulsory health insurance. Rubinow, born in Russia of Jewish parentage, had emigrated to the United States in 1893 at the age of 18. Within a remarkably short time he obtained the M.D. degree at New York University and was practicing in New York. An early interest in economics and social insurance grew to such proportions that he abandoned practice after a few years, and by 1913 he had published an authoritative book on social insurance.[73] In 1914 he received a Ph.D. degree from Columbia, and until he died in 1936, he worked actively in the fields of social insurance and health economics.

Lambert's background was in striking contrast to Rubinow's. Born in comfortable circumstances in New York, he graduated from Yale in 1884 and from the College of Physicians and Surgeons (Columbia) in 1888. A cardiologist by inclination, he was Professor of Clinical Medicine at Cornell for thirty-three years, and was Teddy Roosevelt's personal physician, hunting companion, and confidant. He was also very active in AMA politics, serving (between 1904 and 1920) in some of its most important offices including the presidency. Lambert, a staunch Progressive politically,* became interested in health insurance early in his career and in late 1916 delivered an address entitled *Medical Organization Under Health Insurance* before a joint session of the American Sociologic Society, the American Association for Labor Legislation, and other liberal groups.

---

*The leadership of the Progressive Party, as studied by Chandler,[74] was upper middle class. Most had earlier been Republicans and most were businessmen, lawyers, editors, or university professors, in that order. Very few were physicians.

The address left no doubt as to where he stood on the health insurance issue, and in comments on the presentation Dr. Frank Billings of Chicago unmistakably identified himself as a supporter of Lambert's views.[75] Billings, having served as President of the AMA in 1903, was one of the most prominent physicians and medical academicians of the day. His reputation was unassailable, and his support was very meaningful especially within the ranks of the AMA membership. But his comments got him into an embarrassing position within the AMA a few years later.

In mid-1916 the Committee on Social Insurance of the Association for Labor Legislation, with Lambert and Rubinow participating, had produced a Model Health Insurance Bill, an activity to which the AMA lent its counsel.[76]

In its opening sentence, the model bill rejected the term "sickness insurance" in favor of *health insurance*, ". . . because it calls attention to the main object of the act, the conservation of health. . . ." The bill proposed that the cost of insurance be distributed on a sliding scale between employer, employee, and the state, with special provision for employees in unusually low income brackets. Benefits included medical and nursing care (in- and out-patient), medical and surgical supplies for a limited time, cash payments during illness for up to 26 weeks, maternity benefits, and burial coverage. Participation was compulsory with certain exceptions. Carriers were to be mutual associations supervised by the state. No federal involvement was proposed.*[77]

The AMA's Progressive Era

To 1915, the AMA had, through its *Journal*, shown only modest interest in the changing social and political climate. But in that year, Alexander Lambert, then chairman of the Associa-

---

*The signal importance of the model bill seems to have been largely forgotten in our own time. Drafted with great care, it avoided some of the defects of European systems and has influenced planners, directly or indirectly, ever since. Neither federal nor state government was involved in its preparation. It was introduced into the New York legislature with Governor Al Smith's endorsement; it passed the Senate but was defeated in the House. Commissions to study the proposal were set up in California, Illinois, New Jersey, Ohio, Pennsylvania, Wisconsin, and others. Some reports were favorable but no legislation resulted.

tion's powerful Judicial Council, addressed the House of Delegates on the subject of health insurance. His report was a detailed account of European health insurance systems, setting them out in a very favorable light; and the House was sufficiently impressed to direct, through a reference committee, that the report be brought by state medical societies to the attention of the rank and file.[78]

A few months later, the *Journal* took favorable notice of the Model Health Insurance Bill of the American Association for Labor Legislation. All American physicians should study the bill carefully, said the *Journal*, its implication being that better health insurance legislation might result if they did so.[79] Early in 1916, a *Journal* editorial, noting the introduction of the model bill into the Massachusetts and New York legislatures, said that the move ". . . marks the inauguration of a great movement which ought to result in an improvement in the health of the industrial population and improve the conditions for medical service among the wage earners."[80]

It is difficult today to believe that such sentiments could ever have appeared in the *Journal of the AMA*, long noted for its ultraconservative views in support of *laissez-faire* medical care. But in late 1915 and early 1916, the *Journal* undoubtedly was reflecting the views of the AMA's leadership. To this point, however, the Association had, except for participating in construction of the model bill, taken no action. It now moved, partly at the suggestion of the Association for Labor Legislation but also at Lambert's urging, to set up its own Committee on Social Insurance. The AMA Board of Trustees, which approved the Committee in February 1916, instructed it ". . . to do everything in [its] power to secure such constructions of the proposed laws [on health insurance] as will work the most harmonious adjustment of the new sociologic relations between physicians and laymen which will necessarily result therefrom. . . ."[81] All of which leaves little doubt that the AMA leadership was convinced that some form of compulsory health insurance, backed by government, was in the offing and could be made to serve a useful social purpose.

Lambert, asked to serve as chairman of the new committee, lost no time in taking action. By mid-1916 the Committee had set up offices in New York, conveniently near to those of the American Association for Labor Legislation, and had employed

Rubinow as executive secretary. Rubinow energetically set to work writing, speaking, and travelling in support of health insurance. In April 1916, he found time to testify in support of a health insurance proposal introduced into Congress by Meyer London,* Socialist representative from New York's east side.[83] In hearings before the House Labor Committee, Rubinow said that he was appearing at the request of the Socialist Party of America to which, he affirmed, he had belonged for twenty years. Later in the hearings he and Samuel Gompers traded verbal blows at some length. Toward the end of the exchange, Rubinow said ". . . most emphatically that in my official position as executive secretary of the social insurance committee of the American Medical Association I am authorized to state that [the AMA] is heartily in support of Mr. London's resolution, and . . . is committed to the general principle of social sickness insurance in this country."[84]

He was, in fact, too emphatic. His authorization most likely came from Lambert, and possibly from other AMA leaders. But it was not a position that had been approved by the House of Delegates. London's resolution was never officially backed or opposed by the AMA. Its defeat, which came in 1917, was due largely to opposition from the insurance industry and from organized labor. The vote was 189 yea, 138 nay, and 106 abstentions; but it needed a two-thirds majority to pass.[85] The affirmative vote was not negligible but the defeat of the resolution was a turning point of sorts. And about this time Ernst Freund, Professor of Law at Chicago, implied that the proponents of health insurance might be pushing a bit too hard. He said that use of public funds to improve health was probably justified ". . . upon any reasonably liberal view of constitutional power," but that compulsory contributions by employers were vulnerable to attack in the courts. "Let the advocates of health insurance agree upon a minimum program and urge the adoption of that. The well-known expansive tendency of relief legislation may be relied upon to take care of the future."[86]

In May 1917, Lambert and Rubinow produced a massive

---

*London, like Rubinow, was born in Russia (1871). He came to the United States in 1891 and served in the 64th, 65th, and 66th Congresses representing the 12th New York District. Also like Rubinow, he was an active supporter of the American Association for Labor Legislation.[82]

report for the House of Delegates spelling out the details of German experience with compulsory health insurance, and describing the transition in other countries from voluntary health insurance to schemes that were partly subsidized by the state and to compulsory insurance. It also condemned "blind opposition, indignant repudiation [and] bitter denunciation of [compulsory health insurance] laws." The House of Delegates, its mood now more cautious, instructed Lambert's Committee to continue its study and to make certain stipulations concerning the protection of the profession's interest.[87]

Counterreactions from the Rank and File

But the political mood of the country, now on the verge of declaring war on Germany, was rapidly moving counter to earlier progressive trends. And within the AMA, Lambert and Rubinow had reckoned without the grass roots. It seemed to have gone unnoticed that the medical profession, once a remarkably unified organization, had begun to develop two important factions. On one side stood men like Billings and Lambert whose education had gone beyond the minimal requirements for the M.D. degree, who had moved from general to specialty practice, and who were prominent in academic medicine and research. It was to such men that, prior to World War I, the leadership of the AMA was frequently entrusted. On the other side was the great body of general practitioners, men whose formal education was often limited, who usually had no connection with academic medicine, and whose long hours of exacting service, day in and day out, kept them relatively isolated from currents of social and professional change. The health insurance issue, combined with the rising tide of political reaction, brought them out of isolation.

Letters critical of Lambert and his committee, mostly moderate in tone, began to appear in the *Journal of the AMA* and in state medical journals early in 1917. But it was Eden V. Delphey, a New York general practitioner, who more than any other, converted moderate criticism to a holy war, and initiated a sharp and permanent swing to the right within organized medicine.*

In March 1917, Delphey wrote that the model health insurance bill, then before the New York legislature (and endorsed by the State Medical Society), would convert physicians into mere cogs in a huge political machine. In May, he addressed a letter to the editor of the *Journal of the AMA* condemning compulsory health insurance ". . . Because it is un-American. Americanism means that the individual amounts to something; paternalism, that the individual is nonimportant but that the state is all important. Even a beneficent paternalism is harmful because it destroys individualism and discourages thrift." He went on to say that very few Americans were without adequate medical care, and that surveys indicating the contrary were worthless because they had been done by "medically unqualified and therefore incompetent persons."[88]

As it turned out, Delphey was obviously saying what a good many of the nation's physicians wanted to hear. Many of them, in retrospect, may have read or heard Lambert's reports in silence, possibly owing to the stature of the man who had produced them. But Delphey's move opened the floodgates of opposition.

From that point on, Lambert and colleagues fought a losing battle. Lambert himself went off to war, and by the time he returned health insurance of all kinds was discredited within the AMA. At its annual meeting in 1919, the House of Delegates heard a final plea for adequate and informed consideration of the health insurance issue, delivered by one of Lambert's colleagues. Lambert himself, now president-elect of the Association but still in Europe, sent a strong statement attacking his opposition and urging continuing study of compulsory health insurance. But it was to no avail; the receptive spirit of 1915 and 1916 was a thing of the past, and the House now created a stalemate in Lambert's small committee by adding outspoken conservatives to it.[89]

Even this was not enough for the conservative faction of the AMA. Thoroughly alarmed at any prospect of health insurance

*Eden Vinson Delphey (1858–1925) graduated from the Medical Department of Columbia College in 1889 and practiced at 171 W. 71st Street for many years.

and determined to close the issue once and for all, conservatives contributed a steady stream of outspoken criticism of
Lambert's Committee to medical publications. Rubinow was
singled out for increasingly vituperative attack. The Association
for Labor Legislation, with which the AMA had maintained
cordial rapport a scant four years earlier, was now characterized as a Bolshevist organization in disguise, and it was claimed
that Rubinow had all along been acting secretly as an agent for
the Labor Legislation group.[90] On this ground, in the midst of
the postwar spy scare and anti-Bolshevist hysteria, Rubinow
was summarily fired, the Committee's reports discredited and
suppressed, and the Committee itself allowed to die. Its last
report to the House of Delegates, given by Victor Vaughan in
1920, was brief and defensive.[91] Rubinow, undaunted, continued to battle for health insurance and exerted a considerable
influence on the planners of New Deal social legislation. But
the AMA never forgave him. It was in its progressive era when
it hired him in 1916; it had taken the opposite tack by the time
it fired him in 1919.*

Repudiation and Backlash

Meantime Delphey was still in full pursuit of the health
insurance demon. Acting as Chairman of the New York State
Medical Society's Committee on Compulsory Health Insurance,
he wrote all state medical societies early in 1920, asking if they
had instructed their delgates to the national House of Delegates
on the health insurance issue. Subsequently he wrote all the
delegates themselves, warning them against ". . . propaganda
for a scheme which could but have a serious and destructive
effect upon the most altruistic profession on earth. . . ."[93]

His efforts and those of the *Journal*, which published a series
of articles by the new member of Lambert's committee condemning health insurance, bore fruit. By a series of maneuvers

---

*Rubinow, chairing a session on health insurance at the Seventh National Confer-
ence on Social Security in 1934, said: ". . . I feel that I am called upon to give a
word of caution, which may partly be explained by my own age. I don't look
forward to waiting another thirty or forty years before these various research
programs . . . culminate in a system. I can't help feeling a little bit depressed . . .
by the fact that so much that has been said here this morning has been said . . .
some twenty years ago. . . ."[92] Rubinow died in September 1936.

in the House of Delegates, opponents of health insurance obtained approval of the following in May, 1920:

> Resolved: that the American Medical Association declares its opposition to the institution of any plan embodying the system of compulsory contributory insurance against illness, or any other plan of compulsory insurance against illness which provides for medical service to be rendered contributors or their dependents provided, controlled, or regulated by the federal government.[94]

The action, in effect, closed the door to any possibility of cooperation between organized medicine and the federal government where compulsory health insurance was concerned but made no specific mention of voluntary insurance. Involvement of local government was not specifically excluded, an omission that was soon to be set right.

The 1920 resolution against federally sponsored health insurance was the basic dogma on which all future action in the field of health insurance was built. But the backlash within the AMA had not yet run its full course. The national climate that developed after World War I was producing some extraordinary social and political results. Congress passed a sequel to the Espionage Act of 1917, permitting wholesale deportation of aliens and forbidding reentry of many already deported.[95] New York State launched an investigation on "revolutionary radicalism" which culminated in the Lusk Report of 1920, recommending Americanization through education.[96] "Within a year after the armistice," said W. J. Ghent, in *The Reds Bring Reaction,* "we were in the midst of a tide of reaction which threatened to sweep away every social achievement gained during . . . the two previous decades. By that time or a bit later the whole fabric of social control had been rent and raveled."[97]

Delphey by now had able associates in carrying forward the repudiation of compulsory health insurance and anything else that threatened to bring medical practice under any sort of regulation. Prominent among them was E. H. Ochsner, a Chicago surgeon, who directed his attacks at health insurance, health centers, and Frank Billings. In 1919 Ochsner was among the many who attacked Lambert's committee and in 1920, writing in the *Illinois Medical Journal*, he had said:

> The mental processes of some of our ultra highbrows are beyond comprehension. . . . Compulsory health insurance is but the entering wedge. If this gets by, the next will be old age pensions and the next unemployment pensions and finally . . . the last act in the tragedy of errors will be revolution, anarchy, and chaos. . . .[98]

A few months later, writing in the same journal, Ochsner disposed of health centers ("the same old baby with a new name and its feet cut off . . ."). Quoting Billings' published comments in favor of health insurance and health centers, he turned to the personal attack: "I wonder, gentlemen, whether we have not a right to conclude that this gentleman [Billings] is no longer a safe adviser for the American medical profession on matters of medical economics?"[99] He then went on to a number of other themes that were then new to professional debate. "When I was on the farm," he wrote, "we had occasionally to deal with skunks and rattlesnakes. . . . There is just one way to deal with a skunk or a rattlesnake and that is a good, dependable, reliable double-barrelled shotgun. I would no more temporize or compromise with any of the schemes so far proposed than I would . . . with a rattlesnake, a skunk, or a hyena. I would hit, shoot, or kill them while they are still in embryo. . . ."

Ochsner seems to have carried his antipathy for Billings one step further. At the seventy-fourth annual meeting of the AMA, convened in Boston in 1921, an unsigned circular attacking Billings and quoting his earlier comments in favor of compulsory health insurance was distributed to the members of the House of Delegates. Billings was required to defend himself and he did so by recanting. "I have declared [Billings said] in published articles that compulsory health insurance was not applicable to the United States and that I am opposed to it. . . ." The House, apparently somewhat embarrassed by it all, accepted Billings' defense and affirmed its confidence in him.[100] It also made a weak but unsuccessful effort to discover the perpetrator of the attacks on Billings. According to Morris Fishbein, editor of the *Journal*, it was probably Ochsner.[101]

In any event, nothing quite like the incident had ever been seen in the House and, although Billings survived the attack, its chief purpose was achieved: no one was likely to bring up health insurance again, except to condemn it, before the House. Lambert, who had served as President of the AMA in 1919–20, had already bowed out of the controversy; his presidential address dealt with various nonpolitical aspects of war medicine.[102]

The Final Action: State Medicine Again

The conservative wing of the AMA was now firmly in the saddle. And while the House of Delegates seems to have been unwilling to censure so eminent a person as Billings, the language and methods used by men like Ochsner and Delphey came to be acceptable provided they were directed against compulsory health insurance. The leadership was, in fact, still preoccupied with the threat of government intervention in health. The Shepherd-Towner Act (providing funds for maternal and child health) had become law[103] despite the Association's disapproval.[104] New legislation providing hospital benefits to veterans at government expense was being discussed. As a consequence, the official policy opposing federally backed health insurance that had been adopted in 1920 was viewed as inadequate to cover all possibilities. The question of state medicine again arose* and the old unofficial definition, describing state medicine as public hygiene was, by action of 25 May 1922, superseded by the following:

> The American Medical Association hereby declares its opposition to all forms of "state medicine" because of the ultimate harm that would come to the public weal through such form of medical practice.
> "State Medicine" is . . . any form of medical treatment provided, conducted, controlled or subsidized by the federal or any state government, or municipality. . . .

*It had come up at the 1921 annual session. Delphey had introduced a resolution defining state medicine as ". . . the practice of medicine by the state by physicians on a salary to the exclusion of all other and individual practice of medicine."[105] His resolution, and several other similar ones, were buried in various committees.

The definition excepted the services provided by the Army, Navy, or Public Health Service and those needed in coping with communicable disease, mental illness, and the health of indigents. It also included a loophole in the form of references to "such other services" as may be under the control of county medical societies provided that the appropriate state society did not disapprove.[106]

The action represented a curious inversion of the unofficial definition of 1871. At that time, state medicine had to do, in the eyes of the Association, mainly with control of communicable disease and the AMA approved of it. But in 1922, state medicine became medical treatment of nonindigent citizens provided by government at any level.

The official actions of 1920 and 1922, both in some sense historical accidents, were the foundation on which the organization built the image it still possesses today. The transformation of the AMA from a more or less flexible professional organization to a strongly partisan one, functioning as a cross between a medieval guild and a modern labor union, was completed within a remarkably short time. The Association largely ignored a chorus of external attacks as well as words of caution from a few of its own leaders. In 1923, incoming president Ray Lyman Wilbur* attempted to moderate the organization's rigid new dogma in his inaugural address: "The social relationships of medicine are so intimate and imperative that they are bound to multiply and continue. We cannot stop them by calling them Bolshevik or socialist or pro-German but we can guide them if we get away from the brake and begin to steer."[107] But the members were by that time in no mood to listen to leaders with the instincts of statesmen. They subsequently sought and found leaders who were not afflicted with doubts as to the wisdom of the policies of the twenties and who followed them to the letter.

---

*Ray Lyman Wilbur (1875–1949) was one of the most distinguished men of his time. He was an accomplished physician, President of Stanford from 1916 to 1943, Secretary of the Interior in Hoover's cabinet (1929–1933), President of the AMA in 1923–24 and President of the Association of American Medical Colleges in 1924.

Social Security and After

Actions of the AMA since the twenties have had the effect of obscuring its record during its progressive era, and the events that led up to it. The tenacity with which AMA leaders have adhered to the policies of the twenties, despite criticism from without and within, has been remarkable indeed.

Even the Great Depression failed to shake the organization's faith in its post-war policies. Any form of interference from outside the profession—but especially from government—was to be condemned. Along these lines, W. G. Morgan, president of the AMA in 1930, lectured the members on paternalism: trade unions represented a sort of group paternalism, voluntary health insurance had its paternalistic aspects, and compulsory health insurance would allow the "paternalistic hand of the government" to throttle and degrade medical practice as it had in Germany and Britain. He also warned against nongovernmental paternalistic tendencies such as the mental hygiene movement.[108] In a similar vein was the AMA's official condemnation in 1932 of the majority report submitted by the Committee on the Costs of Medical Care, a prestigious body chaired by ex-president Wilbur and supported by eight major foundations.* The majority of the Committee's 48 members solidly supported the group practice concept and urged that ".... the costs of medical care be placed on a group payment basis, through the use of insurance, through the use of taxation, or through the use of both these methods."[109] A powerful minority, which included a number of AMA conservatives, disagreed. Its report put the emphasis on "medical care furnished by the individual physician with the general practitioner in a central place," and on insurance schemes only when they can be kept under professional control. It opposed the ". . . adoption by medicine of the technique of big business, that is, mass production." Its first recommendation, drawing its substance from the policy of 1922, urged the discontinuance of government competition in the

---

*The Carnegie Corporation, the Josiah Macy, Jr. Foundation, the Milbank Memorial Fund, the New York Foundation, the Rockefeller Foundation, the Julius Rosenwald Fund, the Russell Sage Foundation, and the Twentieth Century Fund.

practice of medicine except in the special instances contained in the policy.

The AMA officially endorsed the minority view and a *Journal* editorial said that the majority was made up of "the forces representing the great foundations, public health officialdom, social theory—even socialism and communism—inciting to revolution."[110] The long-term effect of the decision and, of lesser importance, of the *Journal*'s extravagant language is a matter of conjecture. But the decision, at the time and in retrospect, indicated clearly that AMA policy-makers found their policies so binding that they could not accept the conclusions of the nation's most able authorities in the health field.*

Things were no different when the federal government began to look into matters of health. When Franklin Roosevelt set up the Committee on Economic Security in 1934, the AMA thought that the Committee's Medical Advisory Subcommittee was not representative.[111] Even broadening the membership of the Subcommittee failed to appease the Association although it moderated its critical tone as a result. But the possibility that the federal government might bring health insurance under study was enough to persuade AMA leaders that an emergency meeting of the House of Delegates was needed. The House convened in February 1935 and it found cause for alarm on several counts.[112] Most menacing was the content of the Wagner-Doughton Economic Security Bill which had been introduced on 17 January. Title IV of the bill called for a Social Insurance Board and one of its duties was to study and make recommendations as to ". . . legislation and matters of administrative policy concerning old-age insurance . . . , health insurance, and related subjects."[113]

That was bad enough. Only slightly less acceptable was the drafting of a second Model Bill by the American Association of Social Security. The proposal, made public on 5 January 1935,

*The Committee (17 practicing physicians and dentists, six public health authorities, six social scientists, ten representatives of health institutions, and nine members representing the public) could hardly have been more carefully chosen. Eight of the 15 practicing physicians, and one Ph.D., wrote the minority report. The two dentists also submitted a minority report. One social scientist submitted a critical personal statement and Edgar Sydenstricker (public health) declined to sign the final report because, in his view, it dealt inadequately with "the fundamental economic question which the Committee was formed . . . to consider." The majority report was supported by 35 of the 48 members.

was a state measure and was to be introduced simultaneously into 43 state legislatures (it reached the New York Legislature on 25 January). It called for compulsory health insurance to be paid for by employers, employees, and state government. The employee's contribution varied from 1 to 3 percent, according to the level of his income. The employer's payment went from 3½ percent for employees making $20 or less a week, to 1½ percent for those receiving $40 or more. The state was to put in 1½ percent.[114] There was a suggestion that the federal government should put up 38 cents for each insured employee but the program was still to be administered by the individual states. To the House of Delegates, the Epstein Bill, named after the executive director of the organization that composed it, was unmitigated evil. The House of Delegates condemned it and reaffirmed its old stand against health insurance backed by government; but it yielded a little with regard to voluntary health insurance.

AMA opposition to Title IV of the Economic Security Bill following the special session of the House of Delegates was, under the circumstances, sufficient to dispose of it. A redraft of the proposal, submitted by Congressman Doughton in April, changed the name and purpose of the Board: it now became the Social Security Board and had no charge relating to health insurance.[115] The new draft passed the House with 372 yeas and 33 nays on 19 April.[116] It was signed into law on 14 August, 1935.[117]

The deletion represented a victory for the AMA* but the passage of the law led to a Supreme Court decision that politically and socially was more important than the law itself. When the law came under attack in 1937, Benjamin Cardozo, speaking for the Court in *Steward Machine Company vs. Davis,* quoted the general welfare clause of the Constitution† as the basis for upholding the law.[119] In a companion decision delivered the same day (*Helvering vs. Davis*), Cardozo, again speaking for the Court, said that the Federal Old Age Benefits

---

*Interaction between the AMA and the Committee on Economic Security is described in detail in a memoir by Edwin Witte, Executive Director of the Committee.[118]

†Article I, Section 8, (1): The Congress shall have the power to lay and collect taxes . . . , to pay the debts and provide for the common defense and general welfare of the United States. . . .

provision (Title II) of the Social Security Law does not contravene the Tenth Amendment* and that Congress may spend money in aid of the general welfare. "Nor," said the Court, "is the concept of the general welfare static. What is critical or urgent changes with time. . . . When money is spent to promote the general welfare, the concept of welfare or the opposite is shaped by Congress, not the states."[120] The decision made no mention of health as such, but the implication with regard to it was clear: Congress might, whenever it was persuaded that the state of the country's general welfare required it, pass legislation guaranteeing the right to health and it might, also by inference, use federal tax funds for the purpose.

Meantime, the AMA was moving largely by improvisation as the occasion seemed to demand but always with the policies of the twenties in mind. In 1920 it had not actually condemned voluntary health insurance but its action left the impression that it might be undesirable. In a special session of the House of Delegates in 1938, the AMA dealt again with voluntary insurance but said that it should be confined ". . . to provision of hospital facilities and should not include any type of medical care." Cash indemnity insurance for such purposes was, however, accepted. Under such policies, the insurance organization pays the patient according to rates specified in the policy; the patient, in turn, pays the physician who sets his own rates. No third party should come between the patient and his physician in the view of the House. Opposition to compulsory health insurance was reaffirmed.[121]

The AMA's intransigent stands had, meantime, not gone unnoticed in some segments of the nation's press. The *New York Times* had taken a dim view of its opposition to the Shepherd-Towner Act[122] and in 1929, a writer in *Forum* said the Association's primary interest was in the financial status of the physician.[123] In the thirties, Michael Rorty, among others, pounded away at the AMA's conservatism in traditionally liberal journals.[124,125] But in 1938, even *Fortune* found the AMA's stands too strong to stomach: ". . . Between the elders [Trustees and Delegates] and Dr. Fishbein the AMA has worked against its own purposes by clinging to ideas that rightly or wrongly

---

*"The powers not delegated to the United States by the Constitution, nor prohibited by it to the States, are reserved to the States respectively, or to the people."

have been discredited and it finds itself within hailing distance of its own downfall."[126]

By this time, few indeed remembered the Association's good work in the nineteenth century or its brief progressive era. A revolt in the ranks led by Dr. [James] Howard Means of Boston in 1938 came to very little,[127] but in September of the same year Attorney General Thurmond Arnold served notice that the AMA had gone too far. "Organized medicine [said Arnold] should not be allowed to extend its necessary and proper control over [professional] standards . . . , to include control over methods of payment for services involving the economic freedom and welfare for consumers and the legal rights of individual doctors."[128] A short time later, the AMA was indicted by a federal grand jury charging violation of the Sherman Anti-Trust Act. The AMA and the Medical Society of the District of Columbia were subsequently convicted and nominal fines were imposed.[129] But the most significant result of the sequence was an opinion, handed down by the U.S. Court of Appeals for the District of Columbia, which held that, under the circumstances of the indictment, the medical profession was unmistakably conducting itself as a trade and not as a profession.[130] And while the message got through to some members of the profession,[131] AMA leaders altered their tactics but not their policies.

Compulsory Health Insurance: Modern Times

The introduction by Senator Robert Wagner* of an amendment to the social security law in February 1939 marked the beginning of a long and bitter battle between the AMA and the Senator. The amendment, called the National Health Act of

---

*Robert Ferdinand Wagner (1877–1953) was born in Germany and came to the United States at an early age. He and Franklin Roosevelt were elected to the New York State Senate about the same time (1910) Wagner served in the U.S. Senate from 1927 to 1949 and was one of the New Deal's staunchest supporters.

1939, was a relatively mild one and contained no provision for compulsory health insurance.[132] But the AMA opposed it on the ground that it would lead ultimately to complete federal control of medicine. The bill was a principal topic at the meeting of the House of Delegates in May 1939 and a negative report by a reference committee was, in the words of the *Journal*, "adopted . . . without a dissenting vote and even without any attempt at discussion by individual members."[133]

But when Senators Murray and Wagner, and Congressman Dingell, introduced the first of their proposals to create a system for federal compulsory health insurance and federal support of medical education in June 1943,[134] the *Journal*'s language became pugnacious and abusive. "It would," said a *Journal* editorial, "make the Surgeon General of the Public Health Service . . . a virtual Gauleiter of American medicine."[135] Subsequent editorials rhetorically inquired "does the United States need a medical revolution? Does medical education need to be revolutionized?"[136,137] The answers were predictably negative on the grounds that the American health care system was the best in the world and that federal grants to medical schools would install bureaucratic control and destroy standards of excellence. The first Murray-Wagner-Dingell bill came to nothing, but Roosevelt's State of the Union message, delivered in January 1944, affirmed "the right to adequate medical care and the opportunity to achieve and enjoy good health."[138] Over a year later, the Murray-Wagner-Dingell bill was introduced anew (24 May 1945)[139] and the *Journal of the AMA* promptly took note in a hostile editorial attacking the bill and professional groups which supported it. These, said the *Journal*, were "inclined toward communism."[140] A letter from Senator Wagner, pleading for careful study of the bill and constructive suggestions from physicians[141] was published in June and a duel between the Senator and AMA officials ensued. Wagner noted that the AMA ". . . has condemned every proposal which had a chance to deal with our large national needs on an adequate basis." He went on to mention specific criticisms brought by the AMA and hoped that ". . . instead of pursuing a negative policy you will join with those of us who are trying to find constructive solutions to one of America's basic problems."[142]

Senator Wagner's efforts were largely wasted. Commenting at length on his letter, the Secretary of the AMA, Dr. Olin

West, made it clear that the chief bone of contention was still the matter of compulsory health insurance. "They (the Senator and the Social Security Board) refuse to listen to any other proposals. . . ."[143] But he offered no evidence that the AMA was willing to listen to proposals for any but voluntary insurance proposals under control of the profession. At best, it was a matter of the pot calling the kettle black; the polarization with regard to federal health insurance was absolute.

It was otherwise with regard to the use of federal grants-in-aid, via the states, for hospital construction. The proposal had been considered during the New Deal era and had not been opposed by the AMA. Toward the end of the war it was introduced as S.191 (10 January 1945) by Senators Lister Hill of Alabama and Harold H. Burton of Ohio.[144] The House of Delegates accepted the proposal in December but, at the same time, reaffirmed its opposition to compulsory health insurance.[145] The Hill-Burton Bill, somewhat amended, became law on 13 August 1946.[146]

The Murray-Wagner-Dingell proposal never actually came to a vote but was reintroduced several times. In 1945 it was first introduced as an amendment to the Social Security Act, then was introduced as the National Health Act after Truman's health message to Congress.[147] The AMA continued its resolute opposition throughout. The *Journal* carried verbatim accounts of various hearings and, in an editorial in 1946, outdid itself in the Delphey-Ochsner tradition. Commenting on the hearings that began in April, 1946, it referred to ". . . the propaganda of Pepper, the diatribe of Dingell, the weasel words of Wagner, and the modulations of Murray. . . ."[148] The proposal was, in every sense, a "taking over of medicine by the state" that would abolish free choice of physicians and that would inevitably lead to "political degradation of medical practice."[149] At no time was there serious consideration of the possibility that government and the profession might come together to evolve a workable solution to a pressing national problem, something the existence of which the AMA denied altogether.

The climax of the battle came in 1947 and 1948. Senator Murray (joined by Senators Pepper, Chavez, Taylor, McGrath, and Humphrey) reintroduced the bill on 20 May 1947.[150] Shortly thereafter, Secretary Ewing announced his ten-year plan, calling for more health manpower, 600,000 new hospital beds, and compulsory health insurance.[151] In late 1948, the House of Delegates authorized the Board of Trustees to levy a $25 assessment on all members of the AMA and to employ professional public relations counsel to put down the menace of compulsory health insurance.[152] Under the direction of Whitaker and Baxter, a California firm, the campaign turned out to be one of the most expensive lobbying activities the country had ever seen. "The voluntary way is the American way" became the slogan, the threat was creeping socialism, and the American doctor could, Leone Baxter told the House of Delegates, save and preserve the American Way of Life by defeating compulsory health insurance.[153] The House of Delegates, adhering to the letter of the policies of the twenties, said that "compulsory sickness insurance . . . is a variety of socialized medicine or state medicine. . . . It is contrary to the American tradition."[154]

Committee hearings on the Murray-Wagner-Dingell proposal began for the final time on 23 May 1949, the bill having been reintroduced in January, [155] and in April.[156] But by July the *Journal* stopped publishing transcripts of hearings because ". . . both legislators and the medical profession seem to have lost much of their interest."[157,158]* For one reason or another the battle was beginning to subside despite which the AMA's campaign continued for another two years. Not all physicians approved of the assessment or of the Whitaker-Baxter campaign; but their contract was renewed through 1951. Looking back on it all, the AMA's president (Dr. Louis Bauer) said in 1952: "I realize that some members may have disapproved of the employment of Whitaker and Baxter and . . . have disapproved of some of [their] activities." But without them, Dr. Bauer went on, ". . . we should in all probability now be operating under a government-controlled medical care plan."[160]

The Association breathed somewhat easier in late 1952 when Eisenhower won the presidency and announced his opposition to compulsory health insurance. Dingell's reintroduction of the national health insurance bill in 1953[161] caused no great alarm in the ranks of the AMA. But the new administration was

---

*It was at this juncture that the faithful and indefatigable Dr. Morris Fishbein, for years editor of the *Journal* and a major spokesman for the AMA was fired. "For thirty-seven years he had been crying 'wolf,' " said Milton Mayer. "Now," Mayer continued, "he was blamed for bringing on the wolves and was thrown to them."[159]

unable to ignore the health problem altogether. In late 1954, Oveta Culp Hobby, HEW Secretary, proposed a system of spreading health insurance risks, using federal reinsurance funds, as a means of expanding the coverage of those who already had some form of health insurance.[162] It was to no avail. The AMA and some portions of the insurance industry joined in opposing the proposal despite the fact that it had no compulsory feature. The *Journal* for 18 December 1954 listed 14 bills on national health program, including the reinsurance proposal, that were then pending in Congress. The AMA was actively opposed to 12 of them and took no action on the other two, one of which recommended nothing more startling than study of health and accident insurance.[163]*

The AMA thus made it clear that it would not willingly lend its support to any federal health proposal of consequence and that its policies of 1920 and 1922 were still very much intact. However federal planners might define right to health, the AMA still doggedly pursued the view that the individual's right to curative medicine should not be guaranteed by government unless he was indigent. But a new cloud was on the horizon.

Climax: Medicare

The word *Medicare* first came into view when the Medicare Act of 7 June 1956 was passed, relating solely to the dependents of members of the Armed Forces.[165] Even so, it was thought by the *Journal* to carry with it ". . . some danger to the private practice of medicine."[166]

By this time, the focus was on the plight of the aged and in 1957 Congressman Forand (D. Rhode Island) introduced a bill providing hospital and medical care for the aged through Social Security.[167] Other bills were produced and one of them (the Kerr-Mills bill), which did not employ the social security mechanism for financing, was unopposed by the AMA. It became law in 1960.[168] But the matter would not rest. The Kerr-Mills law required that those over 65 who were not indigent should

*Several years earlier, an exasperated Congressman, Andrew Biemiller of Wisconsin, had said for the record: "Apparently the only kind of medical aid bill the AMA would approve is a measure which would place unlimited public funds in the hands of the AMA itself, to dispense as it sees fit after paying its lobbying and propaganda expenses. . . ."[164]

pay $24 annually for health insurance and that the whole program should be administered by the states. This was acceptable to the AMA; but the King-Anderson bill, introduced in early 1961, was unacceptable because it, like the Forand bill, called for financing through the social security mechanism.[169] In any case, AMA leaders considered the situation threatening enough to justify resort to a political action technique it had used once before. In December, 1961, it created the American Medical Political Action Committee (AMPAC) to ". . . stimulate physicians and others to take a more active part in government . . . and to help . . . in organizing for more effective political action."[170] The AMA's own Board of Trustees appointed the nine members of AMPAC's Board of Directors of which Gunnar Gundersen, a former AMA president, was chairman. In practice, AMPAC's chief function was to solicit funds for the support of candidates for national office who accepted the AMA's views on federal health legislation.

The fight over the King-Anderson bill reached a peak when, on 20 May 1962, President Kennedy addressed an overflow crowd, many of them elderly, at Madison Square Garden urging public support for the measure. The AMA responded dramatically the next evening. At a cost estimated at $100,000 it staged its own TV show, taped in the empty auditorium shortly after Kennedy's audience had left. "This is the inside of that same arena," said an announcer, "just a few hours after yesterday's spectacle had ended. . . . The clean-up crews will arrive shortly." Then Dr. Leonard Larson, president of the AMA, took over and introduced the prime speaker, Dr. Edward R. Annis. The line Annis took was basically the theme of the twenties, artfully framed and delivered. "England's nationalized medical program is what they have in mind for us eventually," he maintained. The King-Anderson bill was "a cruel hoax and a delusion," of limited benefits, inordinate cost, and the "forerunner of a different system of medicine for all Americans." His admonition was to go slow by defeating the bill.[171]

It was an expensive but probably effective antic. In July, the King-Anderson bill went down to defeat, although it never came, as such, to a vote.[172] But two years later a similar proposal was passed by the Senate as part of an amendment (the Gore Amendment) to the Social Security law.[173,174] The

House declined to go along and efforts at resolving House and Senate differences failed.

Meantime the AMA produced a proposal to which it attached the title *Eldercare* and which it persuaded Senator Tower of Texas to introduce.[175] It was the first time the AMA had produced a countermeasure of its own design instead of reacting negatively to health bills from other sources. The Eldercare proposal was a relatively comprehensive one but still excluded the social security financing feature. The final result was the present Medicare law, passed in mid-1965, which adopted Eldercare's comprehensiveness in large measure but settled solidly on the social security method of financing.[176] Participation on the part of the elderly was, however, voluntary and in this regard the AMA won a pyrrhic victory. But federally backed health insurance was, despite decades of AMA opposition, finally on the books for an important group of American citizens not all of whom are indigent.

The AMA's hope of defeating the Medicare proposal had suffered a severe blow when, in December 1964, Wilbur Mills reversed his earlier opposition to it.* Hope had almost been abandoned by the time of the annual meeting in June 1965. Various explanations of the Association's failure to block the legislation were offered. Outgoing President Donovan Ward said that on the evening of 21 November 1963, after AMA spokesmen had testified against the Medicare proposal, ". . . we were on our way to the most resounding legislative victory in our history as an organization." But by early afternoon the next day, President John F. Kennedy had been assassinated and a new Chief Executive, beholden (according to Ward) to labor and liberal forces, was in office.[178] The AMA's incoming President, Dr. James Z. Appel, said that the AMA's political fortunes were on the wane because ". . . many members of Congress—acting as political sheep—are not being responsive to the people in this issue." But he counselled against boycott, if the law should pass;[179] and in this he was subsequently supported by the Board of Trustees.[180]

---

*Mills' reasoning, and the means by which the successful Medicare proposal was put together, are described in detail by Harold B. Meyers.[177] The compromise is said to have crystallized in a conference between Mills and Secretary Wilbur Cohen of HEW in March, 1965.

The passage of Medicare and other health legislation thus left the Association's leaders disgruntled and bewildered but not openly rebellious. And in 1968, another incoming president inquired in his inaugural address: "Will we learn the lessons of our experience, particularly those that led to the laws affecting health that were passed by the 89th Congress?" He followed his question by a plea for enlightened guidance by the Association of the federal health planning process; steering rather than braking.[181] It was basically the same plea that had been made, and ignored, 45 years earlier by Ray Lyman Wilbur; and it was his son, Dwight L. Wilbur, who eloquently restated it in 1968. . . .

Since 1965, new proposals for major federal health legislation have been noticeably lacking. The succession of health and health-related laws enacted by the 89th Congress in 1965 left the country gasping. Implementation of the new laws has been difficult, partly owing to the shortage of administrative personnel and trained professionals.

But the hiatus is approaching its end.

Summary and Prospects for the Seventies

Neither the federal government nor the AMA is irreversibly committed to its precedents; nor is either likely to be uninfluenced by them. Since the first quarantine law was enacted in 1796, the federal definition of the right to health has been steadily broadened. But except for the short-lived vaccination law of 1813, federal health legislation did not begin to approach a guarantee of adequate health services to individual American citizens until comparatively modern times. With the passage of the Social Security Law in 1935, and the Cardozo decision two years later, a new climate was created. The several health bills introduced by Senator Robert Wagner and colleagues beginning in 1939 followed in due course. The passage of the Medicare-Medicaid Law and other health legislation in 1965 brought the process to its present state.

Since its founding in 1848, the AMA has played a key role in the development and passage of health legislation. Prior to the passage of Social Security, the federal government and the AMA, for the most part, saw comfortably eye-to-eye. As long as the definition of the right to health was a conservative one— encompassing the health of the millions but not curative medicine for the individual—the AMA was, in fact, ahead of government, federal and state. The Model Health Insurance Bill of 1916, which the AMA helped to draft, was the real beginning of conflict. It embodied compulsory health insurance, financed by tripartite contributions: employee, employer, and state (but not federal) government. The Association's policies of 1920 and 1922 declared the proposal, and most others in which government control and financing are involved, to be anathema. The stage was then set for the battles over Social Security, the various Wagner bills, and those having to do with health care for the elderly. In the course of the long struggle, the AMA has ceded very little. The Kerr-Mills Law, which the Association approved, focussed on the states, held the federal government more or less at arm's length, and did no great violence to the AMA's view that only the indigent should receive personal health services at taxpayer's expense. But the Forand Bill and its successors put the federal government in the central position and extended benefits to all eligibles, regardless of economic status. In this sense Medicare was a watershed; it breached the AMA's 1922 definition of state medicine solidly and definitely. The extension of the Medicare system to virtually all citizens (and the revision or elimination of the state-oriented Medicaid provision), or possibly a new law having the same effect, is the prospect of the seventies.

Few organizations in American history have been so thoroughly dissected and criticized as the AMA. Some of the analyses are scholarly and relatively dispassionate;[182-185] others are strident and doctrinaire. Many have predicted that unless the AMA changes its ways, it is headed for oblivion. But the Association has ignored them all and has doggedly gone its conservative way. It is a remarkably durable institution; dire prophecies of oblivion, some dating back many decades, show little sign of becoming fact. But the Association's tactics have changed remarkably. Gone are the editorial polemics against the federal government in the *Journal*, and so are full extracts of the Minutes of the House of Delegates. The Association's *American Medical News* and *Today's Health* both reflect its political and social point of view; but reports are likely to be more reportorial and less overtly propagandistic than formerly. Nor is there any suggestion that the spectacular Madison Square Garden countermeasure of 1962 will be repeated in the foreseeable future. Yet the Delphey-Ochsner style has not completely disappeared. It cropped up recently in a letter to the editor of the *American Medical News* when an AMA constituent described the *News* as a "blatant organ of the left-wing conspiracy."[186]

It is hardly that. But in the face of mounting pressure for national health insurance, the AMA has put forward its own plan to which it applies the title *Medicredit*.[187,188] The proposal is based on a scale of federal income tax credit to encourage the voluntary purchase of health insurance from existing organizations, private and semipublic. It would not alter the existing fee-for-service system nor does it contain specific inducements for physicians to locate in low-income or rural areas. It is basically a voluntary financing measure, not one that is designed to create a new health care system. At the opposite pole is a proposal backed by the Committee for National Health Insurance. It calls for compulsory health insurance for everyone and embodies the tripartite (employer, employee, and government) financing system put forward by the Model Bill of 1916.* It would virtually abolish fee-for-service practice and private health insurance plans. It would provide "financial and other" incentives to physicans willing to form medical care groups and to those who move into various low-income areas. It would assign highest priority in payment of funds collected by the system to salaried physicians in institutions, to those working in group practice prepayment units, and to physicians who agree to "accept capitation payments for the care of a defined population."[189]

It is difficult to see how more features that have traditionally been repugnant to the AMA could be incorporated into a single health insurance proposal. The Association's strenuous opposition to some features of the Committee's proposal is a certainty. It is not likely, however, to go back to the tactics of the

---

*Forty percent would come from federal tax revenues, 35 percent from a tax on employer payrolls, and 25 percent from a tax on individual adjusted gross income.

forties, fifties, and early sixties. For one thing, the Association's approach to the public is more sophisticated than it was then. For another, the AMA's political arm (AMPAC) is said to exert more direct influence on the White House than was the case in earlier administrations.[190] But nothing that took place at the 1970 AMA Convention suggests that the AMA is as yet ready to reconsider all the present implications of its policies of the twenties.[191]

The dilemma the AMA faces in the early seventies is, in many respects, more stringent than that faced by the present Administration in Washington. The latter is as yet committed to nothing, beyond the recognition by the President of a health crisis. It can move in many directions, according to its sense of public opinion and the mood of Congress. But the AMA still labors under the self-imposed strictures of the twenties and the disadvantages under which it must now work are formidable. It must, on the one hand, continue to represent the interests of its members; and it must, on the other hand, participate in the creation of a system that will finally guarantee the right to health of all American citizens. The Association is not wrong in pointing out the dangers inherent in a health care system that is controlled absolutely by government; it could as well point out the obvious dangers of complete control by the consumer. But it cannot continue to confuse professional control of health care standards with professional control of the system itself.

To play its vital role in the guarantee of the right to health in the seventies, the AMA needs to reconsider its own precedents. Those of 1920 and 1922, developed in time of great political stress, stand today in sharp contrast to the enlightened and relevant precedents of earlier times. The policies of the twenties, more than anything else, have brought the Association to its present dilemma.

Its future may well depend on how convincingly it can rewrite— or expunge—those policies and on whether or not the House of Delegates' resolution of 1969 really means what it seems to say: It is the basic right of every citizen to have available to him adequate health care.

NOTES

1. Rouse, Milford O., Inaugural Address: To Whom Much Has Been Given. *JAMA* 201:169–171, 17 July 1967.
2. AMA Convention news. *New York Times.* 18 July 1969, p. 21.
3. Capen, Edward Warren, *The Historical Development of the Poor Law of Connecticut.* New York: Columbia University Press, 1905.
4. *Records of the Governor and Company of the Massachusetts Bay in New England*, 1642–1649 2:237, March 1647–8. Boston: William White, 1853.
5. Gordon, Maurice Bear, *Aesculapius Comes to the Colonies.* Ventnor, N.J.: Ventnor Publishers, Inc., 1949.
6. *Gazette of the United States.* 11 September 1793, p. 535.
7. Washington, George, Letter to the Attorney General; Mt. Vernon, 30 September 1793. In: *Writings of Washington* 33:107–109. Washington: U.S. Govt. Printing Office, 1940.
8. *Gazette of the United States.* 2 April 1794, pp. 2–3.
9. An Act to Authorize the President of the United States in Certain Cases to Alter the Place for Holding a Session of Congress. Third Cong., 1st Sess. *Pub. Stat. at Large U.S.* 1:353, 3 April 1794.
10. *Gazette of the United States.* 29 April 1796, p. 2.
11. Dexter, Franklin B., *Biographical Sketches of the Graduates of Yale College* 3:619–620, 1903. New York: H. Holt and Company, 1885–1913.
12. Lyman, William, Comment in House of Representatives. Fourth Cong., 1st Sess. Cong. Rec. (Ann. Cong.), 11 May 1796, p. 1348.
13. An Act Relative to Quarantine. Fourth Cong., 1st Sess. *Pub. Stat. at Large U.S.* 1:474, 27 May 1796.
14. Allen, William H., *The Rise of the National Board of Health. Ann. Amer. Acad. Polit. and Soc. Sci.* 15:51–68, January–May, 1900.
15. An Act Respecting Quarantine and Health Laws. Fifth Cong., 3rd Sess. *Pub. Stat. at Large U.S.* 1:619, 25 February 1799.
16. An Act Concerning Aliens, Fifth Cong., 2nd Sess. *Pub. Stat. at Large U.S.* 1:570–572, 25 June 1798.
17. An Act in Addition to the Act, Entitled "An Act for the Punishment of Certain Crimes Against the United States." Fifth Cong., 2nd Sess. *Pub. Stat. at Large U.S.* 1:596–597, 14 July 1798.

18. Gibbons vs. Ogden. *Reports of Cases Argued and Adjudged by the Supreme Court of the United States* (Wheaton); February term 9:1–222, 1824, p. 203. .

19. Martin, Henry A., Jefferson as a Vaccinator. *North Carolina Med. J.* 7:1–34, January, 1881.

20. An Act to Diffuse the Benefits of Inoculation for the Cow Pox. *Laws of the Commonwealth of Massachusetts From February 28, 1807 to February 28, 1814.* 1(n.s.): 167, 6 March 1810.

21. An Act to Encourage Vaccination. Twelfth Cong., 2nd Sess. *Pub. Stat. at Large U.S.* 2:806–807, 27 February 1813.

22. Report of the Select Committee . . . to Inquire Into the Propriety of Repealing the Act of 1813, to Encourage Vaccination, Accompanied With a Bill to Repeal the Act, Entitled "An Act to Encourage Vaccination." Seventeenth Cong., 1st Sess. *House Report* No. 93, 13 April 1822.

23. An Act to Repeal the Act Entitled "An Act to Encourage Vaccination." Seventeenth Cong., 1st Sess. *Pub. Stat. at Large U.S.* 3:677, 4 May 1822.

24. An Act to Enforce Quarantine Regulations. Twenty-second Cong., 1st Sess. *Pub. Stat. at Large U.S.* 4:577–578, 13 July 1832.

25. Keating, J. M. *A History of the Yellow Fever. The Yellow Fever Epidemic of 1878 in Memphis, Tenn.* Memphis: The Howard Association, 1879, pp. 327–443.

26. *The 1970 World Almanac and Book of Facts.* New York: Newspaper Enterprise Asso., Inc., 1969, p. 254.

27. *Evening Post* (New York). 6 May 1846, p. 2.

28. *Proceedings of the National Medical Conventions Held in New York, May 1846, and in Philadelphia, May, 1847.* Philadelphia: T. K. and P. G. Collins, Printers, 1847.

29. Davis. N. S., *History of the American Medical Association From Its Organization up to January, 1855.* Philadelphia: Lippincott, Grambo, and Co., 1855.

30. Chapman, Nathaniel, President's Address. *Trans. Amer. Med. Asso.* 1:7–9, 1848.

31. Memorial to Congress on Adulterated Drugs and Medicines. *Trans. Amer. Asso. Med.* 1:335, 4 May 1848.

32. An Act to Prevent the Importation of Adulterated and Spurious Drugs and Medicine. Thirtieth Cong., 1st Sess. *Pub. Stat. at Large U.S.* 9:237–239, 26 June 1848.

33. Reed, Charles, President's Address. *JAMA* 36:1599–1606, 8 June 1901.

34. Editorial: The Medical Association. *New York Times*, 6 May 1858, p. 1.
35. Editorial: American Medical Association. A Little Business and a Large Row. *New York Times*, 7 May 1858, p. 1.
36. Editorial: Medical Ethics. *New York Times*, 9 June 1882, p. 4.
37. Davis, Nathan Smith, Resolution at the Eighteenth Annual Meeting, *Trans. Amer. Med. Asso.* 18:33–34, 1867.
38. Logan, Thomas M., Report of the Committee on a National Health Council. *Trans. Amer. Med. Asso.* 23:46–51, 9 May 1872.
39. Richardson, T. G., Presidential Address, Twenty-Ninth Annual Meeting. *Trans. Amer. Med. Asso.* 29:93–111, 1878, p. 111.
40. Commissioners of the Sanitary Survey, *Report of a General Plan for the Promotion of Public and Personal Health . . .* [Lemuel Shattuck]. Boston: Dutton and Wentworth, 1850, p. 10.
41. An Act to Reorganize the Marine Hospital Service and to Provide for the Relief of Sick and Disabled Seamen. Forty-first Cong., 2nd Sess. *Pub. Stat. at Large U.S.* 16:169–170, 29 June 1870.
42. Yellow Fever at Rio de Janeiro. *New York Times*, 17 April 1878, p. 8.
43. Desolation in the South. *New York Times*, 5 September 1878, p. 1.
44. An Act to Prevent the Introduction of Contagious or Infectious Diseases Into the United States. Forty-fifth Cong., 2nd Sess. *Pub. Stat. at Large U.S.* 20:37–38, 29 April 1878.
45. American Public Health Association. Reports and Resolutions Relating to Sanitary Legislation. Presented at Its Meeting in Richmond, Va., November 19–22, 1878. *Rep. Amer. Pub. Health Asso.* 5:101, 1879.
46. Resolution Calling for More Stringent Quarantine Laws to Be Enacted by Congress. *Trans. Amer. Med. Asso.* 8:37–38, 2 May 1855.
47. *Senate Report* No. 734; to Accompany S.1784. Forty-fifth Cong., 3rd Sess. 7 February 1879.
48. Cabell. J. L., A Review of the Operations of the National Board of Health. *Rep. Amer. Pub. Health Asso.* 8:71–101, 1883.
49. An Act to Prevent the Introduction of Infectious or Contagious Diseases Into the United States, and to Establish a

National Board of Health. Forty-fifth Cong., 3rd Sess. *Pub. Stat. at Large U.S.* 20:484–485, 3 March 1879.

50. An Act to Prevent the Introduction of Contagious or Infectious Diseases Into the United States. Forty-sixth Cong., 1st Sess. *Pub. Stat. at Large U.S.* 21:5–7, 2 June 1879.

51. Debate on Quarantine Act of 2 June 1879. Forty-sixth Cong., 1st Sess. *Cong. Rec.* 9(2):1637–1650, 27 May 1879.

52. Billings, John Shaw, Reports and Resolutions Relating to Sanitary Legislation. *Amer. J. Med. Sci.* 78:471–479, October, 1879.

53. Editorial: The National Board of Health and the American Public Health Association. *Boston Med. and Surg. J.* 107:450–451, 9 November 1882.

54. An Act Granting Additional Quarantine Powers and Imposing Additional Duties Upon the Marine-Hospital Service. Fifty-second Cong., 2nd Sess. *Pub. Stat. at Large U.S.* 27:449–452, 15 February 1893.

55. Morgan's Louisiana and Texas Railroad and Steamship Company vs. Board of Health of the State of Louisiana and the State of Louisiana. *U.S. Supreme Court Reps.* (Lawyers Edition) 30:237–243, 10 May 1886.

56. Faulkner, Harold U., *The Decline of Laissez-faire*, 1897–1917. New York: Harper and Row, 1951.

57. An Act Making Appropriations for Sundry Civil Expenses of the Government for the Fiscal Year Ending June Thirtieth, 1902, and for Other Purposes. Fifty-sixth Cong., 2nd Sess. *Pub. Stat. at Large U.S.* 31:1137, 3 March 1901.

58. An Act to Change the Name of the Public Health and Marine Hospital Service to the Public Health Service, to Increase the Pay of Officers of Said Service, and for Other Purposes. Sixty-second Cong., 2nd Sess. *Pub. Stat. at Large U.S.* 37(1):309, 14 August 1912.

59. Hofstadter, Richard, *The Age of Reform: From Bryan to F.D.R.* New York: Alfred Knopf, 1955, 328 pp.

60. An Act for Preventing the Manufacture, Sale, or Transportation of Adulterated or Misbranded or Poisonous or Deleterious Food, Drugs, Medicines, and Liquors, and for Regulating Traffic Therein, and for Other Purposes. Fifty-ninth Cong., 1st Sess. *Pub. Stat. at Large U.S.* 34(1):768:772, 30 June 1906.

61. An Act to Amend Section Eight of the Food and Drugs Act Approved June Thirtieth, Nineteen Hundred and Six. Sixty-second Cong., 2nd Sess. *Pub. Stat. at Large U.S.* 37(1):416–417, 23 August 1912.

62. Resolution on Official Policy of the Association. *Trans. Amer. Med. Asso.* 4:39, 9 May 1851.

63. Official Minutes of the General Sessions, Report of the Transactions of the Reorganization Committee on Revision of Constitution and By-laws. *JAMA* 36:1643–1648, 8 June 1901.

64. Editorial: The House of Delegates. *American Medicine* 3:1030, 21 June 1902.

65. Frankel, Lee K., and Dawson, Miles M., *Workman's Insurance in Europe.* New York: Charities Publication Committee, 1910.

66. Editorial: Socializing the British Medical Profession. *JAMA* 59:1890–1891, 23 November 1912.

67. Brandeis, Louis D., Workingman's Insurance—The Road to Social Efficiency. *Proc. Conf. of Charities and Corrections*, 38th Annual Session, 8 June 1911, pp. 156–162.

68. *A Contract With the People.* Platform of the Progressive Party Adopted at its First National Convention. Chicago, 7 August 1912. New York: Progressive National Committee, 1912.

69. Wilson, Woodrow, First Inaugural Address as President of the United States, 4 March 1913. *The Public Papers of Woodrow Wilson. The New Democracy, vol. 1.* New York: Harper and Brothers, 1926.

70. Warbasse, James P., The Socialization of Medicine. *JAMA* 63:264–266, 18 July 1914.

71. Rubinow, Isaac M., Social Insurance and the Medical Profession. *JAMA* 64:381–386, 30 January 1915.

72. American Association for Labor Legislation. Annual Business Meeting, December 1912. *Amer. Labor Legislation Rev.* 3:121, 1913.

73. Rubinow, I.M., *Social Insurance, With Special Reference to American Conditions.* New York: Henry Holt and Company, 1913.

74. Chandler, Alfred D., The Origins of Progressive Leadership. In *The Letters of Theodore Roosevelt.* Vol. 8, Elting Morrison, ed. Cambridge: Harvard University Press, 1954, pp. 1462–1465.

75. Lambert, Alexander, Medical Organization Under Health Insurance. *Amer. Labor Legislation Rev.* 7:36–50, March, 1917.

76. Editorial: Industrial Insurance. *JAMA* 66:433, 5 February 1916.

77. Health Insurance: Tentative Draft of an Act. *Amer. Labor Legislation Rev.* 6:239–268, June, 1916.
78. Minutes of House of Delegates: Report of the Judicial Council of the House of Delegates [21 June]. *JAMA* 65:73–92, 3 July 1915.
79. Current Comment: A Model Bill for Health Insurance. *JAMA* 65:1824, 20 November 1915.
80. Editorial: Cooperation in Social Insurance Investigation. *JAMA* 66:1469–1470, 6 May 1916.
81. Minutes of House of Delegates: Report of Committee on Social Insurance. *JAMA* 66:1951–1985, 17 June 1916.
82. Rogoff, Hillel, *An East Side Epic; the Life and Work of Meyer London.* New York: Vanguard Press, 1930.
83. House Joint Resolution 159: For the Appointment of a Commission to Prepare and Recommend a Plan for the Establishment of a National Insurance Fund, and for the Mitigation of the Evil of Unemployment. Sixty-fourth Cong., 1st Sess. *Cong. Rec.* 53:2856, 19 February 1916.
84. *Hearings Before the Committee on Labor (HR)*, Commission to Study Social Insurance and Unemployment. April 6 and 11, 1916. Sixty-fourth Cong., 1st Sess. Washington: U.S. Govt. Printing Office, 1916.
85. Debate on National Insurance. Sixty-fourth Cong., 2nd Sess. *Cong. Rec.* 54(3):2650–2654, 5 February 1917.
86. Freund, Ernst, Constitutional and Legal Aspects of Health Insurance. *Nat. Conf. Social Work* 1917:553–558.
87. Minutes of House of Delegates, Reports of Committee on Social Insurance Regarding Invalidity, Old Age, and Unemployment Insurance, and a General Summary Concerning Social Insurance. *JAMA* 68:1721–1755, 9 June 1917.
88. Delphey, Eden V., Arguments Against the "Standard Bill" for Compulsory Health Insurance. *JAMA* 68:1500–1501, 19 May 1917.
89. Minutes of House of Delegates, Report of the Council on Health and Public Instruction. *JAMA* 72:1750–1751, 14 June 1919.
90. Fishbein, Morris, *History of the American Medical Association.* Philadelphia: W. B. Saunders Company, 1947, p. 318.
91. Minutes of House of Delegates, Report of Committee on Social Insurance. *JAMA* 74:1241–1242, 1 May 1920.
92. Wanted—A Health Insurance Program. In *Social Security in the United States*, 1934, p. 112. New York: American Association for Social Security, 1934.

93. Delphey, Eden V., Report of the Committee on Compulsory Health and Workmen's Compensation Insurance of the Medical Society of the County of New York. *New York State J. Med.* 20:394–396, December, 1920.

94. Minutes of House of Delegates, Report of Reference Committee on Hygiene and Public Health (27 April). *JAMA* 74:1319, 8 May 1920.

95. An Act to Deport Certain Undesirable Aliens and to Deny Readmission to Those Deported. Sixty-sixth Cong., 2nd Sess. *Pub. Stat. at Large U.S.* 41(1):593–594, 10 May 1920.

96. Lusk, Clayton R. (Chairman), *Revolutionary Radicalism. . . . Report of the Joint Legislative Committee* [Lusk Report], 4 vols. Albany: J. B. Lyon Co., 1920.

97. Ghent, W. J., *The Reds Bring Reaction.* Princeton: Princeton University Press, 1923.

98. Ochsner, Edward H., Compulsory Health Insurance, a Modern Fallacy. *Illinois Med. J.* 38:77–80, August, 1920.

99. Ochsner, Edward H.: Some Medical Economics Problems. *Illinois Med. J.* 39:406–413, May, 1921.

100. Minutes of House of Delegates for 9 June 1921. *JAMA* 76:1757–1758, 18 June 1921.

101. Fishbein, Morris, *History of the American Medical Association.* Philadelphia: W. B. Saunders Company, 1947, pp. 324–325.

102. Lambert, Alexander, Medicine, a Determining Factor in War. Presidential Address. *JAMA* 72:1713–1721, 14 June 1919.

103. An Act for the Promotion of the Welfare and Hygiene of Maternity and Infancy, and for Other Purposes (P.L.67–97). Sixty-seventh Cong., 1st Sess. *Pub. Stat. at Large U.S.* 42(1):224–226, 23 November 1921.

104. Editorial: Federal Care of Maternity and Infancy. The Shepherd-Towner Bill. *JAMA* 76:383, 5 February 1921.

105. Minutes of House of Delegates: Various Resolutions. *JAMA* 76:1756–1757, 18 June 1921.

106. Minutes of House of Delegates 25 May 1922. Supplementary Report of Reference Committee on Legislation and Public Relations. *JAMA* 78:1715, 3 June 1922.

107. Wilbur, Ray Lyman, Human Welfare and Modern Medicine. Inaugural Address. *JAMA* 80:1889–1893, 30 June 1923.

108. Morgan, William G., The Medical Profession and the Paternalistic Tendencies of the Times. President's Address. *JAMA* 94:2035–2042, 28 June 1930.

109. Committee on the Costs of Medical Care, *Medical Care for the American People: The Final Report.* Chicago: University of Chicago Press, 1932 (Publication No. 28).

110. Editorial: The Committee on the Costs of Medical Care. *JAMA* 99:1950–1952, 3 December 1932.

111. Editorial: The Conference on Economic Security. *JAMA* 103:1624–1625, 24 November 1934.

112. Minutes of the Special Session of the House of Delegates of the American Medical Association, Chicago, 15–16 February 1935. *JAMA* 104:747–753, 2 March 1935.

113. The Economic Security Act (S.1130). Seventy-fourth Cong., 1st Sess. *Cong. Rec.* 79(1):549–556, 17 January 1935.

114. Model Bill Maps Health Insurance. *New York Times*, 6 January 1935, Sec. 2, p. 2.

115. A Bill (H.R. 7260) to Provide for the General Welfare by Establishing a System of Federal Old-Age Benefits, . . . to Establish a Social Security Board; etc. Seventy-fourth Cong., 1st Sess. *Cong. Rec.* 79(5):5079, 4 April 1935.

116. Debate on Social Security Act. Seventy-fourth Cong., 1st Sess. *Cong. Rec.* 79(6):6069–6070, 19 April 1935.

117. An Act to Provide for the General Welfare by Establishing a System of Federal Old-Age Benefits . . . ; to Establish a Social Security Board; etc. Seventy-fourth Cong., 1st Sess. *Pub. Stat. at Large U.S.* 49(1):620–648, 14 August 1935.

118. Witte, Edwin E., *Development of Social Security Act.* Madison: University of Wisconsin Press, 1962.

119. Steward Machine Co. *vs.* Davis, Collector of Internal Revenue. *United States Reports.* 301:548–618, 24 May 1937.

120. Helvering, Commissioner of Internal Revenue, *et al. vs.* Davis. *United States Reports* 301:619–646, 24 May 1937.

121. Minutes of House of Delegates: Report of Reference Committee on Consideration of the National Health Program. *JAMA* 111:1215–1217, 24 September 1938.

122. Editorial: Evidently Change Is Needed. *New York Times*, 7 February 1921, p. 10.

123. Harding, T. Swann, How Scientific Are Our Doctors? *Forum* 81:345–351, June, 1929.

124. Rorty, James, Whose Medicine? *Nation* 143:42–44, 11 July 1936.

125. Rorty, James, Medicine's Misalliance. *Nation* 146:666–669, 11 June 1938.

126. The American Medical Association. *Fortune* 18:88–92, 150, 152, 156, 160, 162, 164, 166, 168, November, 1938.

127. Stephenson, H., Revolt in the AMA. *Current History* 48:24–26, June, 1938.

128. Arnold, T., Department of Justice: Statement About Group Health Insurance Case. *Current History* 49:49–50, September, 1938.

129. Minutes of House of Delegates: Report of Board of Trustees, *JAMA* 116:2791–2792, 21 June 1941.

130. United States *vs.* American Medical Assn., *et al.*, U.S. Court of Appeals for the District of Columbia. No. 7488. *Federal Reporter*, Series 2 110:703–716, 4 March 1940.

131. Morgan, Hugh J., *Professio. Ann. Int. Med.* 28:887–891, May, 1948.

132. National Health Act of 1939 (S.1620). Seventy-sixth Cong., 1st Sess. *Cong. Rec.* 84(2):1976–1982, 28 Feburary 1939.

133. Minutes of House of Delegates: Report of Reference Committee on Consideration of Wagner National Health Bill [17 May]. *JAMA* 112:2295–2297, 3 June 1939.

134. Social Security Act Amendment of 1943. Unified National Social Insurance (S. 1161). Seventy-eighth Cong., 1st Sess. *Cong. Rec.* 89(4):5260–5262, 3 June 1943.

135. Editorial: Wagner-Murray-Dingell Bill for Social Security. *JAMA* 122:600–601, 26 June 1943.

136. Editorial: Does the United States Need a Medical Revolution? *JAMA* 123:418, 16 October 1943.

137. Editorial: Does Medical Education Need to Be Revolutionized? *JAMA* 123:484, 23 October 1943.

138. Roosevelt, Franklin D., Message From the President of the United States on the State of the Union. Seventy-eighth Cong., 2nd Sess. *Cong. Rec.* 90(1):55–57, 11 January 1944, p. 57.

139. Social Security Amendments of 1945 (S. 1050). Seventy-ninth Cong., 1st Sess. *Cong. Rec.* 91(4):4920–4927, 24 May 1945.

140. Editorial: The Wagner-Murray-Dingell Bill (S. 1050) of 1945. *JAMA* 128:364–365, 2 June 1945.

141. Wagner, Robert F., The Wagner-Murray-Dingell Bill [Letter to the Editor]. *JAMA* 128:461, 9 June 1945.

142. The Wagner-Murray-Dingell Bill. Senator Wagner Comments on the Journal Editorial. . . . *JAMA* 128:672–673, 30 June 1945.

143. Editorial: Senator Wagner's Comments. *JAMA* 128:667–668, 30 June 1945.

144. A Bill . . . to Authorize Grants to the States for Surveying Their Hospitals . . . and for Planning Construction of Additional Facilities, and to Authorize Grants to Assist in Such Construction . . . (S.191). Seventy-ninth Cong., 1st Sess. *Cong. Rec.* 91(1):158, 10 January 1945.

145. Minutes of House of Delegates, Report of Reference Committee on Legislation and Public Relations. *JAMA* 129:1200–1201, 22 December 1945.

146. An Act to Amend the Public Health Service Act to Authorize Grants to the States for Surveying Their Hospitals . . . and for Planning Construction of Additional Facilities, and to Authorize Grants to Assist in Such Construction (P.L.79–725). Seventy-ninth Cong., 2nd Sess. *Pub. Stat. at Large U.S.* 60(1):1040–1049, 13 August 1946.

147. National Health Act of 1945 (S. 1606). Seventy-ninth Cong., 1st Sess. *Cong. Rec.* 91(8):10793–10795, 19 November 1945.

148. Editorial: Senate Hearings on the National Health Program. *JAMA* 130:1016, 13 April 1946.

149. Editorial: The Hearings on the Wagner-Murray-Dingell Bill. *JAMA* 131:1424, 24 August 1946.

150. National Health Insurance and Public Health Act (S.1320). Eightieth Cong., 1st Sess. *Cong. Rec.* 93(4):5516–5522, 20 May 1947.

151. Editorial: Mr. Ewing's Ten Year Health Program. *JAMA* 138:297–298, 25 September 1947.

152. Minutes of House of Delegates: Report of Reference Committee on Legislation and Public Relations [1 December 1948]. *JAMA* 138:1241, 25 December 1948.

153. Baxter, Leone: Address to House of Delegates. *JAMA* 140:694–696, 25 June 1949.

154. Minutes of House of Delegates: Statement of Policy of American Medical Association. *JAMA* 138:1171, 18 December 1948.

155. A Bill to Provide a National Health Insurance and Public Health Program (S.5). Eighty-first Cong., 1st Sess. *Cong. Rec.* 95(1):38, 5 January 1949.

156. A Bill to Provide a Program of National Health Insurance and Public Health and to Assist in Increasing the Number of Adequately Trained Professional and Other Health Personnel (S. 1679). Eighty-first Cong., 1st Sess. *Cong. Rec.* 95(4):4946, 4959–4962, 25 April 1949.

157. Washington Letter: Compulsory Insurance Chief Issue as Hearings Open. *JAMA* 140:481–482, 4 June 1949.

158. Editorial: Hearings on Health Legislation. *JAMA* 140:962, 16 July 1949.

159. Mayer, Milton, The Rise and Fall of Dr. Fishbein. *Harper's Magazine* 199:76–85, November, 1949.

160. The President's Page [Louis H. Bauer], The Chicago Meeting. *JAMA* 149:843, 28 June 1952.

161. A Bill to Provide a Program of National Health Insurance and Public Health, etc. (H.R.1817). Eighty-third Cong., 1st Sess. *Cong. Rec.* 99(1):434, 16 January 1953.

162. Hobby, Oveta Culp, Address of HEW Secretary Before House of Delegates, AMA. *JAMA* 156:1506–1508, 18 December 1954.

163. Organization Section: Legislative Review. *JAMA* 156:1514, 18 December 1954.

164. American Medical Association Opposes All Progressive Legislation. New Rival for NAM. Eighty-first Cong., 2nd Sess. *Cong. Rec.* 96(10):13904–13918, 30 August 1950.

165. An Act to Provide Medical Care for Dependents of Members of the Uniformed Services, and for Other Purposes (P.L.84–569). Eighty-fourth Cong., 2nd Sess. *Pub. Stat. at Large U.S.* 70:250–254, 7 June 1956.

166. Editorial: Morale and Medicine. *JAMA* 163:119, 12 January 1957.

167. A Bill to Amend the Social Security Act . . . so as to Increase the Benefits Payable Under the Federal Old-Age, Survivors, and Disability Insurance Program, to Provide Insurance Against the Costs of Hospital, Nursing Home, and Surgical Services, etc. (H.R.9467). Eighty-fifth Cong., 1st Sess. *Cong. Rec.* 103(12):16173, 27 August 1957.

168. An Act to Extend and Improve Coverage under the Federal Old-Age, Survivors and Disability Insurance System . . . ; to Provide Grants to the States for Medical Care for Aged Individuals of Low Income; . . . etc. (P.L.86–778). Eighty-sixth Cong., 2nd Sess. *Pub. Stat. at Large U.S.* 74:924–997, 13 September 1960.

169. A Bill to Provide for Payment for Hospital Services, Skilled Nursing Home Services, and Home Health Services Furnished to Aged Beneficiaries Under the Old-Age Survivors and Disability Insurance Program (H.R.4222). Eighty-seventh Cong., 1st Sess. *Cong. Rec.* 107(2):2136, 13 Feburary 1961.

170. Medical News: Delegates Endorse Kerr-Mills and AM-PAC, Criticize "Public Airing of Disagreements," *JAMA* 178(11):31, 16 December 1961.

171. Kihss, Peter, AMA Rebuttal to Kennedy Sees Aged Care Hoax. *New York Times*, 22 May 1962, p. 1.
172. Public Welfare Amendments of 1962 (H.R.10606). Eighty-seventh Cong., 2nd Sess. *Cong. Rec.* 108(10):13848–13873, 17 July 1962.
173. Social Security Amendments of 1964. Gore Amendment (No. 1256). Eighty-eighth Cong., 2nd Sess. *Cong. Rec.* 110 (16):21113–21122, 31 August 1964.
174. Social Security Amendments of 1964 (H.R.11865). Eighty-eighth Cong., 2nd Sess. *Cong. Rec.* 110(16):21351–21354, 2 September 1964.
175. A Bill to Amend Titles I and XVI of the Social Security Act to . . . [Authorize] Any State to Provide Medical Assistance for the Aged . . . Under Voluntary Private Health Insurance Plans and to Amend the Internal Revenue Code of 1954 to Provide Tax Incentives to Encourage Prepayment Health Insurance for the Aged . . . (S.820). Eighty-ninth Cong., 1st Sess. *Cong. Rec.* 111(2):1461, 28 January 1965.
176. An Act to Provide a Hospital Insurance Program for the Aged Under the Social Security Act With a Supplementary Benefits Program and an Expanded Program of Medical Assistance . . . etc. Eighty-ninth Cong., 1st Sess. *Pub. Stat. at Large U.S.* 79:286–423, 30 July 1965.
177. Meyers, Harold B., Mr. Mills' Elder-medi-better Care. *Fortune* 71:166–168, 196, June, 1965.
178. Ward, Donovan F., Remarks of the President [20 June 1965]. *JAMA* 193:23–25, 5 July 1965.
179. Appel, James Z., Inaugural Address. We the People of the United States—Are We Sheep? [20 June 1965]. *JAMA* 193:26–30, 5 July 1965.
180. Special Announcement: Board of Trustees Action. *JAMA* 193:689, 23 August 1965.
181. Wilbur, Dwight L., Emphasize Steering Instead of the Brake. Inaugural Address. *JAMA* 205:89–91, 8 July 1968.
182. Hyde, David R., Wolff, Payson, Gross, Anne, and Hoffman, Elliott Lee, The American Medical Association: Power, Purpose, and Politics in Organized Medicine. *Yale Law J.* 63:937–1022, May, 1954.
183. Garceau, Oliver, *The Political Life of the American Medical Association.* Cambridge: Harvard University Press, 1941.
184. Burrow, James G., *AMA Voice of American Medicine.* Baltimore: Johns Hopkins Press, 1963.

185. Rayack, Elton, *Professional Power and American Medicine: The Economics of the American Medical Association.* Cleveland: World Publishing Company, 1967.

186. Greely, Horace, Jr., M.D., Letter to the Editor. *Amer. Med. News* 12:5, 3 November 1969.

187. National Health Care—The Gathering Storm. *Amer. Med. News* 12:1; 8–9, 27 October 1969.

188. Watt, Linda, NHI Is Nigh. *Today's Health* 48:26–29; 71, July, 1970.

189. Committee for National Health Insurance: Press Release. Washington, D.C., 7 July 1970.

190. Washington Rounds. *Med. World News* 11:10f, 19 June 1970.

191. AMA, 70. *Med. World News* 11:19–21, 10 July 1970.

DRGs and the Ethical Reallocation of Resources

Robert M. Veatch

THE utilization review committee of a major teaching hospital found that one cardiologist's patients suffering acute myocardial infarctions consistently had hospitalization expenses far exceeding those of his colleagues' patients. While the average stay for such patients at the hospital was 13.1 days, this physician's patients stayed on average 18.2 days. The average cost of hospitalization at this institution for acute myocardial infarction was $10,257, while this physician's patients averaged costs of $14,132. The physician in question was thus an *outlier*—one whose patients consistently showed substantial deviation from mean resource consumption.

The hospital received DRG (diagnosis related groups) prospective payment for Medicare patients. The patients being reviewed were those falling into DRG 122, "acute myocardial infarction without complications, discharged alive." The cost overruns from one member of the staff could jeopardize the financial stability of the entire program. The problem was whether and to what extent the committee should review the physician's costs with the goal of bringing him into line with other physicians.

This case study, synthesized from the experience of three hospitals, provides a concrete example of the problems raised by cost containment, especially of the prospective payment system in which the hospital is reimbursed a set amount according to the DRG in which the patient falls.

From *Hastings Center Report*, 1986, Vol. 16, no. 3. Reprinted by Permission of the Author and The Hastings Center.

A frequent working assumption in utilization review is that the average amount of care given for a diagnosis group is the ideal amount of care. There is no reason to assume this, but deviations from the average are likely to require justification. Let us assume that the utilization review committee with the case described has reviewed this physician's cases and determined that there were no special social or medical factors such as age, severity of disease, or complications that provide an immediate explanation of the deviation from the average. Should the hospital, stimulated by the DRG system, exert pressure on this physician to reduce the extent of his care and, if so, on what ethical grounds? While considerable attention is being given to the technical aspects of operating the DRG system,[1] to ways of categorizing patients to produce a fair reimbursement,[2] and even to the impact that prospective payment will have on health care,[3] little analysis has been offered of the general ethical issues of cost containment.

Some responses that hospitals could make to cut costs are ethically suspect. A hospital could, for example, adopt more rigorous intake screening and transfer costly patients more aggressively. Since criteria for admission, especially for nearly hopeless cases, are ambiguous and the practice of deciding not to resuscitate is gaining strength, a hospital could probably conceal cost-saving decisions under the cloak of judgments not to admit or resuscitate. Suppose a hospital has found that in DRG 386 (extreme prematurity, neonates), it will lose $1,000 per patient at current average costs. It could close its neonatal unit, cutting the loss, or it could raise the minimum birth weight at which resuscitation would be attempted, thus systematically eliminating the babies who, if they survive, would be expected to generate the highest costs. While these strategies might eliminate the loss, neither is the response that the DRG system was intended to produce.

The DRG system or any other financing arrangement should be an opportunity to allocate resources ethically. Patients will not be treated fairly if too few *or too many* resources are committed to them. While the weightings for DRG groups were originally based on empirical findings, they should be adjusted so they reflect an ethically acceptable portion of resources for each group. The weights should be seen as a scale of the relative claims of patients in different categories.

There are four ethical principles that relate to the level of care given to patients. The first two are patient-centered. These are the principles of *patient-centered beneficence* (that one's actions should benefit the patient), and *autonomy* (that the patient's right to self-determination should be respected). These two principles would remain valid considerations even if they happened to increase costs. They are thus only indirectly related to cost containment. Honoring them may nevertheless reduce costs.

The two other principles operate at the social level. These are *full beneficence* (that resources should be used to do the most good), and *justice* (that resources should be distributed to provide all with an equal opportunity for health). Unlike the patient-centered principles, these are directly relevant to cost containment. As long as public funds are limited, these two questions arise: How can we do the most good with the resources available, and who should receive the benefits?

Patient-Centered Principles

A rigorous application of traditional ethical principles that focus exclusively on the individual patient—the patient's welfare and right to self-determination—may reduce costs.

Patient-Centered Beneficence

The first ethical principle that may reduce care and in turn reduce costs is a modified version of the traditional professional ethics of physicians. In the classical codes such as the Hippocratic Oath, the physician's duty is to benefit the patient according to his or her ability and judgment. This is patient-centered beneficence. One strong criticism of these codes is that individual physicians using their own judgment to try to benefit patients will sometimes be mistaken; in such cases, they may actually hurt patients. The outlier physician problem may be an example of this. The well-meaning physician may wrongly conclude that extensive care is required when, in fact, some of that care could do more harm than good.

Some argue that we should at least modify the Hippocratic Oath so that in cases where physicians can be shown to be wrong in assessing the patient's welfare, they should not try to benefit the patient according to their own ability and judgment, but should yield to the best objective estimate of the patient's welfare. This modified form would require physicians to serve the interests of their patients according to the best evidence that is available, not depending solely on their own judgments. The result would still be patient-centered beneficence, but now on a more objective basis. Especially in cases where the physician's personal judgment is substantially different from the best possible judgment, rational patients would not want a physician to try to benefit them according to the physician's own judgment—at least not without careful and detailed consent.

The notion of "objective welfare" is a difficult one, however. While the Hippocratic tradition commits the physician to serving the patient's welfare, physicians are not equipped to assess all the elements involved. Welfare is a complex concept. It includes social, economic, aesthetic, and spiritual components as well as organic ones. Surgery, for example, will have medical consequences—it will have an impact on morbidity and mortality—but it will also have impacts on the social, psychological, aesthetic, and economic well-being of the patient. A peer review panel should be capable of assessing the medical consequences of health care interventions, but two additional tasks are necessary before those consequences can be determined to improve the patient's welfare.

First, the medical consequences of treatment need to be evaluated: for example, if an intervention involved a slight increase in survival probability at the cost of great suffering and inconvenience, it would have to be determined whether those consequences would be beneficial or harmful. Second, the medical consequences of treatment, once evaluated, must be weighed against the other consequences. In neither of these tasks are physicians uniquely expert. Any specialized group including physicians or utilization review groups may assign unique values to medical consequences of treatment. (They may give unusual emphasis to mortality over morbidity, for example.) They may also relate medical consequences to nonmedical ones uniquely. (They may be willing to pay an unusually high economic or aesthetic price to improve mortality or morbidity risks.)

A peer review system can be expected to determine only what is *medically* beneficial on the basis of the values of health professionals. The best health professional assessment of what is medically beneficial is probably a reasonable approximation of what other people would find medically beneficial. We might, therefore, adopt a policy that limits medical care to interventions that are medically beneficial and use the health professional assessment of what is medically beneficial as an approximation.

Aggregate Net Medical Benefit as a Function of Days of Stay

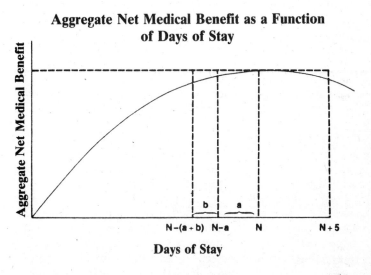

Days of Stay

Figure 1

The care provided in the myocardial infarction example can be divided into several components. Figure 1 illustrates these components with regard to the days of hospital stay. It shows schematically the aggregate net medical benefit of hospitalization plotted against the number of days of stay. The first day of stay is typically the most beneficial. Each succeeding day offers less benefit, until a maximum is reached (here represented as occurring at day N). After that, some net harm might occur (taking into account the iatrogenic risks and possible psychological harm of remaining in the hospital), represented by the slight downturn in the curve. In order for a utilization review committee to examine such a problem, it must have some notion of the medically ideal stay (N). This raises all the problems just discussed about using groups of professional physicians to determine even medical welfare alone. If these problems can be overcome, some estimate of a medical ideal will be established. This estimate will probably be close to the average days of stay, but not necessarily identical.

If the ideal (N) for DRG 122 was thought by the utilization review committee to be about thirteen days (assuming no complicating factors), its members would see their outlier physician as providing five days too much care. Those five days would do the patient no net medical good and might do some harm. Using the modified Hippocratic ethic, the committee might exert pressure to reduce care *in order to benefit the patient.* The unmodified Hippocratic ethic leads the physician to provide $N + 5$ days of care; modified, it drives care back toward N days. The reduction is justified by patient welfare, not by cost-saving.

Autonomy

The Hippocratic ethic has been challenged not only by those seeking more objective grounds for determining medical welfare, but more radically by those advocating the principle of autonomy. Many have concluded that the patient, who may have values and beliefs quite different from those of the medical community, has the right to refuse medical care even if that care is determined as objectively as possible to be in the patient's best medical interests. Patients may evaluate the medical consequences differently, or they may trade off the medical and other benefits and costs differently. They may, for example, place strong value on being at home with family, having home-cooked meals, being away from others who are ill, or simply having privacy. Patients may prefer to sacrifice their welfare for the welfare of their families. While none of these is a medical value, each might be taken into account in deciding about whether to consent to care.

The days approaching the Nth day of stay are interesting in this regard. Patients may prefer to reject some part of the proposed care. In our example they might rather be home on the Nth day. They might consider some marginal increment (shown as *a* in Figure 1) expendable. If they should so choose, autonomy supports their right to reject the care—in our example, to leave the hospital early.

Of course, if patients are given freedom to choose, for every patient who chooses to go home a day early there may be one who chooses to stay a day longer. Those choosing $(N + a)$ days will cancel out those choosing $(N - a)$. While autonomy requires letting patients refuse care, however, it does not require that they be permitted to get care beyond some accepted standard. In this sense the implications of the principle are asymmetrical.

Care on average might well be reduced somewhat if hospitals rigorously affirmed the right of patients to decline treatment— even treatment that is medically beneficial. The basis for doing so would not be cost containment but an ethical principle focused exclusively on the patient. The result, however, would be a pleasant side effect of reducing costs even below what the standard of objective medical interests would require.

Beyond the Patient's Perspective

The patient-centered principles provide two independent grounds for reducing costs, but these changes alone may not be sufficient. In the myocardial infarction case, the reimbursement was slightly below $7,000. If the outlier physician's patients were on average reduced to the average length of stay of the patients of the other physicians, costs for patients in DRG 122 would average $9,104. The hospital would still lose money.

One response of clinicians is to accuse the DRG system itself of forcing physicians to compromise quality of care. They might be willing to eliminate care that is doing harm and even care that autonomous patients are refusing, but they cannot tolerate eliminating care that is beneficial and desired by the patient. Yet that seems to be precisely what the DRG system requires. The result is the demand that reimbursement be adjusted so that the ideal care (N days) or ideal care adjusted for patient autonomy ($N - a$ days) can be delivered, if not to even more radical demands that the entire system be scrapped.

A more careful analysis requires close examination of the ethics of providing all care that meets the criteria of patient-centered beneficence and autonomy. Would it be ethical to eliminate marginally beneficial care that is very expensive in relation to the benefits that it provides? Some increment of care (shown as b in Figure 1)—would be medically beneficial and would be desired by patients, but nevertheless it might not be ethically justified, because other uses of these resources might ethically carry more weight. If autonomy reduces the average length of stay for myocardial care patients by a days, then this new factor may reduce care by an additional b days, thus bringing the length of stay down to $[N - (a + b)]$.

To determine which, if any, of the marginally beneficial yet expensive care should be eliminated between the $[N - (a + b)]$ and the $(N - a)$ points, we should ask: Would a reasonable person planning health insurance want such care included, assuming that it would increase premiums and that those funds could otherwise be used on some other worthwhile social or personal projects? Surely, at least some such care would be eliminated. From this point of view, the reimbursement for various diagnostic groups ought to be set so that adequate care is given but marginally beneficial, desired, expensive care is eliminated. Each DRG weight should be a measure of the ethical claims of persons in the group. The weighting should be set so that it drives care below the ideal level and down to the ethically justified $[N - (a\ b)]$ level. A social ethic of resource allocation will give us the appropriate weight on which to base fair reimbursement.

Two social ethical principles are available for deciding when care should be provided. Each provides a basis for deciding questions such as what the relative weights for DRG groups ought to be. One is the principle of full beneficence; the other is the principle of justice.

Full Beneficence

Planners might be inclined to ask the classical utilitarian question: How do the net benefits from using resources in this manner compare with those of using the resources in some other manner? The ethical principle of beneficence presses decision makers to maximize the net good done by their actions. The use of the full beneficence principle differs from the Hippocratic patient-oriented principle by requiring that the benefits and harm to all parties, and not only to the patient, be taken into account. This is the ethical principle underlying cost-benefit analysis and cost-effectiveness analysis as they are normally practiced.

In our example, at some point further days of stay become marginally beneficial while still about as expensive as earlier hospital days. If the net benefit of using the resources for these days is compared with other possible medical or even nonmedical uses of the resources, the marginally beneficial days will lose. If this strategy were used by the insurance planners to set the relative DRG weights, the goal would be to arrange the weights so that the amount of good done in the system as a whole would be maximized. The marginal expenditures in each DRG group ought to be producing the same marginal increments of good.

If it turns out that the existing DRG weights are not accomplishing this goal, a utilization review committee or a hospital administration might consider cost shifting from one group to another in order to maximize the total amount of good a DRG group is doing as a whole. Thus if the acute myocardial infarction group (DRG 122) gets only $7,000 reimbursement per patient but the local experts consider that $9,100 worth of care is ideal, someone at the local level might ask whether the marginal dollars spent on other DRGs could more effectively be used for myocardial infarction patients. They would not want to appropriate funds to bring that care all the way up to the $9,100 mark, of course, because as that ideal point is approached the benefits get smaller and smaller until the point is reached where they are negligible and the funds could be used more effectively for some other purpose.

Thus the principle of full beneficence has major implications for national and local decision making. However, it may turn out that there are good reasons not to allow this principle to be overriding, especially not to permit local decision makers to shift costs. We shall look more closely at the reasons for avoiding local cost shifting later.

There are two common objections to using the principle of full beneficence for making these cost-benefit decisions. First, many object that the problems of quantification are enormous. For example, comparing the benefits of the eleventh day of hospitalization after a myocardial infarction with those of a comparable dollar investment in nursing home care for an Alzheimer's patient is extremely difficult. If benefits could be measured in a single statistic such as mortality rate, the comparison would be easier, but a rich notion of benefit includes not only preventing death but relieving suffering, avoiding psychological trauma, and so forth. At best all that can be given is a rough approximation.

Though this argument should add humility to the cost-benefit analyst's work, it is not very convincing. In every policy decision some such comparisons have to be made. The defenders of systematic efforts to compare costs and benefits rightly point out that the only alternative to quantifying alternative outcomes is to leave important decisions to intuition or chance.

The second objection is much more serious. When all benefits and harms are aggregated and then compared, the standard methods of cost-benefit analysis mask variations in distribution. One course of action may produce enormous benefits to some persons and only harm to others, while an alternative course may spread the benefits and burdens more evenly. Aggregating benefits and harms results in losing this ethically interesting information.

As a way of avoiding unjust distribution, some have urged that we shift to cost-effectiveness analysis, in which a program goal is preselected and planners simply compare the costs of alternative ways of accomplishing the goal.[4] It turns out, however, that protecting against differences in distribution is not that easy. Whenever two alternatives for accomplishing a goal are compared, the distribution of benefits may be different. Consider a study of the cost-effectiveness of two alternative ways for screening British school girls for bacteriuria (a condition where bacteria are present in the urine).[5] One method involved sending each girl home with a kit containing instructions for obtaining a urine sample. The other method involved obtaining the sample in school under the supervision of a nurse. The study reported that the first method was significantly more cost-effective. While the obvious conclusion seemed to be that the first method should be used in order to maximize the benefits per unit of cost, there was a fascinating complication. That method was much better for detecting cases in middle-class girls than in lower-class girls. The reason seems clear. The familial support network, educational level, and social resources necessary to follow the instructions and return a good sample were more likely to be present in the middle-class homes. What originally appears to be a choice between two methods of accomplishing a single goal (finding cases of bacteriuria) can be reformulated as a choice between two different goals (finding the most cases per pound invested regardless of social class, or giving girls of all social classes an equal chance of having their cases found).

If full beneficence and the techniques of cost-benefit and cost-effectiveness analysis are used to determine the appropriate DRG weights, then benefits may be distributed very unevenly among patients. It is theoretically possible that the most efficient way to maximize net medical benefits in the Medicare system is to assign very high weights to certain groups and very low weights to other groups. This result may be efficient but unfair. Full beneficence should therefore not be regarded as the sole principle of morality. To say this is not to rule out the validity of the principle altogether, of course. All things being equal, maximizing good consequences does seem to be morally required. But to ensure fairness we need to turn to a principle of justice.

Justice

Just as autonomy provides an alternative to patient-centered beneficence at the individual level, so there may be a principle at the social level that forces us to look beyond mere accumulation of good consequences.

If the DRG system were ever extended to include a category for bacteriuria screening in schoolgirls, the planners would have to determine whether they wanted only enough funds to screen most efficiently (regardless of social class) or enough funds to screen in a manner that equalized the chances for all schoolgirls. To make this determination, they would have to consider the principle of justice along with mere maximizing of good consequences.

The meaning of the principle of justice has been open to serious scholarly debate, especially in the fifteen years since the publication of John Rawls's *A Theory of Justice*.[6] Those attempting to identify justice as a principle independent of either autonomy or beneficence emphasize equity or fairness in distribution, normally including in their definition a notion of equality. A pure egalitarian understanding of the principle of justice would have us arrange the distribution of resources so that it produces opportunities for equality of welfare. In the health care sphere the goal would be to ensure that everyone has the chance to be as healthy as anyone else. Insofar as justice is the operative principle, we would want the DRG weights to be assigned in such a way that funds were available to give people in different diagnostic groups equal opportunities for health.

Objections to the Egalitarian Approach

Three objections are raised to the egalitarian interpretation of justice as applied to health care. First, it is not clear whether an egalitarian should strive for opportunities for equality of health status or equality of welfare more generally. The latter seems at least as plausible, and in an ideal world the egalitarian would in fact strive for overall equality. As a practical matter, however, the principle of justice might be easier to apply if health were treated separately from other goods.

Second, the egalitarian interpretation does not deal with the relationship between justice and the other principles we have been considering. What should happen, for example, if striving for equal opportunities for health requires giving enormous weight to DRG 386 (extreme prematurity, neonate), but doing so turns out to be a very inefficient way of maximizing aggregate net benefits?

To answer this question, those involved in making cost-containment decisions need a theory that relates the various principles. Our medical ethics of treatment refusal has led many to the conclusion that at the patient-centered level the principle of autonomy takes absolute precedence over patient benefit. If one extends that relationship to the social level, justice would have priority status over full beneficence. That would mean, for example, that no amount of social benefit would ever justify inflicting enormous harm on individuals, such as was done in the Nazi experiments. What then should be the relationship between the principles of justice and autonomy? One plausible answer is that here we must revert to a balancing strategy with no one principle having priority. Often, the proper weighting becomes clearer in the context of a real life dilemma. In any case, this balancing problem is not unique to egalitarians.

A third and more serious objection often raised against the egalitarian position involves the relationship of justice to patient demand. It is often argued that egalitarianism is impractical because it generates an infinite demand. Certain patients are very poorly off, and on the basis of egalitarian theories of justice, they would get high priority. But they would generate virtually infinite demands, breaking the bank and leaving somewhat more healthy people without any health care at all.

Several responses are available to this important argument. First, egalitarian justice itself sets some limits. If a person with a serious, uncorrectable handicap such as blindness generated an infinite demand, eventually that person would take so many resources that others in the society would be deprived of even the basics of health care. But, as the others' opportunities for health declined, eventually they would become worse off than the blind person, and on the basis of justice they would then take priority over the blind person.

Another limit comes from the principle of autonomy. In certain cases it might be prudent for the least well off not to exercise their right to opportunity for equality. For example, in certain cases the least well off might waive their claims in order to keep others healthy enough to render them needed aid.

A third limit is found in the possibility that promises have been made to those who are not least well off. If promise-keeping is a duty on a par with justice, then some balancing is required, and at least in some circumstances it would be in order to keep promises of health care resources already made to those who are not least well off.

Finally, if these three means of overcoming the infinite demand problem are not satisfactory, one might have to revert to the idea that full beneficence can be balanced against justice, with each having an equal force. Doing so would easily explain why some resources would go to those who are better off. Making this move, however, opens some doors very wide— doors that seem to justify behaviors such as slavery and Nazi research—at least in principle. These are doors that are better kept closed if possible.

The Role of Clinicians in Cost Containment

We now have an ethical framework for thinking about cost containment decisions such as those related to DRGs. Patient welfare and autonomy give us a relatively easy basis for curtailing expenditures. Two additional ethical principles (maximizing aggregate net benefits and creating equal opportunities for people to be as healthy as others) provide further grounds for limiting care and lead to somewhat different decisions. Although the two social principles often lead to identical decisions, they are in fact very different and occasionally (such as in the bacteriuria example) lead to very different policies and very different DRG weightings. Several problems arise in the application of social principles to DRGs and cost containment.

One problem is the role of clinicians. When DRG reimbursement will not cover the average costs, a typical strategy is to encourage clinicians to be more cost-conscious. Bulletin board posters may be displayed, for example, showing the costs of equipment and each procedure. Since cuts based on either patient welfare or autonomy would not require such cost-awareness, the strategy of encouraging cost-consciousness must be rooted in the ethical concerns of justice and full beneficence.

Consider what would happen if the utilization review committee encouraged each clinician to be more cost-conscious and to eliminate procedures that seemed marginal. Each physician would probably shift the level of care somewhat. The outlier physician now hospitalizing patients for eighteen days might cut that number to seventeen, and the physician at the other end of the spectrum might reduce his care somewhat as well. The result would be a slight drop in average cost, but the outlier overtreating physician would still be providing excess care and the undertreating physician reducing care even further.

There are more subtle problems with this strategy. Physicians, in effect, would be determining what is a reasonable reduction below ideal care for their patients. Such an assessment would require comparing the health care under consideration with other goods that could be obtained with the resources.

Clinicians would have to draw on their own beliefs and values to make these comparisons. Yet, as we have seen, professionals may make atypical judgments. Just as military officers may overvalue defense appropriations or philosophers may overvalue philosophy, dedicated health care professionals may overvalue health care. Most probably clinicians asked to determine a reasonable level of care would opt for more care than lay people would choose.

Even more serious is the potential impact on the underlying ethics of the clinician. Asking the physician to be cost-conscious, to eliminate marginally beneficial care, would require a major shift in traditional professional ethics. The Hippocratic ethic is already being challenged when autonomy is added to patient-centered beneficence, but the physician can make this shift while still retaining a patient-centered ethic. Asking physicians to be cost-conscious, however, would be asking them to abandon their central commitment to their patients. In effect they would be asked to remove the Hippocratic Oath from their waiting room walls and replace it with a sign that reads, "Warning all ye who enter here. I will generally work for your rights and welfare, but if benefits to you are marginal and costs are great, I will abandon you in order to protect society." It is not clear that either physicians or lay people want clinicians to take that stand.

The alternative may be no more attractive. We might grant to clinical professionals a special "role-specific" ethic, one that specifies special duties for special roles.[7] Just as parents or defense attorneys have special moral duties (to be advocates for their children or their clients) so clinical professionals might be asked to be advocates for their patients and exclude resource allocation and social welfare from their normal clinical agenda. Just as there are exceptions in extreme cases in which parents or defense attorneys must take the welfare of others into account, so too there may have to be exceptions for clinicians—such as when psychiatrists are expected to break confidence in order to warn that their patients are planning to commit murder. For the general rule, however, clinicians could be given the role of agents for their patients. Cost containment would not normally be on their agenda.

If cost containment is not on the clinicians' agenda, it would have to be on someone else's. Since these choices of maximizing net benefits or distributing benefits equally are fundamentally nonmedical, it is appropriate that they be made by the general public. Thus for DRG weighting the society as a whole, working through its representatives, should decide the relative merit of the claims of the members of various diagnostic groups. If health professionals are among those making these social decisions about ethics, they should be there not as clinicians but in some other capacity. If clinicians' evaluations of the relative importance of health care and other goods are atypical, then they should not be represented in such a policy-making body in numbers that exceed their membership in the general population.

This decision-making strategy has already come about for DRG 103—heart transplants. The weighting for DRG 103 is 0.000. It was not based on the medical judgment that heart transplants would never do any Medicare recipient any good or that all rational candidates would exercise their autonomy to refuse such care, but on the judgment that it would cost the Medicare system a great deal. (The official explanation, however, is that heart transplants are still experimental.) The decision was made that other uses of the funds were of higher priority. Surely it would make no sense to ask the individual cardiac surgeon or even cardiac surgeons as a group to determine whether heart transplants deserved the weighting they received.

The choice for clinicians is an awkward one. They must either adopt an ethical perspective involving full beneficence and justice and in the process give up their commitment to focus only on patients or accept a special role-specific duty of being a patient advocate and in the process yield any role in resource allocation and cost containment. I am increasingly convinced that the latter alternative is preferable although not without its problems. If that move is made, then the clinician should have no direct role in eliminating marginally useful care for cost-containment purposes. The planners of prospective payment systems should make judgments about the relative merit of the claims of people in various groups, taking into account the claims of justice, for those in other medical groups and for those who have needs that are not medical.

Utilization review committees comprised of clinicians face the same problems as individual clinicians. If they make judgments about reducing marginally beneficial care, they will bring to bear atypical constellations of values. In this role, they will have to abandon their patient-centered orientation in order to promote social efficiency or fairness. While there is nothing logically inconsistent about asking clinicians to adopt one ethic in their patient care and another in their committee work (assuming they do not serve on committees that review their own patients), the psychological transition back and forth between patient-centered clinician and societally centered committee member would be very difficult. Moreover, insofar as the committee establishes general policies that seek to eliminate marginally beneficial care (for example, a day limit on ordinary acute myocardial infarction hospitalization without formal review), the committee members would be generating policy decisions that would affect their own patients. They could not work toward such an end while remaining loyal to their patients.

Another difficulty is that different local committees would almost certainly make different trade-offs. One committee might reduce days of stay by one day, while another would do so by two days. It is unfair to let subjective variations of this sort compromise patients' interests at the margin by differing amounts. If cuts are to be made, it would be fairer to make them more nearly uniform. The weighting for DRG 122 should be set uniformly so that the reimbursement would fund, for example, X days below ideal care.

The Implications of Cost-Shifting

The weighting of DRGs has important implications for the morality of shifting costs from one DRG to another. If a hospital finds that it has a loss in one DRG and a profit in another, it has several options. It could eliminate the services for the losing group, increasing profits in the process. If it finds that option morally objectionable, it might simply let one service subsidize the other.

The problem is that this practice systematically circumvents the allocation that was envisioned when weights were assigned. The weights make sense only if they reflect a fair resource distribution among the DRG as judged by a group authorized to represent society in making these judgments. Cost-shifting between groups—even if it is done on a nonprofit basis—circumvents this judgment. It is unfair to the group that generates a profit to have those resources used at the local hospital's discretion for care of some other group whose patients will then be getting care at a level above that envisioned by those who assign the DRG weights. Cost-shifting from one DRG to another is difficult, if not impossible, to justify ethically.

Assuming that a hospital is committed to cost-shifting and still discovers that the costs of patients in DRG 122 far exceed reimbursement, even after eliminating useless care and care refused by patients, how should the institution go about reducing costs?

It is indeed unusual—a measure of society's faith in the medical community—that the Medicare system simply sets a reimbursement level without specifying how much care should be delivered for that money. It is unimaginable that the administrators of the food stamp program would give a grocery store a fixed-dollar reimbursement per family and tell the grocery store manager to provide the family with an adequate, unspecified amount of food that the manager considers reasonable. Yet that is what the Medicare system is doing to hospitals. Only enormous faith in the integrity and dedication of administrators and clinicians makes such a system thinkable. The hospital is held in check only by malpractice laws, the fear of bad publicity, and the institution's own moral integrity and good will. Eventually there may have to be some broader societal participation in deciding how much care ought to be delivered for the reimbursement set for a given DRG group. In the meantime, local hospitals have been left with that task. It is, therefore, important to understand the ethical basis for such decisions.

Once a DRG weight is assigned and the hospital knows its resource limits, then the resources must be allocated among patients within that DRG. Among patients the goal can be either to maximize the benefit per unit of resources invested or to give patients an equal opportunity for health. If the goal is to maximize aggregate benefit (measured in mortality and morbidity statistics), then the sicker and more elderly patients may get low priority, because they consume more resources in producing comparable benefits. For example, if a young patient and an elderly patient are being treated for a comparable disease, the elderly person may require a longer stay in the hospital. If, however, the goal is equality of opportunity for health, then it is irrelevant that more days of stay are invested in older, sicker patients and that aggregate mortality and morbidity statistics are not as good because of this allocation. An egalitarian view of justice clearly calls for the latter view.

A reasonable approach might be to set some general limits on care that cannot be exceeded without review. If reimbursements are adequate to pay for ten days of stay on average, slightly fewer than ten days might be set as the limit, leaving the balance plus any unused resources from those leaving early to be allocated on the basis of need. In theory a group reflecting the broad profile of the society ought to set the limits, but in reality that would probably be impractical. Local groups of administrators with clinical knowledge, like those making up utilization review committees, can be vested with this public authority provided they realize that their task is to make essentially nonmedical value judgments on behalf of the society.

There is an additional problem: How will each patient consume his or her allotment of resources? There is no reason based on justice why each patient must expend his or her resources on exactly the same mix of services. One patient might want to trade in one of his or her allotted days of stay for something nearer the ideal amount of monitoring and testing. Taking into account increased psychological satisfaction the switch may even result in a slight increase in welfare. According to the principle of autonomy, such switching is clearly justified.

While justice would not require the same mix for each patient, however, it might be impractical to permit patients to choose different mixes. Administering such "intra-patient" resource shifts would be extremely difficult. Just educating the patient sufficiently to make knowledgeable decisions would be hard (although every patient may need much of this knowledge in order to give informed consent to treatment). Another pragmatic problem is that making such a shift might leave the patient much worse off medically. While this would not matter to a lover of autonomy, provided the patient is not using up more than his or her just share of the resources, it could present a more complex problem. The patient who has become sicker because of such a shift would have had the opportunity for health and refused it. Therefore, he or she would have less of a claim on medical resources than other comparably sick patients. Two possible solutions come to mind. First, anyone choosing to shift resources at the intra-patient level would have to buy an insurance policy to cover the costs of any additional care needed as a result of that free choice. Second, and probably more practical: intra-personal shifts would be banned, not on the grounds that they jeopardize patient welfare or that people should not be free to choose, but on the grounds that they would create enormous social problems.

A Medical Ethics of the Future

DRGs and the concern about cost containment provide an intriguing opportunity to reassess the ethics of medicine. Some patient-centered concerns may give us adequate leverage for curtailing costs, at least if patient benefit is considered objectively and supplemented with the patient's autonomy. These alone, however, will probably not be adequate. Important cost-curtailing decisions may follow. Therefore newer, more socially oriented ethical principles will have to be incorporated into our medical ethic. While a fuller commitment to beneficence is the more obvious candidate for an expanded ethic, justice may be the more legitimate principle for assigning weights to DRGs and making other cost-containment decisions. DRG weights should be viewed as a scale of the relative ethical claims of patients in the different diagnostic groups. If these social principles become a central part of a medical ethics of the future, we shall have to decide whether health professionals in their clinical role should incorporate them into their ethics or whether they should be given a special duty to remain patient-centered. A good case can be made for the latter.

NOTES

1. See, for example, U.S. Department of Health and Human Services, Health Care Financing Administration, "Medicare Program: Prospective Payment for Medicare In-Patient Hospital Services: Final Rule," *Federal Register* 49 (January 3,

1984), pp. 234–334; Group on Health Service Policy, Division of Health Policy and Program Evaluation, Department of Health Care Resources, *DRGs and the Prospective Payment System: A Guide for Physicians* (Chicago: American Medical Association, 1983).

2. See, for example, Center for Health Affairs, *Case Approach to DRG Assignment: A Guide For Physicians* (Cleveland: Greater Cleveland Hospital Association, 1984).

3. See Steve Holman, "DRGs: Forcing Physicians Into a Business Role?" *Hospital Physician* 20 (5), 1984, 102, 111.

4. See The Hastings Center, "Values, Ethics, and CBA in Health Care." In *The Implications of Cost-Effectiveness Analysis of Medical Technology*, p. 170. Office of Technology Assessment, Congress of the United States. (Washington, D.C.: Office of Technology Assessment, 1980); Michael S. Baram, "Cost-Benefit Analysis: An Inadequate Basis for Health, Safety, and Environmental Regulatory Decisionmaking," *Ecology Law Quarterly* 8, 3 (1980); 474.

5. Gordon Rich, Norman J. Glass, and J.G. Selkon, "Cost-effectiveness of Two Methods of Screening for Asymptomatic Bacteriuria," *British Journal of Preventive and Social Medicine* 30 (1976), 54–59.

6. John Rawls, *A Theory of Justice* (Cambridge: Harvard University Press, 1971).

7. Robert M. Veatch, *A Theory of Medical Ethics* (New York: Basic Books, 1981), pp. 250–87.

THE HMO Physician's Duty to Cut Costs: A Case Study

Robert M. Veatch and Morris F. Collen

WILLIAM Edwards was thirty-nine when a serious, potentially life-threatening ventricular heart arrhythmia (irregular contractions) was diagnosed during a routine physical examination. The cardiologist first prescribed quinidine, but it failed to control the arrhythmia.

Diisopyramide was successful, but Mr. Edwards complained of severe blurred vision and dry mouth. When the medication was reduced, the side effects disappeared but the arrhythmia returned. At this point the cardiologist decided to combine the diisopyramide with propranolol, a common beta-blocker known to be effective in certain arrhythmias. This controlled the problem, without side effects.

Mr. Edwards continued with this medication regimen for five years until moving to a new town, where he joined a health maintenance organization (HMO). He immediately consulted Dr. Sam Forester, a cardiologist.

Dr. Forester agreed that medication was needed, but he was concerned about diisopyramide, since severe problems had been reported in some patients. Moreover, Mr. Edwards and his original physician had never tried the obvious approach of using propranolol alone.

Both Dr. Forester and Mr. Edwards concluded that there were also risks in shifting to the single drug. Although it was generally safer than diisopyramide and probably should have

From *Hastings Center Report,* 1985, vol. 15, no. 4. Reprinted by permission of the authors and the Hastings Center.

been tried originally, there was a small chance of a fatal heart attack. On balance both agreed that the status quo was slightly better for the patient.

Dr. Forester then noticed the financial ledger for Mr. Edwards's care, which included the cost of the medication paid for in full by the HMO. The yearly cost of the diisopyramide was $430; the propranolol cost $26. He realized that even a significant increase in propranolol dosage, something that would involve little risk, would still reduce the HMO's medication bill by about $400.

Should Dr. Forester consider a change in medication, taking into account cost-saving for the HMO, or should he work solely on the basis of the welfare of the patient? If he should take into account the costs to the HMO, should he try to persuade the patient to agree to the change or should he simply refuse to authorize any further prescriptions for the diisopyramide? Does Mr. Edwards have any moral obligation to take costs to the HMO into account in choosing a medication regimen?

Commentary
by Robert M. Veatch

The traditional professional ethics of physicians—reflected in the Hippocratic Oath, the Declaration of Geneva, and elsewhere—is that the physician should always strive to do what he or she thinks will benefit the patient.

In this case that traditional ethical commitment is challenged. In effect, the question is: Should the physician divert his attention from the single-minded pursuit of the patient's welfare where the institution's or other subscribers' interests would be served by slightly compromising the patient? Specifically a very small, but real increment of benefit is purchased for a very substantial cost. Does the patient-benefit principle apply in such cases?

Two ethical options are available, neither of which is very attractive. First, we could amend the Hippocratic commitment so that physicians should, at least in certain circumstances, take into account the welfare of others. We might give the physician the mandate to try to maximize total benefits instead of simply benefit to the patient.

That strategy produces at least two serious problems, however. First, physicians (like any other special social group) have unique notions about the comparative value of resource expenditures. In deciding whether to use Medicaid funds to pay for drugs, for example, a physician should have to compare the value of providing the drugs with the value of some remote nonmedical uses of the money. Asking health professionals to take these social trade-offs into account could introduce serious biases.

Second, if physicians include benefits to others in their calculations, patients have to be told that their physicians have conflicting agendas. The Hippocratic Oath would have to be removed from the waiting room wall and replaced with a sign that says, "Warning all ye who enter here. The physician will at times abandon your interests in order to benefit others and save them money." It is not clear that rational patients or physicians in an HMO would prefer this new mandate.

The other alternative is to give the HMO physician—in fact all clinicians—a special role-related ethic that exempts them from the general ethical duty to promote fair and reasonable distribution of resources. They would then be free to single-mindedly pursue the welfare along with the rights of the patient.

Then, however, someone else must decide to eliminate marginally beneficial care. Surely, in planning the HMO or insurance coverage, no rational persons would want all such care included. Assuming marginal care was eliminated for others as well as themselves, they would opt for a lower premium so they could spend the money on something they valued more. Mr. Edwards would reasonably prefer not to have the diisopyramide and other marginal treatments covered, if he could spend the savings somewhere else.

The most acceptable arrangement, therefore, would actively involve members of the HMO plan in decisions about whether certain marginal medical services are covered. Members might, for example, exclude heart transplant coverage, as Medicare does. They might decide to cover routine physical exams only every five years for people between twenty and forty even though they might reasonably benefit marginally from more frequent exams. They might cover only ten days of hospitalization for myocardial infarction even though a few more days would be marginally beneficial. These decisions should be made by the patients (the subscribers), however. Clinicians should not be put in the position of ruling on how much to compromise their patients.

The drug case poses an interesting problem. To the extent that the decision can be handled as a policy matter, it should be—like the physical exam frequency. Judgments like the one in the diisopyramide case, however, do not lend themselves to policy. No obvious solution is apparent. Administrators, especially in profit-making HMOs, are not in any better position to make such decisions than clinicians.

An ethics committee comprising a representative sample of patients might be given the authority to rule based on the facts presented by the HMO professionals. In doing so the group would be acting as agents for their fellow subscribers with a mandate to eliminate marginally beneficial care. Theoretically, they might be asked to eliminate all care where the cost exceeded the benefit. That, however, would create serious tensions among members and would be unfair to the sickest members, exactly the group that has the greatest claim of justice for care, even inefficient care. If this ethics committee of HMO members cannot make these judgments, we may be forced to the bizarre conclusion that no one is in an ethical position to decide to eliminate such care.

That brings us to the role of Mr. Edwards. Does he have any moral responsibility to consider that the best drug regimen for him is one that offers only marginally more benefit for a much greater cost? Surely, it is both moral and prudent for Mr. Edwards to take all of this into consideration in endorsing, promoting, or participating in collective arrangements by which members establish policies that eliminate marginally beneficial, expensive care.

Does he have any obligation, however, to suggest eliminating his diisopyramide—in order that others may benefit from the savings? I am not convinced he has a strict moral obligation to do so. Such a contribution to his fellow subscribers seems supererogatory.

I am thus forced to conclude that, although the expensive drug should be eliminated, neither Mr. Edwards nor Dr. Forester is the proper person to make that decision. Surely the administrators of the HMO are in no better position to do so. If that decision can be made ethically at all, it should be made by the HMO members as a whole—at the policy level if possible, and by a committee of the members if not.

Commentary
by Morris F. Collen

In almost every patient encounter, a health care practitioner must consider first the quality of care he or she is prescribing—that is, whether a particular clinical decision will achieve an accurate diagnosis and/or bring about the desired benefit; and second, the costs resulting from this decision to the patient and/or to the organization financing the care. Thus, a very common problem in the practice of medicine is balancing the quality with the costs of medical care.

The physician often provides professional services on a fee-for-service basis to a patient with a disease for which there are alternative acceptable methods of treatment. The physician always considers the relative effectiveness of each treatment mode and should also consider the comparative total costs associated with each treatment. The physician should attempt to assess whether the patient can afford the most expensive treatments, and should discuss with the patient the comparative costs and effectiveness of the alternative treatments available, ideally to arrive at a mutually agreeable decision. As the fee-for-service practitioner knows, if the costs for the prescribed treatment exceed the immediate financial resources of the patient, then payment of the physician's fee may be delayed. Thus the financial success of fee-for-service practitioners is intimately linked to the financial solvency of their private patients.

Similarly, if the patient has prepaid for medical care services in a health maintenance organization, the HMO physician knows that the immediate cost consequences of his or her clinical decision will have a direct impact on the HMO's finances. Furthermore, if the overall HMO costs exceed those that had been budgeted by the HMO for the year, then in the following year the prepayment dues (premiums), as direct costs to the patient and to all other subscriber-members of the HMO, will proportionately need to increase to restore the HMO's positive economic balance. If the HMO excessively increases its annual premiums, it will no longer be competitive with other health insurance programs in the community, its membership will likely decrease, and it will need to compensate by reducing personnel or decreasing the comprehensiveness of its prepaid services. Thus the financial success of the HMO physician is intimately linked to the financial solvency of his or her HMO.

Only under arrangements where the patient has no obligation to pay for any medical treatment (as in the Veterans' Administration hospitals or a charity clinic) and where the physician's salary is independent of revenues generated from professional services can individual physicians consider the effectiveness of care without taking into account the treatment costs. However, increasing budgetary restraints and public support for cost containment are introducing economic questions even into these medical practice arrangements.

Thus, in any doctor-patient encounter, under any financing arrangement, the doctor has some financial incentive—in addition to a moral obligation—to consider both the quality and the costs of the care being prescribed and to attempt to arrive at a good balance that can be justified and defended to other physicians, and the doctor should try to persuade the patient to agree to that treatment which is acceptably effective at the lowest cost. Rarely, in a case such as this one, is any treatment 100 percent effective in curing the disease, so rarely is the choice clear-cut or simple. The physician should not refuse to authorize a treatment that the physician and the patient agree is best. Finally, physicians should be prepared to defend their judgment before their peers in the community within which they practice; and before a jury in court if their decision varies from the community's standard of practice.

SECTION III

MEDICAL ETHICS: PRINCIPLES OF AUTONOMY, TRUTHTELLING, CONFIDENTIALITY

The Values Underlying Informed Consent

President's Commission for the Study of Ethical Problems in Medical and Behavioral Research, 1982

WHAT are the values that ought to guide decisionmaking in the provider-patient relationship or by which the success of a particular interaction can be judged? The Commission finds two to be central: promotion of a patient's well-being and respect for a patient's self-determination.[1] They are in many ways compatible, but their potential for conflict in actual practice must be recognized.[2]

Serving the Patient's Well-Being

Therapeutic interventions are intended first and foremost to improve a patient's health. In most circumstances, people agree in a general way on what "improved health" means. Restoration of normal functioning (such as the repair of a fractured limb) and avoidance of untimely death (such as might occur without the use of antibiotics to control life-threatening infections in otherwise healthy persons) are obvious examples. Health care is, in turn, usually a means of promoting patients' well-being. The connection between a particular health care decision and an individual's well-being is not perfect, however. First, the definition of health can be quite controversial: does wrinkled

From *Making Health Care Decisions*, President's Commission for the Study of Ethical Problems in Medical and Behavioral Research, 1982.

skin or uncommonly short stature constitute impaired health, such that surgical repair or growth hormone is appropriate? Even more substantial variation can be found in ranking the importance of health with other goals in an individual's life. For some, health is a paramount value; for others—citizens who volunteer in time of war, nurses who care for patients with contagious diseases, hang-glider enthusiasts who risk life and limb—a different goal sometimes has primacy.

Absence of Objective Medical Criteria

Even the most mundane case—in which there is little if any disagreement that some intervention will promote health—may well have no objective medical criteria that specify a single best way to achieve the goal. A fractured limb can be repaired in a number of ways; a life-threatening infection can be treated with a variety of antibiotics; mild diabetes is subject to control by diet, by injectable natural insulin, or by oral synthetic insulin substitutes. Health care professionals often reflect their own value preferences when they favor one alternative over another; many are matters of choice, dictated neither by biomedical principles or data nor by a single, agreed-upon professional standard.

In the Commission's survey it was clear that professionals recognize this fact: Physicians maintained that decisional authority between them and their patients should depend on the nature of the decision at hand. Thus, for example, whether a pregnant woman over 35 should have amniocentesis was viewed as largely a patient's decision, whereas the decision of which antibiotic to use for strep throat was seen as primarily up to the doctor. Furthermore, on the question of whether to continue aggressive treatment for a cancer patient with metastases in whom such treatment had already failed, two-thirds of the physicians felt it was not a scientific, medical decision, but one that turned principally on personal values. And the same proportion felt the decision should be made jointly (which 64 percent of the doctors claimed it usually was).

Patient's Reasonable Subjective Preferences

Determining what constitutes health and how it is best promoted also requires knowledge of patients' subjective preferences. In pursuit of the other goals and interests besides health that society deems legitimate, patients may prefer one type of medical intervention to another, may opt for no treatment at all, or may even request some treatment when a practitioner would prefer to follow a more conservative course that involved, at least for the moment, no medical intervention. For example, a slipped disc may be treated surgically or with medications and bed rest. Which treatment is better can be unclear, even to a physician. A patient may prefer surgery because, despite its greater risks, in the past that individual has spent considerable time in bed and become demoralized and depressed. A person with an injured knee, when told that surgery has about a 30 percent chance of reducing pain but almost no chance of eliminating it entirely, may prefer to leave the condition untreated. And a baseball pitcher with persistent inflammation of the elbow may prefer to take cortisone on a continuing basis even though the doctor suggests that a new position on the team would eliminate the inflammation permanently. In each case the goals and interests of particular patients incline them in different directions not only as to how, but even as to whether, treatment should proceed.

Given these two considerations—the frequent absence of objective medical criteria and the legitimate subjective preferences of patients—ascertaining whether a health care intervention will, if successful, promote a patient's well-being is a matter of individual judgment. Societies that respect personal freedom usually reach such decisions by leaving the judgment to the person involved.

The Boundaries of Health Care

This does not mean, however, that well-being and self-determination are really just two terms for the same value. For example, when an individual (such as a newborn baby) is unable to express a choice, the value that guides health care decisionmaking is the promotion of well-being—not necessarily an easy task but also certainly not merely a disguised form of self-determination.

Moreover, the promotion of well-being is an important value even in decisions about patients who can speak for themselves because the boundaries of the interventions that health professionals present for consideration are set by the concept of well-being. Through societal expectations and the traditions of the professions, health care providers are committed to helping patients and to avoiding harm. Thus, the well-being principle circumscribes the range of alternatives offered to patients: informed consent does not mean that patients can insist upon anything they might want. Rather, it is a choice among medically accepted and available options, all of which are believed to have some possibility of promoting the patient's welfare, including always the option of no further medical interventions, even when that would not be viewed as preferable by the health care providers.

In sum, promotion of patient well-being provides the primary warrant for health care. But, as indicated, well-being is not a concrete concept that has a single definition or that is solely within the competence of health care providers to define. Shared decisionmaking requires that a practitioner seek not only to understand each patient's needs and develop reasonable alternatives to meet those needs but also to present the alternatives in a way that enables patients to choose one they prefer. To participate in this process, patients must engage in a dialogue with the practitioner and make their views on well-being clear. The majority of physicians (56 percent) and the public (64 percent) surveyed by the Commission felt that increasing the patient's role in medical decisionmaking would improve the quality of health care.[3]

Since well-being can be defined only within each individual's experience, it is in most circumstances congruent to self-determination, to which the report now turns.

Respecting Self-Determination

Self-determination (sometimes termed "autonomy") is an individual's exercise of the capacity to form, revise, and pursue personal plans for life.[4] Although it clearly has a much broader application, the relevance of self-determination in health care decisions seems undeniable. A basic reason to honor an individual's choices about health care has already emerged in this report: under most circumstances the outcome that will best promote the person's well-being rests on a subjective judgment about the individual. This can be termed the instrumental value of self-determination.

More is involved in respect for self-determination than just the belief that each person knows what's best for him- or herself, however. Even if it could be shown that an expert (or a computer) could do the job better, the worth of the individual, as acknowledged in Western ethical traditions and especially in Anglo-American law, provides an independent—and more important—ground for recognizing self-determination as a basic principle in human relations, particularly when matters as important as those raised by health care are at stake. This noninstrumental aspect can be termed the intrinsic value of self-determination.

Intrinsic Value of Self-Determination

The value of self-determination readily emerges if one considers what is lost in its absence. If a physician selects a treatment alternative that satisfies a patient's individual values and goals rather than allowing the patient to choose, the absence of self-determination has not interfered with the promotion of the patient's well-being. But unless the patient has requested this course of conduct, the individual will not have been shown proper respect as a person nor provided with adequate protection against arbitrary, albeit often well-meaning, domination by others. Self-determination can thus be seen as both a shield and a sword.

Freedom from Interference Self-determination as a shield is valued for the freedom from outside control it is intended to provide. It manifests the wish to be an instrument of one's own and "not of other men's acts of will."[5] In the context of health care, self-determination overrides practitioner-determination even if providers were able to demonstrate that they could (generally or in a specific instance) accurately assess the treatment an informed patient would choose. To permit action on the basis of a professional's assessment rather than on a patient's choice would deprive the patient of the freedom not to be forced to do something—whether or not that person would agree with the choice. Moreover, denying self-determination in this way risks generating the frustration people feel when their desires are ignored or countermanded.

The potential for dissatisfaction in this regard is great. In the Commission's survey, 72 percent of the public said that they would prefer to make decisions jointly with their physicians after treatment alternatives have been explained. In contrast, 88 percent of the physicians believe that patients want doctors to choose for them the best alternative. Despite these differences in perception, only 7 percent of the public reports dissatisfaction with their doctors' respect for their treatment preferences.[6]

Creative Self-Agency As a sword, self-determination manifests the value that Western culture places on each person having the freedom to be a creator—"a subject, not an object."[7] Within the broad framework of personal characteristics fixed during the years of development, individuals define their own particular values.[8] In these ways, individuals are capable of creating their own character and of taking responsibility for the kind of person they are. Respect for self-determination thus promotes personal integration within a chosen life-style.

This is an especially important goal to be nourished regarding health care. If it is not fostered regarding such personal matters, it may not arise generally regarding public matters. The sense of personal responsibility for decisionmaking is one of the wellsprings of a democracy. Similarly, when people feel little real power over their lives—in the economy, in political affairs, or even in their daily interactions with other people and institutions—it is not surprising that they are passive in encounters with health care professionals.

If people have been able to form their own values and goals, are free from manipulation, and are aware of information relevant to the decision at hand, the final aspect of self-determination is simply the awareness that the choice is their own to make. Although the reasons for a choice cannot always be defined, decisions are still autonomous if they reflect someone's own purposes rather than external causes unrelated to the person's "self." Consequently, the Commission's concept of health care decisionmaking includes informing patients of alternative courses of treatment and of the reasoning behind all recommendations. Self-determination involves more than choice; it also requires knowledge.

The importance of information to self-determination emerged in the Commission's study of treatment refusals in hospitals. There it was found that, regarding routine treatments, information was frequently so lacking that patient self-determination was compromised.

> Often patients were not told what treatment or procedure had been ordered for them, much less asked to decide whether or not to accept it. The purpose of the procedure was frequently obscure and the risks commonly went unmentioned. Presentation of alternatives was extraordinarily rare. The main concern of the patients we interviewed was not to select the best treatment from those available, but to find out what was being selected for them and why.[9]

Implications of Self-Determination

Despite the importance of self-determination, its exercise is sometimes impermissible and at other times impossible. That is, society sometimes must impose restrictions on the range of acceptable patient choices; at other times, patients either cannot, or at least do not, exercise self-determination.

External Limitations Two restrictions are recognized on the range of patient decisions that should be respected. First, some objectives are so contrary to the public interest or the interests of others that society bars the use of medical interventions toward these ends. For example, physicians may not assist patients in criminal activity (such as defacing fingertips so they will not leave identifiable fingerprints). The professional norms or moral integrity of health care professionals (individually, or collectively in health care institutions) may also conflict with the desires of a patient. When this occurs, the practitioner must first reexamine his or her own beliefs and preconceptions. If the proposed intervention would actually compromise the provider's integrity or standards, the patient will either have to accept the limitation on available interventions or seek another health care provider. Finally, a particular treatment preferred by a patient occasionally calls on very scarce resources that society (or some legitimate resource-controlling segment of the health care system) has decided to allocate to another use. Even as a "sword," self-determination does not invest a patient with rights to demand use of resources that have legitimately been allocated to others—as in the case, for example, of a patient who cannot have elective surgery on a desired date because all beds in a hospital are being used by disaster victims.

A second limitation on self-determination arises when a person's decisionmaking is so defective or mistaken that the decision fails to promote the person's own values or goals. This can happen in many ways: Someone could fail to understand relevant information, such as the risks of a particular treatment, or unconsciously distort unpleasant information, such as the frightening diagnosis of cancer, and so forth. For example, a man in the prime of a full and rewarding life who has great plans for the future suddenly suffers a myocardial infarction in the middle of a poker game in which he has already won handsomely. Yet he refuses to permit himself to be transported to a hospital because he wants to play out his hand. The quality of his decisionmaking capacity is certainly in doubt. If his expressed wishes are respected nonetheless, the results in terms of self-determination would be mixed. Self-determination would be promoted in the sense that he has made the decision for himself, as opposed to having someone else make it, but self-determination would be contravened in that the decision is not the one that would best advance the man's apparent wish to live a long, full life.

Self-determination is valuable in both its roles—in letting an individual be his or her own decisionmaker and in securing each person's own goals. In situations where there is a choice of respecting the individual's decision or overriding it—that is, of favoring one aspect of self-determination at the expense of the other—overriding an individual decision is usually justified on the ground of promotion of well-being rather than of respect for self-choice.[10]

The Absence of Contemporaneous Choice Sometimes people anticipate that they will be unable to participate in future decisions about their own health care. A patient, for example, may be under anesthesia during surgery at a time when diagnostic tests force a decision about a further operation. Similarly, patients with an early diagnosis of senile dementia of the Alzheimer's type can expect that their physical functioning might continue long after they are mentally incapable of deciding about care. Through an "advance directive" such people can specify the types of care they want (or do not want) to receive or the person they want to make such decisions if they are unable to do so.[11] Honoring such a directive shows respect for self-determination in that it fulfills two of its three underlying values.

First, following a directive, particularly one that gives specific instructions about types of acceptable and unacceptable interventions, fulfills the instrumental role of self-determination by providing reassurance that a course of conduct promotes the patient's subjective, individual evaluation of well-being. Second, honoring the directive shows respect for the patient as a person. To disregard it would be nearly as great an insult as to disregard the wishes of a patient who expresses them at that time.

An advance directive does not, however, provide self-determination in the sense of active moral agency by the patient on his or her own behalf.[12] Although any discussion between patient and health care professional leading up to a directive would involve active participation and shared decisionmaking, that would have been in the past by the time the decision actually needs to be made about the patient's health care. At that point, there is no "self," in the active, mental sense, to determine what should be done.

Consequently, self-determination is involved when a patient establishes a way to project his or her wishes into a time of anticipated incapacity. Yet it is a sense of self-determination lacking in one important attribute: active, contemporaneous personal choice. Hence a decision not to follow an advance directive may sometimes be justified even when it would not be ethical to disregard a compentent patient's contemporaneous choice.[13]

Active Participation Because patient noninvolvement in treatment decisions occurs frequently in medical care,[14] it is important to understand whether it is compatible with patient self-determination. First and foremost, patients must be aware that they are entitled to make a decision about treatment rather than merely acquiescing in a professional's recommendation. Some patients feel, for example, that making a particular treatment decision will cause them great distress, or that the complexity and uncertainty of certain decisions make them poor decisionmakers and that trusted physicians or family members would be more likely to choose the treatment most in accord with the patients' own goals and values. Alternatively, some patients simply wish others to decide so that they can spend their time and energy on other matters. This, too, could consititute a transfer of the right to decide.

In contrast, some patients defer to physicians because they believe they have no business interfering in the exercise of medical judgment. Such patients do not think they are transferring their "right to decide" to a physician because they do not in the first place believe they have any right to decide about medical treatment. This is not an exercise of self-determination. Rather, self-determination occurs when patients understand decisions are theirs to make—and also to countermand if they are dissatisfied.[15] In other words, self-determination requires that patients either make a choice or actually give the decisionmaking authority to another, not merely fail to act out of fear or ignorance of their rights.[16]

In recognizing that a self-determining person may waive active involvement in each decision, the Commission does not intend to belittle the moral ideal of the free, self-governing person who attempts to make decisions responsibly by applying his or her own values to relevant facts during deliberations about alternative actions. The ideal certainly justifies encouraging patients to play an active part in treatment decisions and argues for structuring medical practices and institutions in ways that facilitate and encourage effective patient participation. Nevertheless, it remains a moral *ideal*—people may strive to meet it but will often fall short of it. The principle of self-determination, the bedrock on which the Commission's concept of shared decision-making in health care rests, is best understood as respecting people's right to define and pursue their own view of what is good, which is compatible with people freely giving to others the authority to make particular health care decisions for them.

NOTES

1. Although these principles have been discussed in judicial decisions and legal commentary on informed consent, the concern of the Commission with patient-provider communication and with decisionmaking in health care in general causes it to consider the issue in a way that is broader and more complex than the legal doctrine.

2. Pursuit of these two values is constrained in various ways, most notably by society's overall interest in equity, justice, and maximum social welfare. These issues are the central concerns of the Commission's report SECURING ACCESS TO HEALTH CARE. Because these goals need not be central to the decisionmaking process of patients and providers, this report does not take up the complications arising from conflicts between legitimate societal goals and individual patient goals. The Commission's forthcoming report on decisions about life-sustaining therapy explores the relationship between societal and individual concerns in the context of a particular set of health care decisions.

3. Many physicians and patients said they believed an increased patient role would give the patient a better understanding of the medical condition and treatment, would improve physician performance in terms of the honesty and scope of discussion, and would generally improve the doctor-patient relationship. However, a number of physicians claimed that greater patient involvement would improve the quality of care because it would improve compliance and would make patients more cooperative and willing to accept the doctor's judgment.

4. Gerald Dworkin, *Autonomy and Informed Consent* (1982).

5. Isaiah Berlin, *Two Concepts of Liberty*, in FOUR ESSAYS ON LIBERTY, Clarendon Press, Oxford (1969) at 118–38.

6. This finding should be viewed cautiously since it is well known that surveys overstate the extent of actual satisfaction, as measured during on-site interviews immediately following doctor-patient encounters.

7. Berlin *supra* note 4.

8. This is not to deny, of course, people's interdependence nor the ways in which each person's values are influenced by others. But people either incorporate or reject such influences into their own conception of what is good. In this view, self-determination lies in the relation between people's values and their actual desires and actions. An individual is self-

determined or autonomous when that person is the kind of person he or she wants to be. Self-determination does not imply free will in the sense of a will free of causal determination.

9. Paul S. Appelbaum and Loren H. Roth, *Treatment Refusal In Medical Hospitals* (1982). Although this lack of information and resulting patient noninvolvement in decisionmaking seems to have been a cause of treatment refusal, they also occurred in many cases in which patients did not refuse treatment. Nonprovision of relevant information was also observed in the other on-site study.

One caveat must be noted, however. The Appelbaum-Roth team observed house-staff/patient interactions extensively but generally did not have a chance to observe interactions between attending physicians and patients. One would expect that discussions of major treatments and procedures, especially major surgical procedures, which were more often left to the attendings, might correspond more closely to the doctrine of informed consent. However, the investigators' conclusions are probably valid for the discussions about diagnostic procedures, medications, and adjunctive therapies as discussed in the other observational study conducted for the Commission. *See* Charles W. Lidz and Alan Meisel, *Informed Consent and the Structure of Medical Care* (1982), Appendix C, in Volume Two of this Report.

10. Likewise, self-determination is not an adequate guiding principle regarding decisions for persons who suffer permanent or chronic mental impairment, such as those who are severely mentally retarded or demented, who are incapable of forming a set of values or of applying them in particular decisions. The decisions for these patients rest instead on an assessment of what would promote their "best interests" (*ie.*, well-being); *see* pp. 178-80 *infra*.

For an interesting example of some of the difficulties that may exist in determining whether an individual's choice reflects his or her long-term goals and values, *see* Albert R. Jonsen, Mark Siegler, and William J. Winslade, CLINICAL ETHICS, Macmillan Publishing Co., New York (1982) at 78–81.

11. In the Commission's survey, 36 percent of the public reported that they have given instructions to someone about how they would like to be treated if they become too sick to make decisions, although only 23 percent of those instructions are in writing.

12. *See generally* Paul Ramsey. THE PATIENT AS PERSON. Yale University Press, New Haven (1970).

13. In some states, advance directives made pursuant to a statute may achieve "binding" legal effect (subject, usually to considerable room for interpretation). *See* pp. 155–66 *infra*. In such a case, whatever the moral justifications, one may not be legally justified in disregarding the directions.

14. One of the observational studies conducted for the Commission concludes that "on balance the normative patient role in [health care decisionmaking] is one of passive acquiescence." Lidz and Meisel, *supra* note 9, at section 6.

15. A possible exception to this requirement would be an irrevocable grant of decisionmaking power to another, as when Odysseus, wishing both to hear and to resist the lure of the Sirens' call, had himself tied to the mast of his ship and instructed his crew not to release him however much he might entreat them to do so.

16. The critical element is the patient's attitude toward "involvement" in the decision, not the mere existence of some "delegation," for all decisions about matters as complex as medical care require a large measure of delegation. Self-determination is not lacking simply because a patient does not insist that the physician review the reasoning and empirical evidence that led up to the physician's recommendation (and its alternatives, if any), including each standardized laboratory test, each anatomical or metabolic finding, and so forth. Rather, patients' decisions are always the end points of a long series of earlier choices made by physicians and others (where many of the steps in action and reasoning are so ingrained that those involved do not even recognize them for the choices they are). What is at issue, then, is merely the *degree* of delegation of decisionmaking authority by the patient to the professional, not the *fact* of delegation. While some patients want to explore every hypothesis, others want to know only the final recommendation; both may be exercising appropriate self-determination.

Paternalism and Partial Autonomy

Onora O'Neill

Autonomous action, understood literally, is self-legislated action. It is the action of agents who can understand and choose what they do. When cognitive or volitional capacities, or both, are lacking or impaired, autonomous action is reduced or impossible. Autonomy is lacking or incomplete for parts of all lives (infancy, early childhood), for further parts of some lives (unconsciousness, senility, some illness and mental disturbance) and throughout some lives (severe retardation). Since illness often damages autonomy, concern to respect it does not seem a promising fundamental principle for medical ethics. Medical concern would be strangely inadequate if it did not extend to those with incomplete autonomy. Concern for patients' well-being is generally thought a more plausible fundamental principle for medical ethics.

But it is also commonly thought implausible to make beneficence the only fundamental aim of medical practice, since it would then be irrelevant to medical treatment whether patients possessed standard autonomy, impaired autonomy or no capacity for autonomous action. All patients, from infants to the most autonomous, would be treated in ways judged likely to benefit them. Medical practice would be through and through paternalistic, and would treat patients as persons only if beneficence so required.

Recurrent debates about paternalism in medical ethics show

From *Journal of Medical Ethics*, 1984, 10, 173–178. Reprinted by permission of the Author and the *Journal of Medical Ethics*.

that the aim of subordinating concern for autonomy to beneficence remains controversial. The group of notions invoked in
these debates—autonomy, paternalism, consent, respect for persons, and treating others as persons—are quite differently articulated in different ethical theories. A consideration of various
ways in which they can be articulated casts some light on issues
that lie behind discussions of medical paternalism.

1. Paternalism and Autonomy in Result-Oriented Ethics

Most consequentialist moral reasoning does not take patients'
autonomy as a fundamental constraint on medical practice.
Utilitarian moral reasoning takes the production of welfare or
well-being (variously construed) as the criterion of right action.
Only when respect for patients' autonomy (fortuitously) maxi-
mises welfare is it morally required. Paternalism is not morally
wrong; but some acts which attempt to maximise welfare by
disregarding autonomy will be wrong if in fact non-paternalistic
action (such as showing respect for others or seeking their
consent to action undertaken) would have maximised welfare.
Only some 'ideal' form of consequentialism, which took the
maintenance of autonomy as an independent value, could regard the subordination of autonomy to beneficence as wrong.
In utilitarian ethical thinking autonomy is of marginal ethical
importance, and paternalism only misplaced when it reflects
miscalculation of benefits.

This unambiguous picture is easily lost sight of because of an
historical accident. A classical and still highly influential utilitarian discussion of autonomy and paternalism is John Stuart
Mill's *On Liberty*.[1] Mill believed both that each person is the
best judge of his or her own happiness and that autonomous
pursuit of goals is itself a major source of happiness, so he
thought happiness could seldom be maximised by action which
thwarted or disregarded others' goals, or took over securing
them. Paternalists, on this view, have benevolent motives but
don't achieve beneficent results. They miscalculate.

Mill's claims are empirically dubious. Probably many people would be happier under beneficent policies even when these reduce the scope for autonomous action. Some find autonomous pursuit of goals more a source of frustration and anxiety than of satisfaction. In particular, many patients want relief from hard decisions and the burden of autonomy. Even when they don't want decisions made for them they may be unable to make them, or to make them well. The central place Mill assigns autonomy is something of an anomaly in result-oriented ethical thought.[2] It is open to challenge and shows Mill's problem in reconciling liberty with utility rather than any success in showing their coincidence.

2. Paternalism and Autonomy in Action-Oriented Ethics

Autonomy can have a more central place only in an entirely different framework of thought. Within a moral theory which centres on action rather than on results, the preconditions of agency will be fundamental. Since autonomy, of some degree, is a presupposition of agency, an action-centred ethic, whether its fundamental moral category is that of human rights, or of principles of obligation or of moral worth, must make the autonomy of agents of basic rather than derivative moral concern. This concern may be expressed as concern not to use others, but to respect them or 'treat them as persons', or to secure their consent and avoid all (including paternalistic) coercion.

A central difficulty for all such theories is once again empirical. It is obvious enough that some human beings lack cognitive and volitional capacities that would warrant thinking of them as autonomous. But where autonomous action is ruled out, what can be the moral ground for insisting on respect or support for human autonomy?[3] The question is sharply pointed for medical ethics since patients *standardly* have reduced cognitive and volitional capacities.

Yet most patients have some capacities for agency. Their

impairments undercut some but not all possibilities for action. Hence agent-centred moral theories may be relevant to medical ethics, but only if based on an accurate view of human autonomy. The central tradition of debate in agent-centred ethics has not been helpful here because it has tended to take an abstract and inaccurate view of human autonomy. The history of these discussions is revealing.

Enlightenment political theory and especially Locke's writings are classical sources of arguments against paternalism and for respect for human autonomy. Here the consent of citizens to their governments is held to legitimate government action. In consenting citizens become, in part, the authors of government action: the notion of the sovereignty of the people can be understood as the claim that they have consented to, and so authorised, the laws by which they are ruled. In obeying such laws they are not mere subjects but retain their autonomy.

This picture invited, and got, a tough focus on the question 'What constitutes consent?' An early and perennial debate was whether consent has to be *express*—explicitly declared in speech or writing—or can be *tacit*—merely a matter of going along with arrangements. In a political context the debate is whether legitimate government must have explicit allegiance, or whether, for example, continued residence can legitimate government action. A parallel debate in medical ethics asks whether legitimate medical intervention requires explicit consent, recorded by the patient's signing of consent forms, or whether placing oneself in the hands of the doctor constitutes consent to whatever the doctor does, provided it accords with the standards of the medical profession.[4]

The underlying picture of human choice and action invoked by those who advocate the 'informed consent' account of human autonomy is appropriate to a contractual model of human relations. Just as parties to commercial contracts consent to specific action by others, and have legal redress when this is not forthcoming, and citizens consent to limited government action (and may seek redress when this is exceeded), so patients consent to specified medical procedures (and have cause for grievance if their doctors do otherwise). Those who argue that informed consent criteria are not appropriate in medical practice sometimes explicitly reject the intrusion of commercial and contractual standards in medical care.

The contractual picture of human relations is clearly particularly questionable in medicine. We may think that citizenship and commerce are areas where we are autonomous decision-makers, enjoying what Mill would have called 'the maturity of our faculties.' In these areas, if anywhere, we come close to being fully rational decision-makers. Various well-known idealisations of human rationality—'rational economic man', 'consenting adults', 'cosmopolitan citizens', 'rational choosers' —may seem tolerable approximations. But the notion that we could be 'ideal rational patients' cannot stand up to a moment's scrutiny. This suggests that we cannot plausibly extend the enlightenment model of legitimating consent to medical contexts. Where autonomy is standardly reduced, paternalism must it seems be permissible; opposition to medical paternalism appears to reflect an abstract and inaccurate view of human consent which is irrelevant in medical contexts.

3. The Opacity of Consent: A Reversal of Perspective

However, the same picture might be seen from quite a different perspective. Human autonomy is limited and precarious in many contexts, and the consent given to others' actions and projects is standardly selective and incomplete. *All* consent is consent to some proposed action or project *under certain descriptions*. When we consent to an action or project we often do not consent even to its logical implications or to its likely results (let alone its actual results), nor to its unavoidable corollaries and presuppositions. Put more technically, consenting (like other propositional attitudes) is *opaque*. When we consent we do not necessarily 'see through' to the implications of what we consent to and consent to these also. When a patient consents to an operation he or she will often be unaware of further implications or results of that which is consented to. Risks may not be understood and post-operative expectations may be vague. But the opacity of patients' consent is not radically different from the opacity of all human consenting. Even in the most 'transparent', highly-regulated, contractual arrangements, consent reaches only a certain distance. This is recognised whenever contracts are voided because of cognitive or volitional disability, or because the expectations of the 'reasonable man' about the further implications of some activity do not hold up. Medical cases may then be not so much anomalies, with which consent theory cannot adequately deal, as revealing cases which highlight typical limits of human autonomy and consent.[5]

Yet most discussions of consent theory point in the other direction. The limitations of actual human autonomy aren't taken as constraints on working out the determinate implications of respect for autonomy in actual contexts, but often as *aberrations* from ideally autonomous choosing. The rhetoric of the liberal tradition shows this clearly. Although it is accepted that we are discussing the autonomy of '*finite* rational beings', finitude of all sorts is constantly forgotten in favour of loftier and more abstract perspectives.

4. Actual Consent and 'Ideal' Consent

There are advantages to starting with these idealised abstractions rather than the messy incompleteness of human autonomy as it is actually exercised. Debates on consent theory often shift from concern with dubious consent actually given by some agent to a proposed activity or arrangement to concern with consent that would hypothetically be given by an ideally autonomous (rational and free) agent faced with that proposal. This shift to hypothetical consent allows us to treat the peculiar impairments of autonomy which affect us when ill as irrelevant: we can still ask what the (admittedly hypothetical) ideally autonomous patient would consent to. This line of thought curiously allows us to combine ostensible concern for human autonomy with paternalistic medical practice. Having reasoned that some procedure would be consented to by ideally autonomous patients, we may then feel its imposition on actual patients of imperfect autonomy is warranted. But by shifting focus from what has (actually) been consented to, to what would (ideally) be consented to, we replace concern for others' autonomy with concern for the autonomy of hypothetical, idealised agents. This is not a convincing account of what it is not to use others, but rather to treat them as persons.[6]

If we don't replace concern for actual autonomy with concern for idealised autonomy, we need to say something definite about when actual consent is genuine and significant and when it is either spurious or misleading, and so unable to legitimise whatever is ostensibly consented to. Instead of facing the sharp outlines of idealised, hypothetical conceptions of human choosing, we may have to look at messy actual choosing. However, we don't need to draw a sharp boundary between genuine, morally significant consent and spurious, impaired consent which does not legitimate. For the whole point of concern for autonomy and hence for genuine consent is that it is not up to the *initiator* of action to choose what to impose: it is up to those affected to choose whether to accept or to reject proposals that are made. To respect others' autonomy requires that we make consent *possible* for them,[7] taking account of whatever partial autonomy they may have. Medical practice respects patients' autonomy when it allows patients as they actually are to refuse or accept what is proposed to them. Of course, some impairments prevent refusal or acceptance. The comatose and various others have to be treated paternalistically. But many patients can understand and refuse or accept what is proposed over a considerable range. Given some capacities for autonomous action, whatever can be made comprehensible to and refusable by patients, can be treated as subject to their consent—or refusal. This may require doctors and others to avoid haste and pressure and to counteract the intimidation of unfamiliar, technically bewildering, and socially alien medical environments. Without such care in imparting information and proposing treatment, the 'consent' patients give to their treatment will lack the autonomous character which would show that they have not been treated paternally but rather as persons.

5. 'Informed Consent' and Legitimating Consent

There is a long-standing temptation, both in medical ethics and beyond, to find ways in which consent procedures can be formalised and the avoidance of paternalism guaranteed and routinised. But if the ways in which human autonomy is limited are highly varied, it is not likely that any set procedures can guarantee that consent has been given. Early European colonialists who 'negotiated treaties' by which barely literate native peoples without knowledge of European moral and legal traditions 'consented' to sales of land or cession of sovereignty reveal only that the colonialists had slight respect for others' autonomy. Medical practice which relies on procedures such as routine signing of 'consent forms' may meet conditions for avoiding litigation, but does not show concern for human autonomy as it actually exists. Such procedures are particularly disreputable given our knowledge of the difficulties even the most autonomous have in assimilating distressing information or making unfamiliar and hard decisions.

Serious respect for autonomy, in its varied, limited forms, demands rather that patients' refusal or consent, at least to fundamental aspects of treatment, be made possible. The onus on practitioners is to see that patients, as they actually are, understand what they can about the basics of their diagnosis and the proposed treatment, and are secure enough to refuse the treatment or to insist on changes. If the proposal is accessible and refusable for an actual patient, then (but only then) can silence or going along with it reasonably be construed as consent. The notions of seeking consent and respecting autonomy are brought into disrepute when the 'consent' obtained does not genuinely reflect the patient's response to proposed treatment.

6. Partial Autonomy, Coercion and Deception

Once we focus on the limited autonomy of actual patients it becomes clear that consent to *all* aspects and descriptions of proposed treatment is neither possible nor required. Only the ideally, unrestrictedly autonomous could offer such consent. In human contexts, whether medical or political, the most that we can ask for is consent to the more *fundamental* proposed policies, practices, and actions. Patients can no more be asked to consent to every aspect of treatment than citizens can be asked to consent to every act of government. Respect for autonomy requires that consent be possible to *fundamental* aspects of actions and proposals, but allows that consent of trivial and ancillary aspects of action and proposals may be absent or impossible.

Treatment undertaken without consent when a patient could have reached his or her own decisions if approached with care and respect may fail in many ways. In the most serious cases the action undertaken uses patients as tools or instruments. Here the problem is not just that some partially autonomous patient couldn't (or didn't) consent, but that the treatment precluded consent even for ideally autonomous patients. Where a medical proposal hinges fundamentally on coercion or deception, not even the most rational and independent can dissent, or consent. Deceivers don't reveal their fundamental proposal or action; coercers may make their proposal plain enough but rob *anyone* of choice between consent or dissent. In deception 'consent' is spurious because cognitive conditions for consent are not met; in coercion 'consent' is spurious because volitional conditions for consent are not met.

However, some non-fundamental aspects of treatment to which consent has been given may have to include elements of deception or coercion. Use of placebos or of reassuring but inaccurate accounts of expected pain might sometimes be non-fundamental but indispensable and so permissible deceptions.[8] Restraint of a patient during a painful procedure might be a non-fundamental but indispensable and so permissible coercion. But using pa-

tients as unwitting experimental subjects or concealing fundamental aspects of their illness or prognosis or treatment from
them, or imposing medical treatment and ignoring or preventing its refusal, would always use patients, and so fail to respect
autonomy. At best such imposed treatment might, if benevolent, constitute impermissible paternalism; at worst, if non-
benevolent, it might constitute assault or torture.

7. Partial Autonomy, Manipulation and Paternalism

Use of patients is an extreme failure to respect autonomy; it
precludes the consent even of the ideally autonomous, let alone
of those with cognitive or volitional impairments. Respect for
partial autonomy would also require medical practice to avoid
treatment which, though refusable by the ideally autonomous,
would not be refusable by a particular patient in his or her
present condition. Various forms of manipulation and of questionable paternalism fail to meet these requirements. Patients
are manipulated if they are 'made offers they cannot refuse',
given their actual cognitive and volitional capacities. For example, patients who think they may be denied further care or
discharged without recourse if they refuse proposed treatment
may be unable to refuse it. To ensure that 'consent' is not
manipulated available alternatives may have to be spelled out
and refusal of treatment shown to be a genuine option. 'Consent' which is achieved by relying on misleading or alarmist
descriptions of prognosis or uninformative accounts of treatment and alternatives does not show genuine respect. Only
patients who are quite unable to understand or decide need
complete paternalist protection. When there is a relationship of
unequal power, knowledge or dependence, as so often between
patients and doctors, avoiding manipulation and unacceptable
paternalism demands a lot.

Avoiding unacceptable paternalism demands similar care. Ma-
nipulators use knowledge of others and their weaknesses to
impose their own goals; paternalists may not recognise either

others' goals, or that they are *others'* goals. Patients, like anyone with limited understanding and capacity to choose, may be
helped by advice and information, and may need help to achieve
their aims. But if it is not the patients' but others' aims which
determine the limits and goals of medical intervention, the intervention (even if neither deceptive nor coercive) will be unac-
ceptably paternalistic. Handicapped patients whose ways of life
are determined by others may not be deceived or coerced—but
they may be unable to refuse what others think appropriate for
them. This means that patients' own goals, medical and nonmedical, and their plans for achieving these, are constraints on any
medical practice which respects patients' autonomy. Since return
to health is often central to patients' plans, this constraint may
require little divergence from the treatment that paternalistic
medical practice would select, except that patients would have
to be party to fundamental features of their treatment. But where
patients' goals differ from doctors' goals—perhaps they value
quality of life or avoiding pain or dependence more than the
doctor would—respect for the patient requires that these goals
not be overridden or replaced by ones the patient does not share,
and that the patient's own part in achieving them not be set aside.

Debates on medical paternalism often assume that the goals
of medical action can be determined independently of patients'
goals. But in action-oriented ethical thinking morally required
goals are not given independently of agents' goals. Paternalism
in this perspective is simply the imposition of others' goals,
(perhaps those of doctors, nursing homes or relatives) on patients. These goals too must be taken into account if we are to
respect the autonomy of doctors, nursing homes, and relatives.
But imposing their goals on patients capable of some autonomy
does not respect patients. The contextually sensitive, action-
oriented framework discussed here does not reinstate a contractual or consumer-sovereignty picture of medical practice, in
which avoiding deceit and coercion is all that respect requires.
On the contrary, it insists that judgements of human autonomy
must be contextual, and that what it takes to respect human
autonomy will vary with context. When patients' partial autonomy constrains medical practice, respect for patients may demand action which avoids not only deceit and coercion but also
manipulation and paternalism; but where autonomy is absent
there is no requirement that it be respected.

8. Respecting Limited Autonomy

Medical paternalism has been considered within three frameworks. Within a result-oriented framework of the standard utilitarian type it is not only permissible but required that concern for human autonomy be subordinated to concern for total welfare. Within an action-oriented framework that relies on an abstract, 'idealising' account of human autonomy, medical practice is too readily construed as ruling out all paternalism and permitting only treatment that would be consented to by 'idealised' autonomous agents. Within an action-oriented framework that takes account of the partial character of human autonomy, we can sketch patterns of reasoning which draw boundaries in given contexts between permissible and impermissible forms of paternalism. This account yields no formula, such as the requirement to avoid coercion, and deception may be thought to yield for abstract approaches. But the inadequacies of that formula for guiding action when impairment is severe speak in favour of a more accurate and contextual view of human autonomy.

By trying to incorporate concern for actual, partial capacities for autonomous action into an account of respect for patients and medical paternalism we find that we are left without a single boundary-line between acceptable and unacceptable medical practice. What we have are patterns of reasoning which yield different answers for different patients and for different proposals for treatment. One patient can indeed be expected to come to an informed and autonomous (if idiosyncratic) decision; another may be too confused to take in what his options are. A third may be able to understand the issues but too dependent or too distraught to make decisions. Attempts to provide uniform guidelines for treating patients as persons, respecting their autonomy and avoiding unacceptable medical paternalism are bound to be insensitive to the radical differences of capacity of different patients. A theory of respect for patients must rely heavily and crucially on actual medical judgements to assess patient's current capacities to absorb and act on information given in various ways. But it does not follow that 'professional judgement' or 'current medical standards' *alone* can provide appropriate criteria for treating patients as persons. For if these do not take the varying ways in which patients can exercise autonomy as constraints on permissible treatment, they may institutionalise unjustifiable paternalism. Professional judgement determines what constitutes respect for patients only when guided by concern to communicate effectively what patients can understand and to respect the decisions that they can make.

9. Issues and Contexts

Sections 1, 2 and 3 above discussed some ways in which treatment of autonomy, paternalism and respect for patients are articulated in result-oriented ethics and in action-oriented approaches which take an abstract view of cognition and volition, and hence of autonomy. The alternative account proposed in sections 4 to 8 is that only consideration of the determinate cognitive and volitional capacities and incapacities of particular patients at particular times provides a framework for working out boundaries of permissible medical paternalism. If such judgements are contextual, there is no way to demarcate unacceptable paternalism in the abstract. The following headings only point to contexts in which these issues arise and have to be resolved. Which resolutions are justifiable will depend not only on following a certain pattern of reasoning but on the capacities for autonomous action particular patients have at the relevant time.

A. Temporarily Impaired Capacity for Autonomy

If respect for autonomy is morally fundamental, restoring (some) capacities is morally fundamental. Survival is necessary for such restoration; but not sufficient. If patients' autonomy constrains practice, survival can never be foregone in favour of autonomy, but it is an open question whether survival with no or greatly reduced capacities for autonomy can be a permissible goal. Risky surgery may sometimes reasonably be imposed for the sake of restoring capacities, even when mere survival would be surer without surgery.

Temporary loss of autonomy offers grounds for paternalistic intervention to restore autonomy—but not for all paternalistic interventions. It might be better for an unconscious sportsman if advantage were taken of his temporary incapacity to perform some non-urgent operation or to make some non-medical intervention in his affairs. But if restoration of autonomy is likely, an action-oriented ethic offers no ground for such paternalism.

B. Long Term or Permanent Impairment of Autonomy

This is the standard situation of children, and so the original context of paternalism. Those with long and debilitating illnesses, physical as well as mental, may suffer very varied impairments of autonomy. Hence consideration of parental paternalism may illuminate these cases. While the law has to fix an age to end minority, parents have to adapt their action to a constantly altering set of capacities for autonomous action. Choices which cannot be made at one stage can at another; autonomy develops in one area of life and lags in another.[9] Unfortunately, medical trajectories may not be towards fuller capacities. Medical and other decisions may then have to be to some extent imposed. But there is no general reason to think that those who are unable to make some decisions are unable to make any decisions, and even when full return of capacities is unlikely, patients, like children, may gain in autonomy when an optimistic view is taken of their capacities.

C. Permanent Loss of Autonomy

Here decisions have (eventually) to be made that go beyond what is needed for restoring (some) autonomy. Sometimes medical staff and relatives may be able to make some use of a notion of hypothetical consent. But what they are likely to be asking is not 'What would the ideally autonomous choose in this situation?', but rather 'What would this patient have chosen in this situation?' If this can be answered, it may be possible to maintain elements of respect for the particular patient as he or she was in former times. But usually this provides only vague indications for medical or other treatment, and respect for absent autonomy can be at best vestigial.

D. Lifelong Incapacity for Autonomy

For those who never had or will have even slight capacities for autonomous action the notion of respect is vacuous. There is no answer to the hypothetical question 'What would he or she have chosen if able to do so?' and the hypothetical question 'What would the ideally autonomous choose in this situation?' may have no determinate answer. Here, unavoidably, paternalism must govern medical practice indefinitely and the main questions that arise concern the appropriate division of authority to make paternalistic decisions between relatives and medical staff and legally appointed guardians.

NOTES

1. Mill J S. On liberty. In: Warnock M, ed. *Utilitarianism and on liberty, etc.* London: Fontana, 1972.
2. This had been a recurrent criticism of Mill from Stephen J F, *Liberty, equality, fraternity*, London: Smith, Elder, 1873, to Dworkin G. Paternalism. *The monist* 1972; 56: 64–84 and reprinted in Sartorius R, ed. *Paternalism*. Minneapolis: University of Minnesota Press, 1983: section IV.
3. Broader worries mushroom here too: what grounds the moral status of non-autonomous humans in action-oriented ethics? For recent discussion see Haksar V. *Liberty, equality, perfectionism*. Oxford: Clarendon Press, 1979; Clark S. *The moral status of animals*. Oxford: Clarendon Press, 1977; Dennett D Conditions of personhood. In: Rorty A, ed. *The identity of persons*. Berkeley and Los Angeles: University of California Press, 1976, and reprinted in Dennett D. *Brainstorms*. Hassocks, Sussex: The Harvester Press, Ltd 1979.
4. Here US and British practice differ. US legislation and debates often stress the need to secure informed consent from patients (or their guardians). Cf. dicussions and bibliography in Veatch R M. *Case studies in medical ethics*. Cambridge Mass: Harvard University Press, 1977. British law holds that 'what information should be disclosed, and how and when, is very much a matter of professional judgement',

and that 'there is no ground in English law for extending the limited doctrine of informed consent outside the field of property rights'. See Sidaway v Board of Governors of the Bethlem Royal Hospital and the Maudsley Hospital and Others, Law Report, *The Times*, 1984 Feb 24. However, medical paternalism may be more practised in the US than it is praised by those who write on medical ethics. See Buchanan A E Medical paternalism. *Philosophy and public affairs* 1978; 7:371–390, and reprinted in Sartorius, see reference 2.

5. For further comments on the limitations of 'normal' abilities see Wikler D. *Paternalism and the mildly retarded*. Reprinted in Sartorius, see reference (2).

6. A point made long since by Isaiah Berlin in Two concepts of liberty. *Four essays on liberty*. Oxford: OUP, 1969.

7. For the interpretation of Kantian ethics offered here see also O'Neill O. Kant after virtue. *Inquiry* 1984; 26: 387–405; Consistency in action. In: Potter N, Timmons M, eds. *New essays in ethical universalizability*. Dordrecht, the Netherlands: Reidel publishing company, forthcoming, and Between consenting adults, unpublished.

8. Bok S. *Lying: moral choice in public and private life*. New York: Harvester Press, Random House, 1978: 234. Bok points out that sometimes the use of placebos may be more than ancillary, (61–68), and also discusses fundamental forms of deception such as hiding from the patient that the illness is terminal. On the latter point see also Kubler-Ross E. *On death and dying*. New York: Macmillan 1969, and the bibliography in Veatch, reference 4.

9. For discussions of some distinctive features of children's partial autonomy see Leites E. Locke's liberal theory of fatherhood; Slote M A. Obedience and illusions and Katz S N, Schroeder W A, Sidman L. Emancipating our children—coming of legal age in America. In: O'Neill O, Ruddick W, eds. *Having children: philosophical and legal reflections on parenthood*. New York: OUP, 1979.

Dilemmas of "Informed Consent" in Children

Anthony Shaw, M.D.

NUMEROUS articles have been written about "rights" of patients. We read about "right to life" of the unborn, "right to die" of the elderly, "Bill of Rights" for the hospitalized, "Declaration of Rights" for the retarded, "right of privacy" for the pregnant, and of course, "right to medical care" for us all.

Whatever the legitimacy of these sometimes conflicting "rights" there is at present general agreement that patients have at least one legal right: that of "informed consent"— i.e., when a decision about medical treatment is made, they are entitled to a full explanation by their physicians of the nature of the proposed treatment, its risks and its limitations. Once the physician has discharged his obligation fully to inform* an adult, mentally competent patient, that patient may then accept or reject the proposed treatment, or indeed, may refuse any and all treatment, as he sees fit. But if the patient is a minor, a parental decision rejecting recommended treatment is subject to review when physicians or society disagree with that decision.

The purpose of this paper is to consider some of the moral and ethical dilemmas that may arise in the area of "informed consent" when the patient is a minor. The following case reports, all but two from my practice of pediatric surgery, raise questions about the rights and obligations of physicians, par-

*I agree with Ingelfinger[1] that "educate" is a better concept here than "inform."

From *New England Journal of Medicine*, Oct. 25, 1973, No. 17, 885–889. Reprinted by permission of *The New England Journal of Medicine*.

ents, and society in situations in which parents decide to withhold consent for treatment of their children.

Instead of presenting a full discussion of these cases at the end of the paper, I have followed each case presentation with a comment discussing the points I wish to make, relating the issues raised by that case to those raised in some of the other cases, and posing the very hard questions that I had to ask myself in dealing with the patients and parents. At present the questions are coming along much faster than the answers.

Case Reports

A. Baby A was referred to me at 22 hours of age with a diagnosis of esophageal atresia and tracheoesophageal fistula. The infant, the firstborn of a professional couple in their early thirties, had obvious signs of mongolism, about which they were fully informed by the referring physician. After explaining the nature of the surgery to the distraught father, I offered him the operative consent. His pen hesitated briefly above the form and then as he signed, he muttered, "I have no choice, do I?" He didn't seem to expect an answer, and I gave him none. The esophageal anomaly was corrected in routine fashion, and the infant was discharged to a state institution for the retarded without ever being seen again by either parent.

Comment

In my opinion, this case was mishandled from the point of view of Baby A's family, in that consent was not truly informed. The answer to Mr. A's question should have been, "You *do* have a choice. You might want to consider not signing the operative consent at all." Although some of my surgical colleagues believe that there is no alternative to attempting to save the life of every infant, no matter what his potential, in my opinion, the doctrine of informed consent should, under some circumstances, include the right to withhold consent. If the parents do have the right to withhold consent for surgery in a case such as Baby A, who should take the responsibility for pointing that fact out to them—the obstetrician, the pediatrician, or the surgeon?

Another question raised by this case lies in the parents' responsibility toward their baby, who has been saved by their own decision to allow surgery. Should they be obligated to provide a home for the infant? If their intention is to place the baby after operation in a state-funded institution, should the initial decision regarding medical or surgical treatment for their infant be theirs alone?

B. Baby B was referred at the age of 36 hours with duodenal obstruction and signs of Down's syndrome. His young parents had a 10-year-old daughter, and he was the son they had been trying to have for 10 years; yet, when they were approached with the operative consent, they hesitated. They wanted to know beyond any doubt whether the baby had Down's syndrome. If so, they wanted time to consider whether or not to permit the surgery to be done. Within 8 hours a geneticist was able to identify cells containing 47 chromosomes in a bone-marrow sample. Over the next 3 days the infant's gastrointestinal tract was decompressed with a nasogastric tube, and he was supported with intravenous fluids while the parents consulted with their ministers, with family physicians in their home community, and with our geneticists. At the end of that time the B's decided not to permit surgery. The infant died 3 days later after withdrawal of supportive therapy.

Comment

Unlike the parents of Baby A, Mr. and Mrs. B realized that they did have a choice—to consent or not to consent to the intestinal surgery. They were afforded access to a wide range of resources to help them make an informed decision. The infant's deterioration was temporarily prevented by adequate intestinal decompression and intravenous fluids.

Again, some of the same questions are raised here as with Baby A. Do the parents have the right to make the decision to allow their baby to die without surgery?

Can the parents make a reasonable decision within hours or days after the birth of a retarded or brain-damaged infant? During that time they are overwhelmed by feelings of shock, fear, guilt, horror, and shame. What is the proper role of the medical staff and the hospital administration? Can parents make an intelligent decision under these circumstances, or are they simply reacting to a combination of their own instincts and fears as well as to the opinions and biases of medical staff? Rickham[2] has described the interaction of physician and parents in such situations as follows:

> Every conscientious doctor will, of course, give as correct a prognosis and as impartial an opinion about the possible future of the child as he can, but he will not be able to be wholly impartial, and whether he wants it or not, his opinion will influence the parents. At the end it is usually the doctor who has to decide the issue. It is not only cruel to ask the parents whether they want their child to live or die, it is dishonest, because in the vast majority of cases, the parents are consciously or unconsciously influenced by the doctor's opinion.

I believe that parents often *can* make an informed decision if, like the B's, they are afforded access to a range of resources beyond the expertise and bias of a single doctor and afforded sufficient time for contemplation of the alternatives. Once the parents have made a decision, should members of the medical staff support them in their decision regardless of their own feelings? (This support may be important to assuage recurrent feelings of guilt for months or even years after the parents' decision.)

When nutritional and fluid support was withdrawn, intestinal intubation and pain medication were provided to prevent suffering. To what extent should palliative treatment be given in a case in which definitive treatment is withheld? The lingering death of a newborn infant whose parents have denied consent for surgery can have a disastrous effect on hospital personnel, as illustrated last year by the well-publicized Johns Hopkins Hospital case, which raised a national storm of controversy. In this case, involving an infant with mongoloidism and duodenal atresia, several of the infant's physicians violently disagreed with the parents' decision not to allow surgery. The baby's lingering death (15 days) severely demoralized the nursing and house staffs. In addition, it prolonged the agony for the parents, who called daily to find out if the baby was still alive. Colleagues of mine who have continued to keep such infants on gastrointestinal decompression and intravenous fluids for weeks after the parents have decided against surgery have told me of several cases in which the parents have finally changed their minds and given the surgeon a green light! Does such a change of heart represent a more deliberative decision on the part of the parents or merely their capitulation on the basis of emotional fatigue?

After the sensationalized case in Baltimore, Johns Hopkins Hospital established a committee to work with physicians and parents who are confronted by similar problems. Do such medical-ethics committees serve as a useful resource for physicians and families, or do they, in fact, further complicate the decision-making process by multiplying the number of opinions?

Finally, should a decision to withhold surgery on an infant with Down's syndrome or other genetically determined mental-retardation states be allowed on clinical grounds only, without clear-cut chromosomal evidence?

> C. I was called to the Newborn Nursery to see Baby C, whose father was a busy surgeon with 3 teen-age children. The diagnoses of imperforate anus and microcephalus were obvious. Doctor C called me after being informed of the situation by the pediatrician. "I'm not going to sign that op permit," he said. When I didn't reply, he said. "What would you do, doctor, if he were your baby?" "I wouldn't let him be operated on either," I replied. Palliative support only was provided, and the infant died 48 hours later.

Comment

Doctor C asked me bluntly what I would do were it my baby, and I gave him my answer. Was my response appropriate? In this case I simply reinforced his own decision. Suppose he had asked me for my opinion before expressing his own inclination?

Should my answer in any case have simply been, "It's not my baby"—with a refusal to discuss the subject further? Should I have insisted that he take more time to think about it and discuss it further with his family and clergy, like the parents of Baby B? Is there a moral difference between withholding surgery on a baby with microcephalus and withholding surgery on a baby with Down's syndrome?

Some who think all children with mongolism should be salvaged since many of them are trainable, would not dispute a decision to allow a baby with less potential such as microcephalic Baby C to die. Should, then, decisions about life and death be made on the basis of IQ? In a recent article,[3] Professor Joseph Fletcher outlined criteria for what he calls "humanhood"—minimal standards by which we could judge whether a living organism is or is not a human being. These criteria (further defined in Dr. Fletcher's article) include minimal intelligence, self-awareness, self-control, a sense of time, a sense of futurity, a sense of the past, the capability to relate to others, concern for others, communication, control of existence, curiosity, change and changeability, balance of rationality and feeling, idiosyncrasy, and neocortical function. Dr. Fletcher also offers a shorter list of what a human being is not. By trying to arrive at a definition of what we call "human," Doctor Fletcher has, of course, stirred up a hornet's nest. But in so doing, he is not laying down a set of rigid standards but is issuing a challenge that should be a particularly attractive one to the medical profession. Is it possible that physicians and philosophers can agree on a "profile of man" that might afford more rational grounds for approaching problems in biomedical ethics?

> D. In 1972 I wrote in a piece published by the *New York Times*, "Parents of mongoloids have the legal (and, I believe, the moral) responsibility of determining if their child with a potentially deadly but surgically correctable defect should live or die."[4] After reading this article, Mr. D called me for advice concerning his 2-week-old grandson. This infant had been born in a New York hospital with Down's syndrome and with bilateral hydroureteronephrosis secondary to urethral valves, for the correction of which the family had refused surgery. Since the infant was becoming

increasingly uremic, the family was being strongly pressured by the medical staff to consent to surgery. After an absolute refusal to sign, the family was ordered to take the infant home immediately despite the wish for the baby to die in the hospital. At my last conversation with the infant's grandfather, the family and the hospital had reached an impasse about discharge and the infant was dying slowly of uremia.

Comment

In threatening to discharge the dying infant, the medical staff was trying to coerce the family into signing consent for surgery. Aside from the issue of coercion here, is providing facilities for dying patients a proper role for a hospital? The parents refused to take the infant home because of the devastating emotional impact that the dying baby would have on the entire family. The hospital wanted to discharge the infant partly because of the devastating emotional impact that the dying infant was having on the hospital staff. Can we prepare hospital, medical, and paramedical personnel to accept the death of infants under these circumstances without the destruction of morale? Can we realistically expect hospital staff to be able to make such an emotional accommodation no matter how they view the situation from an intellectual standpoint? Finally, if the decision is not to operate, where does one draw the line between palliation of the infant's suffering and active shortening of the infant's life? This, of course, is one of the areas where the question of euthanasia has been raised. To my knowledge, the question of whether Baby D died at home or in the hospital finally became a legal matter to be resolved between the hospital's legal counsel and the family's attorney.

If the medical staff felt strongly that allowing Baby D to die for lack of simple surgery was immoral, why did they not obtain a court order permitting them to operate?

E. A court order *was* obtained for Baby E who was "reported" in *Life* magazine 2 years ago. This infant, with Down's syndrome, intestinal obstruction and congenital heart disease, was born in her mother's car on the way to the hospital. The mother thought that the retarded infant would be impossible for her to care for and would have a destructive effect on her already shaky marriage. She therefore refused to sign permission for intestinal surgery, but a local child-welfare agency, invoking the state child-abuse statute, was able to obtain a court order directing surgery to be performed. After a complicated course and thousands of dollars worth of care, the infant was returned to the mother. The baby's continued growth and development remained markedly retarded because of her severe cardiac disease. A year and a half after the baby's birth, the mother felt more than ever that she had been done a severe injustice.

Comment

Is the crux of this case parental rights versus the child's right to life? Can the issue in this case be viewed as an extension of the basic dilemma in the abortion question? Does this case represent proper application of child-abuse legislation —i.e., does the parents' refusal to consent to surgery constitute neglect as defined in child-abuse statutes? If so, under these statutes does a physician's concurrence in a parental decision to withhold treatment constitute failure to report neglect, thereby subjecting him to possible prosecution?

Baby E's mother voluntarily took the baby home, but had she not done so, could the state have forced her to take the baby? Could the state have required her husband to contribute to the cost of medical care and to the subsequent maintenance of the infant in a foster home or institution?

If society decides that the attempt must be made to salvage every human life, then, as I have written, ". . . society *must* provide the necessary funds and facilities to meet the continuing medical and psychological needs of these unfortunate children."[4]

F. Baby F was conceived as the result of an extramarital relation. Mrs. F had sought an abortion, which she had been denied. F was born prematurely, weighing 1600 g and in all respects normal except for the presence of esophageal atresia and tracheoesophageal fistula. Mrs. F signed the operative consent, and the

surgery was performed uneventfully. Mrs. F fears that
her husband will eventually realize that the baby is not
his and that her marriage may collapse as a result of
this discovery.

Comment

Like those of Mrs. E, Mrs. F's reasons for not wanting her
baby were primarily psychosocial. However, Mrs. F never raised
the question of withholding consent for surgery even though the
survival of her infant might mean destruction of her marriage.
Does the presence of mental retardation or severe physical
malformation justify withholding of consent for psychosocial
reasons (Babies B, C, D, and E), whereas the absence of such
conditions does not (Baby F)? If she had decided to withhold
consent there is no doubt in my mind that I would have obtained
a court order to operate on this baby, who appeared to be
normal beyond her esophageal anomaly. Although I personally
would not have objected to an abortion in this situation for the
sociopsychologic reasons, I would not allow an otherwise normal baby with a correctable anomaly to perish for lack of
treatment for the same reasons. Although those who believe
that all life is sacred, no matter what its level of development,
will severely criticize me for the apparent inconsistency of this
position, I believe it to be a realistic and humane approach to a
situation in which no solution is ideal.

Although my case histories thus far have dealt with the forms
of mental retardation most common in my practice, similar
dilemmas are encountered by other physicians in different
specialties, the most obvious being in the spectrum of hydrocephalus and meningomyelocele. Neurosurgeons are still grap-
pling unsuccessfully and inconsistently with indications for surgery
in this group, trying to fit together what is practical, what is
moral, and what is humane. If neurosurgeons disagree violently
over criteria for operability on infants with meningomyelocele,
how can the parents of such a child decide whether to sign for
consent? Who would say that they *must* sign if they don't want
a child whose days will be measured by operations, clinic visits,
and infections? I have intentionally omitted from discussion in
this paper the infant with crippling deformities and multiple
anomalies who does not have rapidly lethal lesions. Infants with

such lesions may survive for long periods and may require palliative procedures such as release of limb contractures, ventriculoperitoneal shunts, or colostomies to make their lives more tolerable or to simplify their management. The extent to which these measures are desirable or justifiable moves us into an even more controversial area.

I must also point out that the infants discussed in the preceding case reports represent but a small percentage of the total number of infants with mental-retardation syndromes on whom I have operated. Once the usual decision to operate has been made I, of course, apply the same efforts as I would to any other child.

> G. Six-year-old boy G was referred to me because of increasing shortness of breath due to a large mediastinal mass. The parents had refused diagnostic procedures and recommended treatment until the child had become cachectic and severely dyspneic. His liver was enlarged. A thorough in-hospital work-up, including liver biopsy, bone-marrow aspiration, thoracentesis, and mediastinal tomography failed to establish a diagnosis. The child was obviously dying of progressive compromise of his respiratory tract and vena-cava obstruction. His family belonged to a fundamentalist religious sect and firmly believed that the child would be healed by God. They refused to sign permission for exploratory thoracotomy. We spent 2 weeks trying to convince them that, although the boy's chances were slim in any case, his only hope lay in the possibility of our encountering a resectable tumor. When the parents refused to sign permission for surgery, a court order was obtained from the Juvenile Court judge permitting surgery. The next day exploratory thoracotomy was carried out, and a non-resectable neuroblastoma was found. The child died a respiratory death 3 days later. Members of the family subsequently threatened the lives of the physicians and of the judge. A letter of inquiry was subsequently sent to me by their lawyer, implying an intention to sue. However, it was not followed up.

Comment

Some of the same questions are raised here as in the Jehovah's Witness cases. Does the parents' right to practice their religion include the right to deny their child medical or surgical treatment? The fact that I allowed a two-week delay before obtaining the court order indicates my strong feeling that a court order should be the last resort used to obtain parents' co-operation on behalf of their child. We persisted as long as we thought we might obtain such co-operation.

Should a court order be obtained by physicians only when they think their treatment will certainly save the child, or should they obtain an order so long as there is any possibility of helping the child? Were we justified in obtaining the court order and putting the parents and ourselves through such an ordeal when the odds against us of finding a curable lesion were so long? I believe the answer is yes. In making a decision to obtain a court order directing surgery, the physician must balance the risk for the child if surgery is withheld against the risk of surgery itself coupled with the demoralizing consequences for the family if the surgery fails. In G's case, in which his life expectancy without treatment appeared to be measurable in days, I believe that the decision to obtain a court order was appropriate.

Statutes on child abuse and neglect have on occasion been invoked to give a hospital or a physician temporary custody of a child whose parents' religion prevents lifesaving medical care. At the same time some states have worded their child-abuse statutes to avoid appearance of interfering with constitutional guarantees of freedom of religion. For example, in Virginia's child-abuse law,[5] the following statement appears ". . . that a child who is being furnished Christian Science treatment by a duly accredited Christian Science practitioner shall not be considered for that reason alone a physically neglected child for the purposes of this section." However, the law may be invoked when, as a result of the practice of his parents' religion, a child's health can be demonstrated to be in jeopardy. For this reason, such religious exclusion clauses as the one just cited would not, in my opinion, be held applicable in G's case.

Several new questions arise when a child is an adolescent who himself refuses surgery on the basis of his sincere religious conviction. Then, one has to ask whether minors should be allowed to make life-and-death decisions about their own treatment. Should it depend on the degree of maturity of the child, or can one try to write into law an age at which a child's wishes should be seriously taken into consideration in medical decision making? In a sensitively written article Schowalter et al.[6] recently discussed the "agonizing dilemma" created for a hospital staff by a 16-year-old girl with uremia who, with her parents' consent, chose death over continued therapeutic efforts. The authors concluded that ". . . there are instances when a physician should honor an adolescent patient's wish to die." The case in point, although not terminal, had a poor prognosis. Suppose the patient had been a 16-year-old Jehovah's Witness with a ruptured spleen, who appeared to be mature and in full possession of his faculties and who, although he understood he would die without blood, refused to accept it?

> H. Ten-year-old H was brought to the surgical clinic by her mother for removal of some cysts from the scalp. The family is well known to our hospital since most of its members have Gardner's syndrome and most of the senior family members either have enterostomies or have died of cancer of the gastrointestinal tract. H's mother has had rectal bleeding for the past year but has not permitted herself to be examined by a physician. She also would not permit H to have a barium-enema examination or sigmoidoscopy when this question was first raised. However, when excision of the scalp cysts was made contingent upon the mother's permitting evaluation of the child's colon, she consented. The barium-enema study and a proctosigmoidoscopy were negative. The cysts were excised. Since more cysts tend to form, we expect to be able to arrive at a regular quid pro quo that will enable us to continue evaluating the child's colon until such time as the premalignant polyps are detected. We do not know what we will do if polyps begin to proliferate, making colectomy advisable before H achieves legal maturity. In all likelihood, the mother will not willingly permit us to perform major surgery on her child.

Comment

Here we found a substitute for judicial intervention. We called it "making a deal." If the mother had not consented to this bargain, would we have been justified in obtaining a court order for a diagnostic procedure? Would it not then be necessary to put the mother under long-term court supervision so that she would be forced to bring the child for regular diagnostic examinations and for resection when deemed necessary? It seems to me that such judicial intervention is proper when one is dealing with a potentially lethal condition in a young child and would be, I believe, fully sanctioned by the child-neglect laws of most states. Note that there is no question of religious freedom involved here. Should court orders also be sought in situations in which parents refuse treatment for children with diseases or deformities that, if untreated, will result in permanent physical or emotional damage but not death?

Discussion

If an underlying philosophy can be gleaned from the vignettes presented above, I hope it is one that tries to find a solution, humane and loving, based on the circumstances of each case rather than by means of a dogmatic formula approach. (Fletcher has best expressed this philosophy in his book, *Situation Ethics*,[7] and in subsequent articles.[3,8]) This outlook contrasts sharply with the rigid "right-to-life" philosophy, which categorically opposes abortion, for example. My ethic holds that all rights are not absolute all the time. As Fletcher points out, ". . . all rights are imperfect and may be set aside if human *need* requires it." My ethic further considers quality of life as a value that must be balanced against a belief in the sanctity of life.

Those who believe that the sanctity of life is the overriding consideration in all cases have a relatively easy time making decisions. They say that all babies must be saved; no life may be aborted from the womb, and all attempts to salvage newborn life, whatever its quality and whatever its human and financial costs to family and society, must be made. Although many philosophies express the view that "heroic" efforts need not be made to save or prolong life, yesterday's heroic efforts are todays' routine procedures. Thus, each year it becomes possible to remove yet another type of malformation from the "unsalvageable" category. All pediatric surgeons, including myself, have "triumphs"—infants who, if they had been born 25 or even five years ago, would not have been salvageable. Now with our team approaches, staged surgical technics, monitoring capabilities, ventilatory support systems and intravenous hyperalimentation and elemental diets, we can wind up with "viable" children three and four years old well below the third percentile in height and weight, propped up on a pillow, marginally tolerating an oral diet of sugar and amino acids and looking forward to another operation.

Or how about the infant whose gastrointestinal tract has been removed after volvulus and infarction? Although none of us regard the insertion of a central venous catheter as a "heroic" procedure, is it right to insert a "lifeline" to feed this baby in the light of our present technology, which can support him, tethered to an infusion pump, for a maximum of a year and some months?

Who should make these decisions? The doctors? The parents? Clergymen? A committee? As I have pointed out, I think that the parents must participate in any decision about treatment and that they must be fully informed of the consequences of consenting and of withholding consent. This is a type of informed consent that goes far beyond the traditional presentation of possible complications of surgery, length of hospitalization, cost of the operation, time lost from work, and so on.

It may be impossible for any general agreement or guidelines for making decisions on cases such as the ones presented here to emerge, but I believe we should bring these problems out into public forum because whatever the answers may be, they should not be the result of decisions made solely by the attending physicians. Or should they?

NOTES

1. Ingelfinger FJ: Informed (but uneducated) consent. *N Engl J Med* 287:465–466, 1972

2. Rickham PP: The ethics of surgery on newborn infants. *Clin Pediatr* 8:251–253, 1969
3. Fletcher J: Indicators of humanhood: a tentative profile of man, *The Hastings Center Report* Vol 2, No 5. Hastings-on-Hudson, New York, Institute of Society, Ethics and Life Sciences, November, 1972, pp 1–4
4. Shaw A: Doctor, do we have a choice? *New York Times Magazine*, January 30, 1972, pp 44–54
5. Virginia Code, Sect 16.1–217.1 through 16.1–217.4
6. Schowalter JE, Ferholt JB, Mann NM: The adolsecent patient's decision to die. *Pediatrics* 51:97–103, 1973
7. Fletcher JF: *Situation Ethics: The new morality*. Philadelphia, Westminster Press, 1966
8. *Idem:* Ethical aspects of genetic controls: designed genetic changes in man. *N Engl J Med* 285:776–783, 1971

Medical Confidentiality:
An Intransigent and
Absolute Obligation

Michael H. Kottow

THE contemporary expansion of ethics in general and medical ethics in particular harbours the danger of increasing scholasticism to the point where not even pressing practical problems are being offered workable solutions. People involved in health care may end up by distrusting the discipline of ethics, thus increasing the improbability of agreement between pragmatists and analysts.[1] Even traditionally straightforward practices, such as confidentiality, have been subject to extensive review and analysis which have proved incapable of offering committed stances or unequivocal guidelines for action.[2,3] In an effort to illustrate that more stringency is desirable and possible, the status of confidentiality as an exceptionless or absolute commitment is here defended. It should be stated at the outset that I share general scepticism about absolute ethical propositions,[4] and that confidentiality is here not defended as an inviolable moral value—a position that would be self-defeating—but as an interpersonal communications strategy that ceases to function unless strictly adhered to. Confidentiality is a brittle arrangement that disintegrates if misdirected in pursuance of other goals and, since it is a necessary component of medical practice, care should be taken to safeguard its integrity.

From *Journal of Medical Ethics*, 1986, 12:117–22. Reprinted by permission of the author and *The Journal of Medical Ethics*.

Defining Confidentiality

The following definition of confidentiality is used: A situation is confidential when information revealing that harmful acts have been or possibly will be performed is consciously or voluntarily passed from one rationally competent person (confider) to another (confidant) in the understanding that this information shall not be further disclosed without the confider's explicit consent. The harm alluded to may be physical, but moral damage alone may also be the subject matter of a confidential exchange. When this sort of communication occurs in a medical setting it constitutes medical confidentiality.

What Is at Issue in Confidentiality Conflicts?

The main ethical controversy around confidentiality concerns the assessment of whether more harm is done by occasionally breaching confidentiality or by always respecting it regardless of the consequences. As long as the physician gathers private information, that is information that only concerns the confider and harbours no element of past or potential harm, confidentiality will concern exclusively the patient and any disclosure would be nothing but a malicious or at the very least gratuitous act of the physician, of little or no moral significance. It seems redundant to discuss other instances of confidentiality than those involving either the possibility of impending harm or testimonial of past injury, for these are the fundamental cases where dilemmas arise and a breach of confidence must seek justification.

Breaching is defended on the ground that the harm announced in the confidence is severe and can possibly only be averted by the confidant's disclosure.[5,6,7] Exceptionless confidentiality, on the other hand, is upheld by the idea that breaching will relentlessly harm the confider, subjecting her or him to precautionary investigations and constraints of some sort, perhaps even with unavoidable defamatory consequences. The harm purportedly averted is merely potential and all the less likely to occur, the more exorbitant and preposterous the threatener's claims are. After all, excessively vicious menaces may well be uttered by psychotics who are rationally incompetent and therefore not protected by a pledge to confidentiality they can neither honour nor demand. Furthermore, the practice of confidentiality is in itself damaged by breaching because its trustworthiness is disqualified. Ultimately, degrees and probability of harm are so difficult to assess,[8] that they will hardly deliver an intersubjectively acceptable argument for or against confidentiality, except for one; breaching confidentiality cannot be a significant and enduring contribution against harmful actions, for these are no more than potential, whereas the damages caused to the confidant, to the practice of confidentiality and to the honesty of clinical relationships are unavoidable.

Perhaps less elusive is the conflict of rights—and their correlative obligations—which ensue in confidential situations. Confidentiality is an agreement bound by the principle of fairness;[9] it gives the confider the right to expect discretion whereas the confidant has the right to hear the truth, but also the obligation to ensure guardianship of the information received. It could be argued against this right that past victims might be vindicated or potential ones helped by divulging confidential information that seems critical, and that these victims also have a right, namely to vindication or protection. In order for the victim's right to prevail, the confider must involuntarily forfeit her or his right to secrecy, which the confidant will forcefully violate by divulging information against the confider's will. This forfeiture of the confider's right can only occur subsequently to the confidence, for it is triggered by the contents of the confider's disclosure. To avoid the risk of losing the right to secrecy, confiders would have to confide falsely or not at all, a strategy that would erode their legitimate and initially granted right to be impunibly outspoken, distort or reduce confidentiality to lies and irrelevancies, and destroy both the confidant's right to hear the truth and the institution of confidentiality.

Medical Confidentiality

Physicians would appear to be under the *prima facie* obliga-tion to respect the right to secrecy, but also to abide by the right of potential victims to be protected. In cases involving moral conflict they must necessarily override one of these rights. Infringing certain rights for the sake of other rights may be justifiable, but it leaves a sediment of negative feelings of regret, shame or guilt.[10,11] It is an unhealthy and paralysing notion to know that the relationship one enters into with pa-tients may unexpectedly turn into a situation of conflict, in-fringement of rights, and guilt. This guilt may be compounded by the awareness that breaching relates to a family of dubious practices that misuse information obtained by resorting to de-ception or even duress. Of course, confidentiality is enacted in the unfettered environment of medical encounters, but its breach-ing infringes the rights of the confiders, harms them, and abrades confidentiality as an institution, all this in the name of elusive values and hard-to-specify protective and vindicative functions.

In the case where a physician believes the patient's exorbitant threats and alerts the police, a morally questionable principle becomes involved. The patient has sought the clinical encounter and proffered information on the understanding that this is necessary for an efficient therapy and also that the relationship with the physician is protected by a mantle of confidentiality. Confidence is offered and accepted in medical acts, and known to be an indispensable component of the clinical encounter, thus enticing the patient to deliver unbiased, unfiltered, uncensored, and sincerely presented information.[12]

Consequently, it appears contradictory and perverse first to offer confidentiality as an enticement to sincerity, only subse-quently to breach it because the information elicited is so terri-ble it cannot remain unpublicised. Confidence is understood as an unconditional offer, otherwise it would not be accepted, and it appears profoundly unfair to disown the initial conditions once the act of confiding has occurred.

Should one decide to introduce exception clauses, it would only be fair to promulgate them beforehand, allowing every potential confider to know what to expect. But officially sanctioned exceptions would have the undesirable side-effect of creating a second-class kind of medicine for those cases where the patient considers it too risky to assume confidentiality. The communication between patient and physician would in these cases be hampered and would thus render the patient's medical care less than optimal.

Gathering Confidential Material

The covenant of confidentiality only obtains if information is voluntarily and consciously given. No question of confidence arises unless the relationship involves rational, conscious, and free individuals. But subtleties arise in the medical context when incriminating information reaches the physician unintentionally. Does this information fall within the confidence pact in virtue of being part of the clinical encounter? Or does it obey independent rules because it occurred marginally to the intended doctor/patient relationship?

During the clinical encounter a perspicacious physician may find tell-tale signs of matters the patient did not intend to disclose (skin blemishes perhaps caused by alcohol excess, suspiciously pin-point pupils, injection marks). This involuntary information transfer might not seem at first to fall under any confidentiality agreement according to the above presented definition. Nevertheless, it is the product of a conscious interaction between patient and physician. In consulting a doctor, a person implicitly accepts the risk of surrendering more information than intended but at the same time understands herself or himself to be under the protection of confidentiality. Information fortuitously gained within the freely chosen association of the clinical encounter is to be considered confidential and treated in the same way as information voluntarily disclosed by the patient. Everything that happens in the interpersonal relationship of a clinical encounter is confidential.

Are There Exceptions to Confidentiality?

Exceptions to unrelenting confidentiality[6] have been invoked for the sake of the confider (paternalistic breaching in general and medical consultations as a special case thereof), in the name of potentially endangered innocent others, in the name of institutional or public interests, and less explicitly, in cases where the confidant is potentially in danger.

Confidentiality Throughout Time

Confidants may consider the potential harm of divulging information they have had in custody eventually to diffuse after the confider's death, so that a posthumous revelation will not be injurious. The contrary position that harm after death is possible is too weak to support obligations to the dead.[13] A more convincing approach suggests that posthumous disclosures may be harmful to surviving persons. If the death of a famous politician should prompt a physician to uncover his knowledge about the deceased's homosexual inclination, still living patients of the same physician might register with distaste and fear the possibility that private information about them could eventually be disclosed after they died. This suspicion may well be unsettling and therefore harmful to them, especially if they happen to believe in some form of 'after-life', the quality of which would be polluted by indiscretions occurring after their biological death. Also to be considered are the negative effects a disparaging disclosure might have upon surviving family members as well as groups of individuals with whom the deceased had a commonality of interests. Death does not cancel the obligation of confidentiality which remains of import to all survivors within the radius of interests of the deceased.

Paternalistic Breaching

A commonly suggested exemption to confidentiality is that some patients' interests might be better served by physicians' indiscretion.[14] Harming confiders for their own purported good is like forcing therapeutic decisions on patients for the sake of their health care. Such stern paternalism has nothing to recommend it, for it is generally agreed that autonomous individuals are not to be compelled into undergoing medical procedures they have explicitly rejected. If rationally competent patients refuse a medical procedure that would do them good, the physician is not authorised to insist, let alone proceed. Rationally competent individuals are allowed to take decisions against their own interests and this does not make them irrational, as some have misleadingly suggested.[15] Why, then, should confidentiality function differently? If patients wish certain knowledge to be kept confidential even if this course of action injures their own interests, they are entitled to do so and no one, not even the physician, has the right to breach confidentiality in the name of patients' welfare.

Medical Consultations

Multi-professional care seems to offer plausible alibis to breach confidentiality for the sake of the confider.[16] It has been argued that patients negotiate confidentiality with their primary care physician and that if additional professionals are involved in the patient's care they are to report to the confidant physician. This position is discarded by those who believe that patients, in as much as their autonomy is respected, are to re-negotiate—or count upon—confidentiality with every physician involved. Such a line of thought has much to recommend it since every physician/patient encounter may unveil unedited information which the patient is willing to discuss in a certain setting but is reluctant to have brought to the attention of the primary-care physician. Consultations and other expansions of a medical care programme do not serve as an excuse to exchange information about patients against their will. If they did, they would be supporting double morality and possibly double-quality medicine, where primary health-care would have a paternalistic format embedded in trust and confidence whilst secondary and tertiary services would operate in a contractual setting. This would not be acceptable, it being preferable that each act of confidence be equally and non-transmittably entrenched in all medical encounters.

Harm to Innocent Others

Another major exception invoked against absolute confidentiality concerns the aversion of damage to uninvolved and innocent third parties. These are the oft-quoted cases of the doctor telling the bride that her fiancé is homosexual, or calling the wife because he is treating the husband for venereal disease. Escalating examples include informing authorities about a confider's intention to kill someone, as well as encounters with terrorists at large.

This postulated exemption to confidentiality is self-defeating. Firstly, if physicians become known as confidence-violators, problem-ridden patients will try to lie, accommodate facts to their advantage or, if this does not work, avoid physicians altogether.[17] Physicians would then be unable to give optimal advice or treatment to the detriment of both the reluctant patients and their threatened environment. It is better to treat and advise the syphilitic husband without informing the wife than not have him come at all for fear of undesired revelations.

Physicians who believe themselves in possession of information that must be disclosed in order to safeguard public interests are contemplating preventive action against the putative malefactor. Like all preventive policies, breaching confidentiality is difficult to analyse in terms of cost/benefits: is the danger real, potential or fictitious? what preventive measure will appear justified? how much harm may these measures cause before they lose justification? Since physicians will rarely be instrumental in deciding or carrying out preventive actions, they have no way of knowing in advance whether taking the risk of honouring confidentiality will eventually prove more or less harmful than breaching it.

If physicians play it safe and commit frequent breaches of confidentiality they will unleash overreacting preventive programmes, at the same time progressively losing credibility as reliable informers. On the other hand, should they remain critical and carefully decide each case on its own merits, they will be equally suspect and unreliable informers, for their conscientiousness and judgement might well deviate from what other authorities, notably the police, consider adequate.

In apparently more delicate cases it could be argued that physicians might subject their co-operation with the authorities to some conditions in order to defuse the dramatic moment. They may suggest that violence be refrained from, that their own intervention be kept secret, that the preventive action be discreet. But certainly, if physicians accept that their confidential relationship with patients is conditional, they must consequently expect authorities to handle their own role as informants in a similarly unpredictable and contingent way. Physicians who breach confidentiality cannot expect to be protected by it just because they have exchanged the confidant for the confider role. Physicians who are known to take confidentiality as a *prima facie* value cannot demand that the authorities they are serving by disclosing information should honour their request for discretion. For similar reasons they must expect some patients to become increasingly inconsiderate or even vicious. By breaking confidentiality, physicians are helping sustain a language of dishonesty and they cannot expect violence-prone patients to refrain from blackmailing, threatening, or otherwise molesting them. As a physician, I would be most unsettled if it became a matter of policy that my colleagues violated confidentiality for the public good, for it would leave me defenceless when confronted with a public offender. No amount of promising would help, since physicians would already have a reputation as unpredictable violators of agreements.

Who should control the policy of confidentiality in medicine anyhow? If public interest demands a catalogue of situations where the physician would be under obligation to inform, medicine becomes subaltern to political design and starts down a treacherous path. Should one prefer to leave the management of confidentiality to the physician's conscience and moral judgment, public interest would not be relying on a consistent and trustworthy source of information. Fear of either political misuse or personal arbitrariness should make us wary of opening the doors of confidentiality for the sake of public interest.

What about possible conflicts between the frailties of public figures and the purported interests of society? National leaders from time to time suffer from disabilities due to old age and the question is raised whether the attending medical team are under an obligation to publish full-fledged clinical reports. It must again be brought to mind that the medical team have been commissioned not to safeguard the public interest but to care for the health of this individual who happens to be influential. Consequently, the medical team's duties remain in the clinical realm, not in the political arena. Furthermore, if the leader in question were in such a precarious situation as to constitute a public danger, his political mismanagement would become obvious to other individuals more qualified to take public decisions and would not require the physicians to play the role of enlightening figures. Observers of the political scene have preferred to suggest constitutional amendments and political measures to cope with this problem, being aware that cajoling physicians out of their commitment to confidentiality is no solution.[18]

Competing Claims
to Confidential Material

This issue refers to conflicts arising from individual interests colliding with those of groups or institutions. It differs from those previously discussed in that here physicians do not necessarily engage in active disclosure but restrict themselves to a one-sided co-operation. The emphasis here is not so much on harm being prevented—although this also plays a major role—but on conflicting parties claiming the physician's loyalty.

Company doctors doing routine examinations of employees are under obligation to report even disparaging findings, for their duty is to the commissioning company. By failing to report an epileptic bus driver or a hypertensive pilot, the doctor is deceiving the company and hindering its efforts to secure safe transportation. If, on the contrary, the same bus driver or pilot goes to the private office of a doctor unconnected with his employer, there would be no excuse for unauthorisedly reporting any findings to the company, for the physician is now being commissioned by the individual, not by the institution, to perform a medical act under the mantle of confidentiality. If this results in the bus driver continuing to work under precarious conditions, it means that the company has not established an efficient medical service to check its drivers and is negligent. Physicians are to declare themselves explicitly and unmistakably loyal to those who engage their services for, again, the legitimate claim to confidentiality lies in the act of entering an agreement, not in the contents of the confided material.

Not even these competing claims of loyalty can be settled unless a robust and relentless position in favour of exceptionless confidentiality is upheld. If a physician owes loyalty to an institution, he has no right to misuse the confidence of his employer in order to honour any personal desire for confidentiality. Conversely, when physicians are committed to the confidential situations that arise in their consulting rooms, they lack the right to infringe this agreement to the benefit of other interests.

Does Risk to the Confidant Justify Breaching?

The situation could arise where the patient's revelations contain threats of harm or disclosure of damage already done directly to the confidant physician, his or her family members, or their interests. Can the physician disclaim the obligation to confidentiality in the name of self-defence? If physicians were morally allowed to breach confidentiality in defence of their own interests it would mean accepting the principle that one can inflict harm upon others for self-interested reasons. It has already been stated that in disclosing confidential information there is no adequate way of comparing amounts of harm inflicted with harm prevented, so it might well occur that a person brought about severe harm to others in an effort to avert a fairly trivial or improbable harm to her or his own interests, comparable to killing a burglar who is running away with some property—perhaps no more than a loaf of bread. Since an unbiased view can hardly be expected from someone who believes his interests to be in jeopardy, legal systems do not tolerate self-administered justice and condemn, albeit with leniency, injuring others in the face of putative menace to self-interests. Physicians may not safeguard their own interests by mishandling patients, so why should they be allowed to cause harm by breaching confidentiality only because they believe or fear their interests to be imperilled?

Although imaginary situations can be concocted that make it awkward to insist on not breaching, the basic attitude should still be to respect confidentiality to the utmost. Admittedly, if the patient's disclosure implies impending harm to the confidant, the moral obligation to the confidential relationship is weakened in its core, but this admission requires a double qualification: firstly, such situations are highly improbable and therefore of little paradigmatic interest; secondly, even if they should obtain, breaching confidentiality should be used as a last, certainly not first, resort to resolve the conflict, precisely because there is no suasive justification for employing confidentiality as a weapon to avert harm.

Concluding Remarks

Confidentiality is a widely recognised implicit warranty of fairness in clinical situations and thus constitutes a technically and morally essential element of efficient medical care. If breaches of confidentiality occur, they do so necessarily after the communication and therefore retroactively introduce unfairness into the clinical encounter. A situation that is potentially, even if only occasionally, unfair can no longer be described as fair, especially if breaching occurs unpredictably. All possible exceptions to an attitude of unrelenting confidentiality lead to morally untenable situations where harm avoided versus harm inflicted is incommensurable, and rights preserved are less convincing than rights eroded. Confidentiality collapses unless strictly adhered to, for even occasional, exceptional, or otherwise limited leaks are sufficient to discredit confidentiality into inefficiency.

The clinical encounter is consistently described as a confidential relationship. If this statement is adhered to, there can be no room for violation without making the initial statement untrue. Nor can the description be qualified—'usually confidential'—or made into a conditional—'confidential unless'—statement, for these half-hearted commitments are, from the confider's point of view, as worthless as no guarantee of confidentiality at all. Confidentiality cannot but be, factually and morally, an all or none proposition. It might perhaps be easier to present a plausible defence of conditional confidentiality, but the ethical atmosphere of the clinical encounter, the autonomy of patients, and the sovereignty of the medical profession are all better served by making confidentiality an unexceptionable element of medicine.

NOTES

1. MacIntyre A. Moral philosophy: what next? In: Hauerwas S, MacIntyre A, eds. *Revisions: changing perspectives in moral philosophy*. Notre Dame/London: University of Notre Dame Press, 1983: 1–15.
2. Thompson I E. The nature of confidentiality. *Journal of medical ethics* 1979; 5: 57–64.
3. Pheby D F H. Changing practice on confidentiality: a cause for concern. *Journal of medical ethics* 1982; 8: 12–18.
4. Anscombe G E M. Modern moral philosophy. In: Anscombe G E M. *Ethics, religion and politics*. Oxford: Blackwell, 1981: 26–42.
5. Walters L. Confidentiality. In: Beauchamp T L, Walters L, eds. *Contemporary issues in bioethics*. Encino/Belmont: Dickenson, 1978: 169–175.
6. *Handbook of medical ethics*. London: British Medical Association 1981.
7. Anonymous. Medical confidentiality [editorial]. *Journal of medical ethics* 1984; 10: 3–4.
8. Carli T. Confidentiality and privileged communication: a

psychiatrist's perspective. In: Basson M D, ed. *Ethics, humanism, and medicine*. New York: Liss, 1980: 245–251.

9. Rawls J. *A theory of justice*. Cambridge, Mass: Belknap Press, 1971: 342–350.

10. Melden A I. *Rights and persons*. Oxford: Balckwell, 1977: 47–48.

11. Morris H. The status of rights. *Ethics* 1981; 92: 40–56.

12. Veatch R M. *A theory of medical ethics*. New York: Basic Books, 1981; 184–189.

13. Levenbook B B. Harming someone after his death. *Ethics* 1984; 94: 407–419.

14. Veatch R M. *Case studies in medical ethics*. Cambridge/London: Harvard University Press, 1977: 131–135.

15. Culver C M, Gert B. *Philosophy in medicine*. New York: Oxford, 1983: 26–28.

16. Siegler M. Medical consultations in the context of the physician-patient relationship. In: Agich G J, ed. *Responsibility in health care*. Dordrecht: Reidel, 1982: 141–162.

17. Havard J. Medical confidence. *Journal of medical ethics* 1985; 11: 8–11.

18. Robins R S, Rothschild H. Hidden health disabilities and the presidency: medical management and political consideration. *Perspectives in biology and medicine* 1981; 24: 240–253.

RESEARCH ETHICS: MEDICAL EXPERIMENTATION AND GENETIC RESEARCH

Philosophical Reflections on Experimenting with Human Subjects

Hans Jonas

EXPERIMENTING with human subjects is going on in many fields of scientific and technological progress. It is designed to replace the over-all instruction by natural, occasional experience with the selective information from artificial, systematic experiment which physical science has found so effective in dealing with inanimate nature. Of the new experimentation with man, medical is surely the most legitimate; psychological, the most dubious; biological (still to come), the most dangerous. I have chosen here to deal with the first only, where the case *for* it is strongest and the task of adjudicating conflicting claims hardest. When I was first asked[1] to comment "philosophically" on it, I had all the hesitation natural to a layman in the face of matters on which experts of the highest competence have had their say and still carry on their dialogue. As I familiarized myself with the material,[2] any initial feeling of moral rectitude that might have facilitated my task quickly dissipated before the awesome complexity of the problem, and a state of great humility took its place. The awareness of the problem in all its shadings and ramifications speaks out with such authority, perception, and sophistication in the published discussions of the researchers themselves that it would be foolish of me to hope that I, an onlooker on the sidelines, could tell those battling in the arena anything they have not pondered themselves. Still, since the matter is obscure by its nature and

From *Experimentation with Human Subjects* by Paul A Freund, ed. Reprinted with permission of George Braziller, Publishers, c. 1969. All rights reserved.

involves very fundamental, transtechnical issues, anyone's attempt at clarification can be of use, even without novelty. And even if the philosophical reflection should in the end achieve no more than the realization that in the dialectics of this area we must sin and fall into guilt, this insight may not be without its own gains.

I. The Peculiarity of Human Experimentation

Experimentation was originally sanctioned by natural science. There it is performed on inanimate objects, and this raises no moral problems. But as soon as animate, feeling beings become the subjects of experiment, as they do in the life sciences and especially in medical research, this innocence of the search for knowledge is lost and questions of conscience arise. The depth to which moral and religious sensibilities can become aroused over these questions is shown by the vivisection issue. Human experimentation must sharpen the issue as it involves ultimate questions of personal dignity and sacrosanctity. One profound difference between the human experiment and the physical (beside that between animate and inanimate, feeling and unfeeling nature) is this: The physical experiment employs small-scale, artificially devised substitutes for that about which knowledge is to be obtained, and the experimenter extrapolates from these models and simulated conditions to nature at large. Something deputizes for the "real thing"—balls rolling down an inclined plane for sun and planets, electric discharges from a condenser for real lightning, and so on. For the most part, no such substitution is possible in the biological sphere. We must operate on the original itself, the real thing in the fullest sense, and perhaps affect it irreversibly. No simulacrum can take its place. Especially in the human sphere, experimentation loses entirely the advantage of the clear division between vicarious model and true object. Up to a point, animals may fulfill the proxy role of the classical physical experiment. But in the end man himself must furnish knowledge about himself, and the comfortable separation of noncommittal experiment and definitive action vanishes. An experiment in education affects the lives of its subjects, perhaps a whole generation of schoolchildren. Human experimentation for whatever purpose is always *also* a responsible, nonexperimental, definitive dealing with the subject himself. And not even the noblest purpose abrogates the obligations this involves.

This is the root of the problem with which we are faced: Can both that purpose and this obligation be satisfied? If not, what would be a just compromise? Which side should give way to the other? The question is inherently philosophical as it concerns not merely pragmatic difficulties and their arbitration, but a genuine conflict of values involving principles of a high order. May I put the conflict in these terms. On principle, it is felt, human beings *ought not* to be dealt with in that way (the "guinea pig" protest); on the other hand, such dealings are increasingly urged on us by considerations, in turn appealing to principle, that claim to override those objections. Such a claim must be carefully assessed, especially when it is swept along by a mighty tide. Putting the matter thus, we have already made one important assumption rooted in our "Western" cultural tradition: The prohibitive rule is, to that way of thinking, the primary and axiomatic one; the permissive counter-rule, as qualifying the first, is secondary and stands in need of justification. We must justify the infringement of a primary inviolability, which needs no justification itself; and the justification of its infringement must be by values and needs of a dignity commensurate with those to be sacrificed.

Before going any further, we should give some more articulate voice to the resistance we feel against a merely utilitarian view of the matter. It has to do with a peculiarity of human experimentation quite independent of the question of possible injury to the subject. What is wrong with making a person an experimental subject is not so much that we make him thereby a means (which happens in social contexts of all kinds), as that we make him a thing—a passive thing merely to be acted on, and passive not even for real action, but for token action whose token object he is. His being is reduced to that of a mere token or "sample." This is different from even the most exploitative situations of social life: there the business is real, not fictitious. The subject, however much abused, remains an agent and thus a "subject" in the other sense of the word. The soldier's case is instructive: Subject to most unilateral discipline, forced to risk mutilation and death, conscripted without, perhaps against, his will—he is still conscripted with his capacities to act, to hold his own or fail in situations, to meet real challenges for real stakes. Though a mere "number" to the High Command, he is not a token and not a thing. (Imagine what he would say if it turned out that the war was a game staged to sample observations on his endurance, courage, or cowardice.)

These compensations of personhood are denied to the subject of experimentation, who is acted upon for an extraneous end without being engaged in a real relation where he would be the counterpoint to the other or to circumstance. Mere "consent" (mostly amounting to no more than permission) does not right this reification. Only genuine authenticity of volunteering can possibly redeem the condition of "thinghood" to which the subject submits. Of this we shall speak later. Let us now look at the nature of the conflict, and especially at the nature of the claims countering in this matter those on behalf of personal sacrosanctity.

II. "Individual Versus Society" as the Conceptual Framework

The setting for the conflict most consistently invoked in the literature is the polarity of individual versus society—the possible tension between the individual good and the common good, between private and public welfare. Thus, W. Wolfensberger speaks of "the tension between the long-range interests of society, science, and progress, on one hand, and the rights of the individual on the other."[3] Walsh McDermott says: "In essence, this is a problem of the rights of the individual versus the rights of society."[4] Somewhere I found the "social contract" invoked in support of claims that science may make on individuals in the matter of experimentation. I have grave doubts about the adequacy of this frame of reference, but I will go along with it part of the way. It does apply to some extent, and it has the advantage of being familiar. We concede, as a matter of course, to the common good some pragmatically determined measure of precedence over the individual good. In terms of rights, we let some of the basic rights of the individual be overruled by the acknowledged rights of society—as a matter of right and moral justness and not of mere force or dire necessity (much as such necessity may be adduced in defense of that right). But in making that concession, we require a careful clarification of what the needs, interests, and rights of society are, for society—as distinct from any plurality of individuals—is an abstract and, as such, is subject to our definition, while the individual is the primary concrete, prior to all definition, and his basic good is more or less known. Thus the unknown in our problem is the so-called common or public good and its potentially superior claims, to which the individual good must or might sometimes be sacrificed, in circumstances that in turn must also be counted among the unknowns of our question. Note that in putting the matter in this way—that is, in asking about the right of society to individual sacrifice—the consent of the sacrificial subject is no necessary part of the *basic* question.

"Consent," however, is the other most consistently emphasized and examined concept in discussions of this issue. This attention betrays a feeling that the "social" angle is not fully satisfactory. If society has a right, its exercise is not contingent on volunteering. On the other hand, if volunteering is fully genuine, no public right to the volunteered act need be construed. There is a difference between the moral or emotional appeal of a cause that elicits volunteering and a right that demands compliance—for example, with particular reference to the social sphere, between the *moral claim* of a common good and society's *right* to that good and to the means of its realization. A moral claim cannot be met without consent; a right can do without it. Where consent is present anyway, the distinction may become immaterial. But the awareness of the many ambiguities besetting the "consent" actually available and used in medical research[5] prompts recourse to the idea of a public right conceived independently of (and valid prior to) consent; and, vice versa, the awareness of the problematic nature of such a right makes even its advocates still insist on the idea of consent with all its ambiguities: an uneasy situation either way.

Nor does it help much to replace the language of "rights" by that of "interests" and then argue the sheer cumulative weight of the interest of the many over against those of the few or the single individual. "Interests" range all the way from the most marginal and optional to the most vital and imperative, and only those sanctioned by particular importance and merit will be admitted to count in such a calculus—which simply brings us back to the question of right or moral claim. Moreover, the appeal to numbers is dangerous. Is the number of those afflicted with a particular disease great enough to warrant violating the interests of the nonafflicted? Since the number of the latter is usually so much greater, the argument can actually turn around to the contention that the cumulative weight of interest is on *their* side. Finally, it may well be the case that the individual's interest in his own inviolability is itself a public interest, such that its publicly condoned violation, irrespective of numbers, violates the interest of all. In that case, its protection in *each* instance would be a paramount interest, and the comparison of numbers will not avail.

These are some of the difficulties hidden in the conceptual framework indicated by the terms "society-individual," "interest," and "rights." But we also spoke of a moral call, and this points to another dimension—not indeed divorced from the social sphere, but transcending it. And there is something even beyond that: true sacrifice from highest devotion, for which there are no laws or rules except that it must be absolutely free. "No one has the right to choose martyrs for science" was a statement repeatedly quoted in the November 1967 *Dædalus* conference. But no scientist can be prevented from making himself a martyr for his science. At all times, dedicated explorers, thinkers, and artists have immolated themselves on the altar of their vocation, and creative genius most often pays the price of happiness, health, and life for its own consummation. But no one, not even society, has the shred of a right to expect and ask these things in the normal course of events. They come to the rest of us as a *gratia gratis data*.

III. The Sacrificial Theme

Yet we must face the somber truth that the *ultima ratio* of communal life is and has always been the compulsory, vicarious sacrifice of individual lives. The primordial sacrificial situation is that of outright human sacrifices in early communities. These were not acts of blood-lust or gleeful savagery; they were the solemn execution of a supreme, sacral necessity. One of the fellowship of men had to die so that all could live, the earth be fertile, the cycle of nature renewed. The victim often was not a captured enemy, but a select member of the group: "The king must die." If there was cruelty here, it was not that of men, but that of the gods, or rather of the stern order of things, which was believed to exact that price for the bounty of life. To assure it for the community, and to assure it ever again, the awesome *quid pro quo* had to be paid over again.

Far should it be from us to belittle, from the height of our enlightened knowledge, the majesty of the underlying conception. The particular *causal* views that prompted our ancestors have long since been relegated to the realm of superstition. But in moments of national danger we still send the flower of our young manhood to offer their lives for the continued life of the community, and if it is a just war, we see them go forth as consecrated and strangely ennobled by a sacrificial role. Nor do we make their going forth depend on their own will and consent, much as we may desire and foster these. We conscript them according to law. We conscript the best and feel morally disturbed if the draft, either by design or in effect, works so that mainly the disadvantaged, socially less useful, more expendable, make up those whose lives are to buy ours. No rational persuasion of the pragmatic necessity here at work can do away with the feeling, a mixture of gratitude and guilt, that the sphere of the sacred is touched with the vicarious offering of life for life. Quite apart from these dramatic occasions, there is, it appears, a persistent and constitutive aspect of human immolation to the very being and prospering of human society—an immolation in terms of life and happiness, imposed or voluntary, of few for many. What Goethe has said of the rise of Christianity may well apply to the nature of civilization in general: *"Opfer fallen hier, / Weder Lamm noch Stier, / Aber Menschenopfer unerhoert."*[6] We can never rest comfortably in the belief that the soil from which our satisfactions sprout is not watered with the blood of martyrs. But a troubled conscience compels us, the undeserving beneficiaries, to ask: Who is to be martyred? in the service of what cause and by whose choice?

Not for a moment do I wish to suggest that medical experimentation on human subjects, sick or healthy, is to be likened to primeval human sacrifices. Yet something sacrificial is involved in the selective abrogation of personal inviolability and the ritualized exposure to gratuitous risk of health and life, justified by a presumed greater, social good. My examples from the sphere of stark sacrifice were intended to sharpen the issues implied in that context and to set them off clearly from the kinds of obligations and constraints imposed on the citizen in the normal course of things or generally demanded of the individual in exchange for the advantages of civil society.

IV. The "Social Contract" Theme

The first thing to say in such a setting-off is that the sacrificial area is not covered by what is called the "social contract." This fiction of political theory, premised on the primacy of the individual, was designed to supply a rationale for the *limitation* of individual freedom and power required for the existence of the body politic, whose existence in turn is for the benefit of the individuals. The principle of these limitations is that their *general* observance profits all, and that therefore the individual observer, assuring this general observance for his part, profits by it himself. I observe property rights because their general observance assures my own; I observe traffic rules because their general observance assures my own safety; and so on. The obligations here are mutual and general; no one is singled out for special sacrifice. Moreover, for the most part, *qua* limitations of my liberty, the laws thus deducible from the hypothetical "social contract" enjoin me from certain actions rather than obligate me to positive actions (as did the laws of feudal society). Even where the latter is the case, as in the duty to pay taxes, the rationale is that I am myself a beneficiary of the services financed through these payments. Even the contributions levied by the welfare state, though not originally contemplated in the liberal version of the social contract theory, can be interpreted as a personal insurance policy of one sort or another—be it against the contingency of my own indigence, be it against the dangers of disaffection from the laws in consequence of widespread unrelieved destitution, be it even against the disadvantages of a diminished consumer market. Thus, by some stretch, such contributions can still be subsumed under the principle of enlightened self-interest. But no complete abrogation of self-interest at any time is in the terms of the social contract, and so pure sacrifice falls outside it. Under the putative terms of the contract alone, I cannot be required to die for the public good. (Thomas Hobbes made this forcibly clear.) Even short of this extreme, we like to think that nobody is entirely and one-sidedly the victim in any of the renunciations exacted under normal circumstances by society "in the general interest"—that is, for the benefit of others. "Under normal circumstances," as we shall see, is a necessary qualification. Moreover, the "contract" can legitimitize claims only on our overt, public actions and not on our invisible private being. Our powers, not our persons, are beholden to the common weal. In one important respect, it is true, public interest and control do extend to the private sphere by general consent: in the compulsory education of our children. Even there, the assumption is that the learning and what is learned, apart from all future social usefulness, are also for the benefit of the individual in his own being. We would not tolerate education to degenerate into the conditioning of useful robots for the social machine.

Both restrictions of public claim in behalf of the "common good"—that concerning one-sided sacrifice and that concerning the private sphere—are valid only, let us remember, on the premise of the primacy of the individual, upon which the whole idea of the "social contract" rests. This primacy is itself a metaphysical axiom or option peculiar to our Western tradition, and the whittling away of its force would threaten the tradition's whole foundation. In passing, I may remark that systems adopting the alternative primacy of the community as their axiom are naturally less bound by the restrictions we postulate. Whereas we reject the idea of "expendables" and regard those not useful or even recalcitrant to the social purpose as a burden that society must carry (since their individual claim to existence is as absolute as that of the most useful), a truly totalitarian regime, Communist or other, may deem it right for the collective to rid itself of such encumbrances or to make them forcibly serve some social end by conscripting their persons (and there are effective combinations of both). We do not normally—that is, in nonemergency conditions—give the state the right to conscript labor, while we do give it the right to "conscript" money, for money is detachable from the person as labor is not. Even less than forced labor do we countenance forced risk, injury, and indignity.

But in time of war our society itself supersedes the nice balance of the social contract with an almost absolute precedence of public necessities over individual rights. In this and similar emergencies, the sacrosanctity of the individual is abrogated, and what for all practical purposes amounts to a near-totalitarian, quasi-communist state of affairs is *temporarily* permitted to prevail. In such situations, the community is conceded the right to make calls on its members, or certain of its members, entirely different in magnitude and kind from the calls normally allowed. It is deemed right that a part of the population bears a disproportionate burden of risk of a disproportionate gravity; and it is deemed right that the rest of the community accepts this sacrifice, whether voluntary or enforced, and reaps its benefits—difficult as we find it to justify this acceptance and this benefit by any normal ethical categories. We justify it transethically, as it were, by the supreme collective emergency, formalized, for example, by the declaration of a state of war.

Medical experimentation on human subjects falls somewhere between this overpowering case and the normal transactions of the social contract. On the one hand, no comparable extreme issue of social survival is (by and large) at stake. And no comparable extreme sacrifice or foreseeable risk is (by and large) asked. On the other hand, what is asked goes decidedly beyond, even runs counter to, what it is otherwise deemed fair to let the individual sign over of his person to the benefit of the "common good." Indeed, our sensitivity to the kind of intrusion and use involved is such that only an end of transcendent value or overriding urgency can make it arguable and possibly acceptable in our eyes.

V. Health as a Public Good

The cause invoked is health and, in its more critical aspect, life itself—clearly superlative goods that the physician serves directly by curing and the researcher indirectly by the knowledge gained through his experiments. There is no question about the good served nor about the evil fought—disease and premature death. But a good to whom and an evil to whom? Here the issue tends to become somewhat clouded. In the attempt to give experimentation the proper dignity (on the problematic view that a value becomes greater by being "social" instead of merely individual), the health in question or the disease in question is somehow predicated on the social whole, as if it were society that, in the persons of its members, enjoyed the one and suffered the other. For the purposes of our problem, public interest can then be pitted against private interest, the common good against the individual good. Indeed, I have found health called a national resource, which of course it is, but surely not in the first place.

In trying to resolve some of the complexities and ambiguities lurking in these conceptualizations, I have pondered a particular statement, made in the form of a question, which I found in the *Proceedings* of the earlier *Dædalus* conference: "Can society afford to discard the tissues and organs of the hopelessly unconscious patient when they could be used to restore the otherwise hopelessly ill, but still salvageable individual?" And somewhat later: "A strong case can be made that society can ill afford to discard the tissues and organs of the hopelessly unconscious patient; they are greatly needed for study and experimental trial to help those who can be salvaged."[7] I hasten to add that any suspicion of callousness that the "commodity" language of these statements may suggest is immediately dispelled by the name of the speaker, Dr. Henry K. Beecher, for whose humanity and moral sensibility there can be nothing but admiration. But the use, in all innocence, of this language gives food for thought. Let me, for a moment, take the question literally. "Discarding" implies proprietary rights—nobody can discard what does not belong to him in the first place. Does society then own my body? "Salvaging" implies the same and, moreover, a use-value to the owner. Is the life-extension of certain individuals then a public interest? "Affording" implies a critically vital level of such an interest—that is, of the loss or gain involved. And "society" itself—what is it? When does a need, an aim, an obligation become social? Let us reflect on some of these terms.

VI. What Society Can Afford

"Can society afford . . . ?" Afford what? To let people die intact, thereby withholding something from other people who desperately need it, who in consequence will have to die too? These other, unfortunate people indeed cannot afford not to have a kidney, heart, or other organ of the dying patient, on which they depend for an extension of their lease on life; but does that give them a right to it? And does it oblige society to procure it for them? What is it that *society* can or cannot afford—leaving aside for the moment the question of what it has a *right* to? It surely can afford to lose members through death; more than that, it is built on the balance of death and birth decreed by the order of life. This is too general, of course, for our question, but perhaps it is well to remember. The specific question seems to be whether society can afford to let some people die whose death might be deferred by particular means if these were authorized by society. Again, if it is merely a question of what society can or cannot afford, rather than of what it ought or ought not to do, the answer must be: Of course, it can. If cancer, heart disease, and other organic, noncontagious ills, especially those tending to strike the old more than the young, continue to exact their toll at the normal rate of incidence (including the toll of private anguish and misery), society can go on flourishing in every way.

Here, by contrast, are some examples of what, in sober truth, society cannot afford. It cannot afford to let an epidemic rage unchecked; a persistent excess of deaths over births, but neither—we must add—too great an excess of births over deaths; too low an average life expectancy even if demographically balanced by fertility, but neither too great a longevity with the necessitated correlative dearth of youth in the social body; a debilitating state of general health; and things of this kind. These are plain cases where the whole condition of society is critically affected, and the public interest can make its imperative claims. The Black Death of the Middle Ages was a *public* calamity of the acute kind; the life-sapping ravages of endemic malaria or sleeping sickness in certain areas are a public calamity of the chronic kind. Such situations a society as a whole can truly not "afford," and they may call for extraordinary remedies, including, perhaps, the invasion of private sacrosanctities.

This is not entirely a matter of numbers and numerical ratios. Society, in a subtler sense, cannot "afford" a single miscarriage of justice, a single inequity in the dispensation of its laws, the violation of the rights of even the tiniest minority, because these undermine the moral basis on which society's existence rests. Nor can it, for a similar reason, afford the absence or atrophy in its midst of compassion and of the effort to alleviate suffering—be it widespread or rare—one form of which is the effort to conquer disease of any kind, whether "socially" significant (by reason of number) or not. And in short, society cannot afford the absence among its members of *virtue* with its readiness for sacrifice beyond defined duty. Since its presence—that is to say, that of personal idealism—is a matter of grace and not of decree, we have the paradox that society depends for its existence on intangibles of nothing less than a religious order, for which it can hope, but which it cannot enforce. All the more must it protect this most precious capital from abuse.

For what objectives connected with the medico-biological sphere should this reserve be drawn upon—for example, in the form of accepting, soliciting, perhaps even imposing the submission of human subjects to experimentation? We postulate that this must be not just a worthy cause, as any promotion of the health of anybody doubtlessly is, but a cause qualifying for transcendent social sanction. Here one thinks first of those cases critically affecting the whole condition, present and future, of the community we have illustrated. Something equivalent to what in the political sphere is called "clear and present danger" may be invoked and a state of emergency proclaimed, thereby suspending certain otherwise inviolable prohibitions and taboos. We may observe that averting a disaster always carries greater weight than promoting a good. Extraordinary danger excuses extraordinary means. This covers human experimentation, which we would like to count, as far as possible, among the extraordinary rather than the ordinary means of serving the common good under public auspices. Naturally, since foresight and responsibility for the future are of the essence of institutional society, averting disaster extends into long-term prevention, although the lesser urgency will warrant less sweeping licenses.

VII. Society and the Cause of Progress

Much weaker is the case where it is a matter not of saving but of improving society. Much of medical research falls into this category. As stated before, a permanent death rate from heart failure or cancer does not threaten society. So long as certain statistical ratios are maintained, the incidence of disease and of disease-induced mortality is not (in the strict sense) a "social" misfortune. I hasten to add that it is not therefore less of a human misfortune, and the call for relief issuing with silent eloquence from each victim and all potential victims is of no lesser dignity. But it is misleading to equate the fundamentally human response to it with what is owed to society: it is owed by man to man—and it is thereby owed by society to the individuals as soon as the adequate ministering to these concerns outgrows (as it progressively does) the scope of private spontaneity and is made a public mandate. It is thus that society assumes responsibility for medical care, research, old age, and innumerable other things not originally of the public realm (in the original "social contract"), and they become duties toward "society" (rather than directly toward one's fellow man) by the fact that they are socially operated.

Indeed, we expect from organized society no longer mere protection against harm and the securing of the conditions of our preservation, but active and constant improvement in all the domains of life: the waging of the battle against nature, the enhancement of the human estate—in short, the promotion of progress. This is an expansive goal, one far surpassing the disaster norm of our previous reflections. It lacks the urgency of the latter, but has the nobility of the free, forward thrust. It surely is worth sacrifices. It is not at all a question of what society can afford, but of what it is committed to, beyond all necessity, by our mandate. Its trusteeship has become an established, ongoing, institutionalized business of the body politic. As eager beneficiaries of its gains, we now owe to "society," as its chief agent, our individual contributions toward its *continued pursuit*. I emphasize "continued pursuit." Maintaining the existing level requires no more than the orthodox means of taxation and enforcement of professional standards that raise no problems. The more optional goal of pushing forward is also more exacting. We have this syndrome: Progress is by our choosing an acknowledged interest of society, in which we have a stake in various degrees; science is a necessary instrument of progress; research is a necessary instrument of science; and in medical science experimentation on human subjects is a necessary instrument of research. Therefore, human experimentation has come to be a societal interest.

The destination of research is essentially melioristic. It does not serve the preservation of the existing good from which I profit myself and to which I am obligated. Unless the present state is intolerable, the melioristic goal is in a sense gratuitous, and this not only from the vantage point of the present. Our descendants have a right to be left an unplundered planet; they do not have a right to new miracle cures. We have sinned against them, if by our doing we have destroyed their inheritance—which we are doing at full blast; we have not sinned against them, if by the time they come around arthritis has not yet been conquered (unless by sheer neglect). And generally, in the matter of progress, as humanity had no claim on a Newton, a Michelangelo, or a St. Francis to appear, and no right to the blessings of their unscheduled deeds, so progress, with all our methodical labor for it, cannot be budgeted in advance and its fruits received as a due. Its coming-about at all and its turning out for good (of which we can never be sure) must rather be regarded as something akin to grace.

VIII. The Melioristic Goal, Medical Research, and Individual Duty

Nowhere is the melioristic goal more inherent than in medicine. To the physician, it is not gratuitous. He is committed to curing and thus to improving the power to cure. Gratuitous we called it (outside disaster conditions) as a *social* goal, but noble at the same time. Both the nobility and the gratuitousness must influence the manner in which self-sacrifice for it is elicited, and even its free offer accepted. Freedom is certainly the first condition to be observed here. The surrender of one's body to medical experimentation is entirely outside the enforceable "social contract."

Or can it be construed to fall within its terms—namely, as repayment for benefits from past experimentation that I have enjoyed myself? But I am indebted for these benefits not to society, but to the past "martyrs," to whom society is indebted itself, and society has no right to call in my personal debt by way of adding new to its own. Moreover, gratitude is not an enforceable social obligation; it anyway does not mean that I must emulate the deed. Most of all, if it was wrong to exact such sacrifice in the first place, it does not become right to exact it again with the plea of the profit it has brought me. If, however, it was not exacted, but entirely free, as it ought to have been, then it should remain so, and its precedence must not be used as a social pressure on others for doing the same under the sign of duty.

Indeed, we must look outside the sphere of the social contract, outside the whole realm of public rights and duties, for the motivations and norms by which we can expect ever again the upwelling of a will to give what nobody—neither society, nor fellow man, nor posterity—is entitled to. There are such dimensions in man with trans-social wellsprings of conduct, and I have already pointed to the paradox, or mystery, that society cannot prosper without them, that it must draw on them, but cannot command them.

What about the moral law as such a transcendent motivation of conduct? It goes considerably beyond the public law of the social contract. The latter, we saw, is founded on the rule of enlightened self-interest: *Do ut des*—I give so that I be given to. The law of individual conscience asks more. Under the Golden Rule, for example, I am required to give as I wish to be given to under like circumstances, but not in order that I be given to and not in expectation of return. Reciprocity, essential to the social law, is not a condition of the moral law. One subtle "expectation" and "self-interest," but of the moral order itself, may even then be in my mind: I prefer the environment of a moral society and can expect to contribute to the general morality by my own example. But even if I should always be the dupe, the Golden Rule holds. (If the social law breaks faith with me, I am released from its claim.)

IX. Moral Law and Transmoral Dedication

Can I, then, be called upon to offer myself for medical experimentation in the name of the moral law? *Prima facie,* the Golden Rule seems to apply. I should wish, were I dying of a disease, that enough volunteers in the past had provided enough knowledge through the gift of their bodies that I could now be saved. I should wish, were I desperately in need of a transplant, that the dying patient next door had agreed to a definition of death by which his organs would become available to me in the freshest possible condition. I surely should also wish, were I drowning, that somebody would risk his life, even sacrifice his life, for mine.

But the last example reminds us that only the negative form of the Golden Rule ("Do not do unto others what you do not want done unto yourself") is fully prescriptive. The positive form ("Do unto others as you would wish them to do unto you"), in whose compass our issue falls, points into an infinite, open horizon where prescriptive force soon ceases. We may well say of somebody that he ought to have come to the succor of B, to have shared with him in his need, and the like. But we may not say that he ought to have given his life for him. To have done so would be praiseworthy; not to have done so is not blameworthy. It cannot be asked of him; if he fails to do so, he reneges on no duty. But *he* may say of himself, and only he, that he ought to have given his life. *This* "ought" is strictly between him and himself, or between him and God; no outside party—fellow man or society—can appropriate its voice. It can humbly receive the supererogatory gifts from the free enactment of it.

We must, in other words, distinguish between moral obligation and the much larger sphere of moral value. (This, incidentally, shows up the error in the widely held view of value theory that the higher a value, the stronger its claim and the greater the duty to realize it. The highest are in a region beyond duty and claim.) The ethical dimension far exceeds that of the moral law and reaches into the sublime solitude of dedication and ultimate commitment, away from all reckoning and rule—in short, into the sphere of the *holy*. From there alone can the offer of self-sacrifice genuinely spring, and this—its source—must be honored religiously. How? The first duty here falling on the research community, when it enlists and uses this source, is the safeguarding of true authenticity and spontaneity.

X. The "Conscription" of Consent

But here we must realize that the mere issuing of the appeal, the calling for volunteers, with the moral and social pressures it inevitably generates, amounts even under the most meticulous rules of consent to a sort of *conscripting*. And some soliciting is necessarily involved. This was in part meant by the earlier remark that in this area sin and guilt can perhaps not be wholly avoided. And this is why "consent," surely a non-negotiable minimum requirement, is not the full answer to the problem. Granting then that soliciting and therefore some degree of conscripting are part of the situation, who may conscript and who may be conscripted? Or less harshly expressed: Who should issue appeals and to whom?

The naturally qualified issuer of the appeal is the research scientist himself, collectively the main carrier of the impulse and the only one with the technical competence to judge. But his being very much an interested party (with vested interests, indeed, not purely in the public good, but in the scientific enterprise as such, in "his" project, and even in his career) makes him also suspect. The ineradicable dialect of this situation—a delicate incompatibility problem—calls for particular controls by the research community and by public authority that we need not discuss. They can mitigate, but not eliminate the problem. We have to live with the ambiguity, the treacherous impurity of everything human.

XI. Self-Recruitment of the Community

To whom should the appeal be addressed? The natural issuer of the call is also the first natural addressee: the physician-researcher himself and the scientific confraternity at large. With such a coincidence—indeed, the noble tradition with which the whole business of human experimentation started—almost all of the associated legal, ethical, and metaphysical problems vanish. If it is full, autonomous identification of the subject with the purpose that is required for the dignifying of his serving as a subject—here it is; if strongest motivation—here it is; if fullest understanding—here it is; if freest decision—here it is; if greatest integration with the person's total, chosen pursuit— here it is. With the fact of self-solicitation the issue of consent in all its insoluble equivocality is bypassed *per se*. Not even the condition that the particular purpose be truly important and the project reasonably promising, which must hold in any solicitation of others, need be satisfied here. By himself, the scientist is free to obey his obsession, to play his hunch, to wager on chance, to follow the lure of ambition. It is all part of the "divine madness" that somehow animates the ceaseless pressing against frontiers. For the rest of society, which has a deep-seated disposition to look with reverence and awe upon the guardians of the mysteries of life, the profession assumes with this proof of its devotion the role of a self-chosen, consecrated fraternity, not unlike the monastic orders of the past, and this would come nearest to the actual, religious origins of the art of healing.

It would be the ideal, but is not a real solution, to keep the issue of human experimentation within the research community itself. Neither in numbers nor in variety of material would its potential suffice for the many-pronged, systematic, continual attack on disease into which the lonely exploits of the early investigators have grown. Statistical requirements alone make their voracious demands; and were it not for what I have called the essentially "gratuitous" nature of the whole enterprise of progress, as against the mandatory respect for invasion-proof selfhood, the simplest answer would be to keep the whole population enrolled, and let the lot, or an equivalent of draft boards, decide which of each category will at any one time be called up for "service." It is not difficult to picture societies with whose philosophy this would be consonant. We are agreed that ours is not one such and should not become one. The specter of it is indeed among the threatening utopias on our own horizon from which we should recoil, and of whose advent by imperceptible steps we must beware. How then can our mandatory faith be honored when the recruitment for experimentation goes outside the scientific community, as it must in honoring another commitment of no mean dignity? We simply repeat the former question: To whom should the call be addressed?

XII. "Identification" as the Principle of Recruitment in General

If the properties we adduced as the particular qualifications of the members of the scientific fraternity itself are taken as general criteria of selection, then one should look for additional subjects where a maximum of identification, understanding, and spontaneity can be expected—that is, among the most highly motivated, the most highly educated, and the least "captive" members of the community. From this naturally scarce resource, a descending order of permissibility leads to greater abundance and ease of supply, whose use should become proportionately more hesitant as the exculpating criteria are relaxed. An inversion of normal "market" behavior is demanded here—namely, to accept the lowest quotation last (and excused only by the greatest pressure of need); to pay the highest price first.

The ruling principle in our considerations is that the "wrong" of reification can only be made "right" by such authentic identification with the cause that it is the subject's as well as the researcher's cause—whereby his role in its service is not just permitted by him, but *willed*. That sovereign will of his which embraces the end as his own restores his personhood to the otherwise depersonalizing context. To be valid it must be autonomous and informed. The latter condition can, outside the research community, only be fulfilled by degrees; but the higher the degree of the understanding regarding the purpose and the technique, the more valid becomes the endorsement of the will. A margin of mere trust inevitably remains. Ultimately, the appeal for volunteers should seek this free and generous endorsement, the appropriation of the research purpose into the person's own scheme of ends. Thus, the appeal is in truth addressed to the one, mysterious, and sacred source of any such generosity of the will—"devotion," whose forms and objects of commitment are various and may invest different motivations in different individuals. The following, for instance, may be responsive to the "call" we are discussing: compassion with human suffering, zeal for humanity, reverence for the Golden Rule, enthusiasm for progress, homage to the cause of knowledge, even longing for sacrificial justification (do not call that "masochism," please). On all these, I say, it is defensible and right to draw when the research objective is worthy enough; and it is a prime duty of the research community (especially in view of what we called the "margin of trust") to see that this sacred source is never abused for frivolous ends. For a less than adequate cause, not even the freest, unsolicited offer should be accepted.

XIII. The Rule of the "Descending Order" and Its Counter-Utility Sense

We have laid down what must seem to be a forbidding role to the number-hungry research industry. Having faith in the transcendent potential of man, I do not fear that the "source" will ever fail a society that does not destroy it—and only such a one is worthy of the blessings of progress. But "elitistic" the rule is (as is the enterprise of progress itself), and elites are by nature small. The combined attribute of motivation and information, plus the absence of external pressures, tends to be socially so circumscribed that strict adherence to the rule might numerically starve the research process. This is why I spoke of a descending order of permissibility, which is itself permissive, but where the realization that it is a *descending* order is not without pragmatic import. Departing from the august norm, the appeal must needs shift from idealism to docility, from high-mindedness to compliance, from judgment to trust. Consent spreads over the whole spectrum. I will not go into the casuistics of this penumbral area. I merely indicate the principle of the order of preference: The poorer in knowledge, motivation, and freedom of decision (and that, alas, means the more readily available in terms of numbers and possible manipulation), the more sparingly and indeed reluctantly should the reservoir be used, and the more compelling must therefore become the countervailing justification.

Let us note that this is the opposite of a social utility standard, the reverse of the order by "availability and expendability": The most valuable and scarcest, the least expendable elements of the social organism, are to be the first candidates for risk and sacrifice. It is the standard of *noblesse oblige*; and with all its counter-utility and seeming "wastefulness," we feel a rightness about it and perhaps even a higher "utility," for the soul of the community lives by this spirit.[8] It is also the opposite of what the day-to-day interests of research clamor for, and for the scientific community to honor it will mean that it will have to fight a strong temptation to go by routine to the readiest sources of supply—the suggestible, the ignorant, the dependent, the "captive" in various senses.[9] I do not believe that heightened resistance here must cripple research, which cannot be permitted; but it may indeed slow it down by the smaller numbers fed into experimentation in consequence. This price—a possibly slower rate of progress—may have to be paid for the preservation of the most precious capital of higher communal life.

XIV. Experimentation on Patients

So far we have been speaking on the tacit assumption that the subjects of experimentation are recruited from among the healthy. To the question "Who is conscriptable?" the spontaneous answer is: Least and last of all the sick—the most available of all as they are under treatment and observation anyway. That the afflicted should not be called upon to bear additional burden and risk, that they are society's special trust and the physician's trust in particular—these are elementary responses of our moral sense. Yet the very destination of medical research, the conquest of disease, requires at the crucial stage trial and verification on precisely the sufferers from the disease, and their total exemption would defeat the purpose itself. In acknowledging this inescapable necessity, we enter the most sensitive area of the whole complex, the one most keenly felt and most searchingly discussed by the practitioners themselves. No wonder, it touches the heart of the doctor-patient relation, putting its most solemn obligations to the test. There is nothing new in what I have to say about the ethics of the doctor-patient relation, but for the purpose of confronting it with the issue of experimentation some of the oldest verities must be recalled.

A. *The Fundamental Privilege of the Sick*

In the course of treatment, the physician is obligated to the patient and to no one else. He is not the agent of society, nor of the interests of medical science, nor of the patient's family, nor of his co-sufferers, or future sufferers from the same disease. The patient alone counts when he is under the physician's care.

By the simple law of bilateral contract (analogous, for example, to the relation of lawyer to client and its "conflict of interest" rule), the physician is bound not to let any other interest interfere with that of the patient in being cured. But manifestly more sublime norms than contractual ones are involved. We may speak of a sacred trust; strictly by its terms, the doctor is, as it were, alone with his patient and God.

There is one normal exception to this—that is, to the doctor's not being the agent of society vis-à-vis the patient, but the trustee of his interests alone: the quarantining of the contagious sick. This is plainly not for the patient's interest, but for that of others threatened by him. (In vaccination, we have a combination of both: protection of the individual and others.) But preventing the patient from causing harm to others is not the same as exploiting him for the advantage of others. And there is, of course, the abnormal exception of collective catastrophe, the analogue to a state of war. The physician who desperately battles a raging epidemic is under a unique dispensation that suspends in a nonspecifiable way some of the strictures of normal practice, including possibly those against experimental liberties with his patients. No rules can be devised for the waiving of rules in extremities. And as with the famous shipwreck examples of ethical theory, the less said about it the better. But what is allowable there and may later be passed over in forgiving silence cannot serve as a precedent. We are concerned with non-extreme, non-emergency conditions where the voice of principle can be heard and claims can be adjudicated free from duress. We have conceded that there are such claims, and that if there is to be medical advance at all, not even the superlative privilege of the suffering and the sick can be kept wholly intact from the intrusion of its needs. About this least palatable, most disquieting part of our subject, I have to offer only groping, inconclusive remarks.

B. The Principle of "Identification" Applied to Patients

On the whole, the same principles would seem to hold here as are found to hold with "normal subjects": motivation, identification, understanding on the part of the subject. But it is clear that these conditions are peculiarly difficult to satisfy with regard to a patient. His physical state, psychic preoccupation, dependent relation to the doctor, the submissive attitude induced by treatment—everything connected with his condition and situation makes the sick person inherently less of a sovereign person than the healthy one. Spontaneity of self-offering has almost to be ruled out; consent is marred by lower resistance or captive circumstance, and so on. In fact, all the factors that make the patient, as a category, particularly accessible and welcome for experimentation at the same time compromise the quality of the responding affirmation that must morally redeem the making use of them. This, in addition to the primacy of the physician's duty, puts a heightened onus on the physician-researcher to limit his undue power to the most important and defensible research objectives and, of course, to keep persuasion at a minimum.

Still, with all the disabilities noted, there is scope among patients for observing the rule of the "descending order of permissibility" that we have laid down for normal subjects, in vexing inversion of the utility order of quantitative abundance and qualitative "expendability." By the principle of this order, those patients who most identify with and are cognizant of the cause of research—members of the medical profession (who after all are sometimes patients themselves)—come first; the highly motivated and educated, also least dependent, among the lay patients come next; and so on down the line. An added consideration here is seriousness of condition, which again operates in inverse proportion. Here the profession must fight the tempting sophistry that the hopeless case is expendable (because in prospect already expended) and therefore especially usable; and generally the attitude that the poorer the chances of the patient the more justifiable his recruitment for experimentation (other than for his own benefit). The opposite is true.

C. Nondisclosure as a Borderline Case

Then there is the case where ignorance of the subject, sometimes even of the experimenter, is of the essence of the experiment (the "double blind"-control group-placebo syndrome). It is said to be a necessary element of the scientific process. Whatever may be said about its ethics in regard to normal subjects, especially volunteers, it is an outright betrayal of trust in regard to the patient who believes that he is receiving treatment. Only supreme importance of the objective can exonerate it, without making it less of a transgression. The patient is definitely wronged even when not harmed. And ethics apart, the practice of such deception holds the danger of undermining the faith in the *bona fides* of treatment, the beneficial intent of the physician—the very basis of the doctor-patient relationship. In every respect, it follows that concealed experiment on patients—that is, experiment under the guise of treatment— should be the rarest exception, at best, if it cannot be wholly avoided.

This has still the merit of a borderline problem. The same is not true of the other case of necessary ignorance of the subject— that of the unconscious patient. Drafting him for nontherapeutic experiments is simply and unqualifiedly impermissible; progress or not, he must never be used, on the inflexible principle that utter helplessness demands utter protection.

When preparing this paper, I filled pages with a casuistics of this harrowing field, but then scrapped most of it, realizing my dilettante status. The shadings are endless, and only the physician-researcher can discern them properly as the cases arise. Into his lap the decision is thrown. The philosophical rule, once it has admitted into itself the idea of a sliding scale, cannot really specify its own application. It can only impress on the practitioner a general maxim or attitude for the exercise of his judgment and conscience in the concrete occasions of his work. In our case, I am afraid, it means making life more difficult for him.

It will also be noted that, somewhat at variance with the emphasis in the literature, I have not dwelt on the element of "risk" and very little on that of "consent." Discussion of the first is beyond the layman's competence; the emphasis on the second has been lessened because of its equivocal character. It is a truism to say that one should strive to minimize the risk and to maximize the consent. The more demanding concept of "identification," which I have used, includes "consent" in its maximal or authentic form, and the assumption of risk is its privilege.

XV. No Experiments on Patients Unrelated to Their Own Disease

Although my ponderings have, on the whole, yielded points of view rather than definite prescriptions, premises rather than conclusions, they have led me to a few unequivocal yeses and noes. The first is the emphatic rule that patients should be experimented upon, if at all, *only* with reference to *their disease*. Never should there be added to the gratuitousness of the experiment as such the gratuitousness of service to an unrelated cause. This follows simply from what we have found to be the *only* excuse for infracting the special exemption of the sick at all—namely, that the scientific war on disease cannot accomplish its goal without drawing the sufferers from disease into the investigative process. If under this excuse they become subjects of experiment, they do so *because*, and only because, of *their* disease.

This is the fundamental and self-sufficient consideration. That the patient cannot possibly benefit from the unrelated experiment therapeutically, while he might from experiment related to his condition, is also true, but lies beyond the problem area of pure experiment. I am in any case discussing nontherapeutic experimentation only, where *ex hypothesi* the patient does not benefit. Experiment as part of therapy—that is, directed toward helping the subject himself—is a different matter altogether and raises its own problems, but hardly philosophical ones. As long as a doctor can say, even if only in his own thought: "There is no known cure for your condition (or: You have responded to none); but there is promise in a new treatment still under investigation, not quite tested yet as to effectiveness and safety; you will be taking a chance, but all things considered, I judge it in your best interest to let me try it on you"—as long as he can speak thus, he speaks as the patient's physician and may err, but does not transform the patient into a subject of experimentation. Introduction of an untried therapy into the treatment where the tried ones have failed is not "experimentation on the patient."

Generally, and almost needless to say, with all the rules of the book, there is something "experimental" (because tentative) about every individual treatment, beginning with the diagnosis itself; and he would be a poor doctor who would not learn from every case for the benefit of future cases, and a poor member of the profession who would not make any new insights gained from his treatments available to the profession at large. Thus, knowledge may be advanced in the treatment of any patient, and the interest of the medical art and all sufferers from the same affliction as well as the patient himself may be served if something happens to be learned from his case. But this gain to knowledge and future therapy is incidental to the *bona fide* service to the present patient. He has the right to expect that the doctor does nothing to him just in order to learn.

In that case, the doctor's imaginary speech would run, for instance, like this: "There is nothing more I can do for you. But you can do something for me. Speaking no longer as your physician but on behalf of medical science, we could learn a great deal about future cases of this kind if you would permit me to perform certain experiments on you. It is understood that you yourself would not benefit from any knowledge we might gain; but future patients would." This statement would express the purely experimental situation, assumedly here with the subject's concurrence and with all cards on the table. In Alexander Bickel's words: "It is a different situation when the doctor is no longer trying to make [the patient] well, but is trying to find out how to make others well in the future."[10]

But even in the second case, that of the nontherapeutic experiment where the patient does not benefit, at least the patient's own disease is enlisted in the cause of fighting that disease, even if only in others. It is yet another thing to say or think: "Since you are here—in the hospital with its facilities—anyway, under our care and observation anyway, away from your job (or, perhaps, doomed) anyway, we wish to profit from your being available for some other research of great interest we are presently engaged in." From the standpoint of merely medical ethics, which has only to consider risk, consent, and the worth of the objective, there may be no cardinal difference between this case and the last one. I hope that the medical reader will not think I am making too fine a point when I say that from the standpoint of the subject and his dignity there is a cardinal difference that crosses the line between the permissible and the impermissible, and this by the same principle of "iden-tification" I have been invoking all along. Whatever the rights and wrongs of any experimentation on any patient—in the one case, at least that residue of identification is left him that it is his own affliction by which he can contribute to the conquest of that affliction, his own kind of suffering which he helps to alleviate in others; and so in a sense it is his own cause. It is totally indefensible to rob the unfortunate of this intimacy with the purpose and make his misfortune a convenience for the furtherance of alien concerns. The observance of this rule is essential, I think, to at least attenuate the wrong that nontherapeutic experimenting on patients commits in any case.

XVI. On the Redefinition of Death

My other emphatic verdict concerns the question of the re-definition of death—that is, acknowledging "irreversible coma as a new definition for death."[11] I wish not to be misunder-stood. As long as it is merely a question of when it is permitted to cease the artificial prolongation of certain functions (like heartbeat) traditionally regarded as signs of life, I do not see anything ominous in the notion of "brain death." Indeed, a new definition of death is not even necessary to legitimize the same result if one adopts the position of the Roman Catholic Church, which here at least is eminently reasonable—namely that "when deep unconsciousness is judged to be permanent, extraordinary means to maintain life are not obligatory. They can be terminated and the patient allowed to die."[12] Given a clearly defined negative condition of the brain, the physician is allowed to allow the patient to die his own death by *any* definition, which of itself will lead through the gamut of all possible definitions. But a disquietingly contradictory purpose is combined with this purpose in the quest for a new definition of death—that is, in the will to *advance* the moment of declar-ing him dead: Permission not to turn off the respirator, but, on the contrary, to keep it on and thereby maintain the body in a state of what would have been "life" by the older definition (but is only a "simulacrum" of life by the new)—so as to get at his organs and tissues under the ideal conditions of what would previously have been "vivisection."[13]

Now this, whether done for research or transplant purposes, seems to me to overstep what the definition can warrant. Surely it is one thing when to cease delaying death, another when to start doing violence to the body; one thing when to desist from protracting the process of dying, another when to regard that process as complete and thereby the body as a cadaver free for inflicting on it what would be torture and death to any living body. For the first purpose, we need not know the exact borderline between life and death—we leave it to nature to cross it wherever it is, or to traverse the whole spectrum if there is not just one line. All we need to know is that coma is irreversible. For the second purpose we must know the borderline with absolute certainty; and to use any definition short of the maximal for perpetrating on a *possibly* penultimate state what only the ultimate state can permit is to arrogate a knowledge which, I think, we cannot possibly have. *Since we do not know the exact borderline between life and death,* nothing less than the maximum definition of death will do—brain death plus heart death plus any other indication that may be pertinent—before final violence is allowed to be done.

It would follow then, for this layman at least, that the use of the definition should itself be defined, and this in a restrictive sense. When only permanent coma can be gained with the artificial sustaining of functions, by all means turn off the respirator, the stimulator, any sustaining artifice, and let the patient die; but let him die all the way. Do not, instead, arrest the process and start using him as a mine while, with your own help and cunning, he is still kept this side of what may in truth be the final line. Who is to say that a shock, a final trauma, is not administered to a sensitivity diffusely situated elsewhere than in the brain and still vulnerable to suffering—a sensitivity that we ourselves have been keeping alive. No fiat of definition can settle this question.[14] But I wish to emphasize that the question of possible suffering (easily brushed aside by a sufficient show of reassuring expert consensus) is merely a subsidiary and not the real point of my argument; this, to reiterate, turns on the indeterminacy of the boundaries between *life and death*, not between sensitivity and insensitivity, and bids us to lean toward a maximal rather than a minimal determination of death in an area of basic uncertainty.

There is also this to consider: The patient must be absolutely sure that his doctor does not become his executioner, and that no definition authorizes him ever to become one. His right to this certainty is absolute, and so is his right to his own body with all its organs. Absolute respect for these rights violates no one else's rights, for no one has a right to another's body. Speaking in still another, religious vein: The expiring moments should be watched over with piety and be safe from exploitation.

I strongly feel, therefore, that it should be made quite clear that the proposed new definition of death is to authorize *only* the one and *not* the other of the two opposing things: only to break off a sustaining intervention and let things take their course, not to keep up the sustaining intervention for a final intervention of the most destructive kind.

XVII. Conclusion

There would now have to be said something about nonmedical experiments on human subjects, notably psychological and genetic, of which I have not lost sight. But I must leave this for another occasion. I wish only to say in conclusion that if some of the practical implications of my reasonings are felt to work out toward a slower rate of progress, this should not cause too great dismay. Let us not forget that progress is an optional goal, not an unconditional commitment, and that its tempo in particular, compulsive as it may become, has nothing sacred about it. Let us also remember that a slower progress in the conquest of disease would not threaten society, grievous as it is to those who have to deplore that their particular disease be not yet conquered, but that society would indeed be threatened by the erosion of those moral values whose loss, possibly caused by too ruthless a pursuit of scientific progress, would make its most dazzling triumphs not worth having. Let us finally remember that it cannot be the aim of progress to abolish the lot of mortality. Of some ill or other, each of us will die. Our mortal condition is upon us with its harshness but also its wisdom—

because without it there would not be the eternally renewed promise of the freshness, immediacy, and eagerness of youth; nor would there be for any of us the incentive to number our days and make them count. With all our striving to wrest from our mortality what we can, we should bear its burden with patience and dignity.

NOTES

Editorial Note: This was a conference sponsored by the National Academy of Arts and Sciences on the ethics of human experimentation held in 1969.
1. In preparation for the Conference from which this volume originated.
2. G. E. W. Wolstenholme and Maeve O'Connor (editors), *CIBA Foundation Symposium, Ethics in Medical Progress: With Special Reference to Transplantation* (Boston, 1966); "The Changing Mores of Biomedical Research," *Annals of Internal Medicine* (Supplement 7), Vol. 67, No. 3 (Philadelphia, September, 1967); *Proceedings of the Conference on the Ethical Aspects of Experimentation on Human Subjects.* November 3–4, 1967 (Boston, Massachusetts; hereafter called *Proceedings*); H. K. Beecher, "Some Guiding Principles for Clinical Investigation," *Journal of the American Medical Association,* Vol. 195 (March 28, 1966), pp. 1135–36; H. K. Beecher, "Consent in Clinical Experimentation: Myth and Reality," *Journal of the American Medical Association,* Vol. 195 (January 3, 1966), pp. 34–35; P. A. Freund, "Ethical Problems in Human Experimentation," *New England Journal of Medicine,* Vol 273 (September 23, 1965), pp. 687–92; P. A. Freund, "Is the Law Ready for Human Experimentation?," *American Psychologist,* Vol 22 (1967), pp. 394–99; W. Wolfensberger, "Ethical Issues in Research with Human Subjects," *World Science,* Vol. 155 (January 6, 1967), pp. 47–51; See also a series of five articles by Drs. Schoen, McGrath, and Kennedy, "Principles of Medical Ethics," which appeared from August to December in Volume 23 of *Arizona Medicine.* The most recent entry in the growing literature is E. Fuller Torrey (editor), *Ethical Issues in Medicine* (New York, 1968), in which the chapter "Ethical Problems in Human Experimentation" by Otto E. Guttentag should be especially noted.

3. Wolfensberger, "Ethical Issues in Research with Human Subjects," p. 48.

4. *Proceedings,* p.29.

5. Cf. M. H. Pappworth, "Ethical Issues in Experimental Medicine" in D. R. Cutler (editor), *Updating Life and Death* (Boston, 1969), pp. 64–69.

6. *Die Braut von Korinth:* "Victims do fall here, /Neither lamb nor steer, /Nay, but human offerings untold."

7. *Proceedings,* pp. 50–51.

8. Socially, everyone is expendable relatively—that is, in different degrees; religiously, no one is expendable absolutely: The "image of God" is in all. If it can be enhanced, then not by anyone being expended, but by someone expending himself.

9. This refers to captives of circumstance, not of justice. Prison inmates are, with respect to our problem, in a special class. If we hold to some idea of guilt, and to the supposition that our judicial system is not entirely at fault, they may be held to stand in a special debt to society, and their offer to serve—from whatever motive—may be accepted with a minimum of qualms as a means of reparation.

10. *Proceedings,* p. 33. To spell out the difference between the two cases: In the first case, the patient himself is meant to be the beneficiary of the experiment, and directly so; the "subject" of the experiment is at the same time its object, its end. It is performed not for gaining knowledge, but for helping him—and helping him in the *act* of performing it, even if by its results it also contributes to a broader testing process currently under way. It is in fact part of the treatment itself and an "experiment" only in the loose sense of being untried and highly tentative. But whatever the degree of uncertainty, the motivating anticipation (the wager, if you like) is for success, and success here means the subject's own good. To a pure experiment, by contrast, undertaken to gain knowledge, the difference of success and failure is not germane, only that of conclusiveness and inconclusiveness. The "negative" result has as much to teach as the "positive." Also, the true experiment is an act distinct from the uses later made of the findings. And, most important, the subject experimented on is distinct from the eventual beneficiaries of those findings: He lets himself be used as a means toward an end external to himself (even if he should at some later time happen to be among the beneficiaries himself). With respect to his own present needs and his own good, the act is gratuitous.

11. "A Definition of Irreversible Coma," Report of the *Ad Hoc* Committee of Harvard Medical School to Examine the Definition of Brain Death, *Journal of the American Medical Association,* Vol 205, No. 6 (August 5, 1968), pp. 337–40.

12. As rendered by Dr. Beecher in *Proceedings,* p. 50.

13. The Report of the *Ad Hoc* Committee no more than indicates this possibility with the second of the "two reasons why there is need for a definition": "(2) Obsolete criteria for the definition of death can lead to controversy in obtaining organs for transplantation." The first reason is relief from the burden of indefinitely drawn out coma. The report wisely confines its recommendations on application to what falls under this first reason—namely, turning off the respirator— and remains silent on the possible use of the definition under the second reason. But when "the patient is declared dead on the basis of these criteria," the road to the other use has theoretically been opened and will be taken (if I remember rightly, it has even been taken once, in a much debated case in England), unless it is blocked by a special barrier in good time. The above is my feeble attempt to help doing so.

14. Only a Cartesian view of the "animal machine," which I somehow see lingering here, could set the mind at rest, as in historical fact it did at its time in the matter of vivisection: But its truth is surely not established by definition.

Research on the Condemned, the Dying, the Unconscious

Paul Ramsey

ABOUT 12 or 14 years ago, an American physician, Jack Kevorkian, M.D., published two books and at least one article on a novel use of people who are condemned to die.[1] One book was entitled *Capital Punishment or Capital Gain?* His was a serious proposal in justification of research on the condemned. Even now when capital punishment finds less favor in our society and has been declared unconstitutional under certain circumstances in the United States, it is worth trying to recover the flavor and anatomy of Kevorkian's argument for purposes of comparison with some defenses currently made of experimentation on the live human fetus.

Capital punishment as it existed in 1959–60, Kevorkian believed, offered a "golden opportunity" for research on human beings to break out of the limits imposed by the need to protect normal volunteers from serious damage. He proposed that "a prisoner condemned to death by due process of law be allowed to submit, by his own free choice, to medical experimentation under complete anesthesia (at the time appointed for administering the penalty) as a form of execution in lieu of conventional methods prescribed by law."[2] In fact, the medical experiment, however extreme, need not be thought of as a form of execution, since "ultimate death could be induced by an overdose of anesthetic given by a layman." That is, an official of the state

From *The Ethics of Fetal Research*, by Paul Ramsey, Yale University Press, 1975
Reprinted from *The Ethics of Fetal Research* by Paul Ramsey with permission of Yale University Press.

would step in to deliver the *coup de grace*. In case the perilous experiment itself pushed the subject over the brink, Kevorkian contended, physicians would still not be executioners because "their aim was not to kill but to learn."

Likewise it might be argued today that, while some physicians assumed the role of a public functionary (in using socio-economic indices) or the role of executor of women's wishes, still those physicians engaged in fetal research have as such the aim not to kill but to learn. The death decreed by an abortion only affords a "golden opportunity" for "capital gain" for humankind.

The experiments made possible in anticipation of execution, in Kevorkian's judgment, promised "much more than the bleak aim of ending a criminal's life." Likewise, it might be argued today that fetal experiments made possible in anticipation of abortion, or as a consequence of abortive actions set in course, promise much more than the bleak aim of ending the fetus's life. If prenatal lives are going to be wasted anyway, why cannot some of that waste be redeemed?

Moreover, the allocation of funds for much "animal work" now in progress in medical research would be rendered "a complete waste of time and money"; one could proceed at once to the "human work." For Kevorkian the decisive point in favor of his proposal was that rapid progress could be made "in those fields where animal work cannot help (for example, anatomy of the human brain)." That, precisely, is a main apology for the necessity of experimentation on fetuses, namely, that there are uniquely prenatal and pediatric diseases and information about human development in its early stages that finally can only be researched by "human work." Human fetuses already condemned by an abortion decision afford us the same unique opportunity which Kevorkian believed capital punishment opened for human experimentation in general.

In Kevorkian's proposed experiments, it could be argued that "to the condemned" his proposal "allows the dignity inherent in being permitted to decide how he is to die." The condemned are rewarded by a "feeling of utility through death." Some "positive significance" is imparted to the death of his victim if he is a murderer; and Kevorkian believed his proposal afforded "a means of restoring some honor to the family of the condemned." The fact that adults condemned to death are capable of choosing to become heroic partners in medical progress is an advantage condemned fetuses do not have. Here the analogy breaks down.

For society, Kevorkian further argued, the "proposed 'judicial euthanasia' for the first time introduces a concept of recompensing into a matter now of pure vengeance." Likewise, apologists for fetal research sometimes argue that there ought to be some recompense, some good to come from the extraordinary number of unborn lives that today are being destroyed.

A religious interpretation or commentary could not fail to notice at this point the significance of the desire to wrest some recompense or redemption out of the condemnation of these human lives. Surely that motivation has grown enormously among the saving and healing professions and in society generally in face of the huge wastage of one form of human life today by abortion. I believe that a load of guilt is the propellant behind much of the acceptance of fetal research, even as the expected benefits are its lure and goal. If not specific moral guilt, then a load of "survivor guilt"; but surely also a generalized moral guilt as well. The wastage of unborn lives needs redemption; something "must" be saved from it. The research gains promise not only benefits; they also can "rectify" and do at least something to redeem the destruction we collectively are causing in pursuit of other social and personal goods.

Finally, however, Kevorkian guards himself against lending support to capital punishment itself. "The pros and cons of capital punishment are not at all involved in my proposal. My only contention is that so long as it is practiced, and wherever it is practiced, there is a far more humane, sensible and profitable way to administer it." Similar things might be said about the practice of abortion.

Despite its facile persuasiveness, I think we should reject Kevorkian's proposal. Even if his scheme had no tendency to strengthen capital punishment as an institution, it would be morally outrageous for other people to profit by research on the condemned. So also, I suggest, it would be morally outrageous for future fetuses or children to be made to benefit from research on sacrificed fetuses. The research subjects are additionally misused if the experimentation is irrelevant to what caused their condemnation to be deemed just and necessary or electable.

*   *   *

The fetal human being, whether from induced or spontaneous abortion or unsalvageable prematurity, is also among the dying. In research upon the dying we should not, even with their consent, impose on them irrelevant experiments. With research into cures for their diseases—even beyond any hope of successfully treating their particular case—we reach the outer limit of ethical research upon the dying. This is based on a human being's sense of identity with his body, even with his dying body. Thus Hans Jonas argues[3] that the terminally ill should be spared "the gratuitousness of service to an unrelated cause." In no case should the dying be told: "Since you are here—in the hospital with its facilities—under our care and observation, away from your job (or, perhaps, doomed) we wish to profit from your being available for some other research of great interest we are presently engaged in." Neither ought we to act as if we are saying to the abortus: "Since you are going to die anyway and are available and under observation, wouldn't it be more significant for you to die as our 'partner' in research of great interest and which may prove profitable to the uncondemned?" Research on the terminally ill, Jonas reasoned, should always be relevant to that patient's illness. In research aimed at learning more about that illness, a "residue of identification is left him that it is his own affliction by which he can contribute to the conquest of that affliction." It is a kind of violation of bodily identity, and a misuse of the dying, even to ask the terminally ill to consent to irrelevant research.

A fortiori, we ought not similarly to abuse the fetal research subject who cannot be asked. In the case of the capitally condemned, it generally would not be proposed to limit nontherapeutic research upon them to the development of more humane methods of capital punishment or the accumulation of medical evidence against capital punishment. Nor is fetal research limited to studies intended to remove pain from future abortion procedures or to gather evidence that a civilized society should limit that dying as much as possible. The experiments are irrelevant to the bodily identity or dying of those singled out for coopted contributions to medical progress. They should be spared such gratuitous service. Relevance is the condition that is lacking, and it alone can morally redeem making use of these dying ones.

Doubtless there is an obligation to develop techniques to increase viability and to prevent or offset certain congenital defects or consequences of prematurity. But there can be no obligation—indeed, it would be positively wrong—to obtain those results by means of abortuses who are hovering between life and death precisely because for them no such rescue or remedies were wanted. Those beneficial results should rather be among the research aims of therapeutic investigations that have as a first purpose the promotion of the survival of fetal patients and premature infants.

The fetal subject is also among the unconscious, with the small and, I suggest, morally irrelevant difference that the fetus has never been conscious. Even that concession can be questioned. How accurate it is depends on one's definition of consciousness and at what stage of gestation experiments are proposed to be done on fetuses. The unborn hears the lower tones of its mother's voice and responds to extrauterine stimuli. The fetus is certainly not in coma. There is good evidence that the fetus feels pain, although pain studies are notoriously difficult to do. Perhaps we ought to do pain studies in connection with abortion, if they can be devised, and disseminate that information to the public. If that is possible, the research would be *relevant* to fetal dying, in the sense explained above, even though no one aimed to use the information for the benefit of the particular dying subjects coopted for that purpose.

If the analogy with unconscious patients is believed to be pertinent to an analysis of the moral aspects of fetal research—or to the extent that it is—the conclusion should be clear. To quote Hans Jonas again: "Drafting him [the unconscious] for non-therapeutic experiments is simply and unqualifiedly not permissible; progress or not, he must never be used, on the inflexible principle that utter helplessness demands utter protection."[4] Research on the unconscious subject must be done only in investigations related (however remotely) to his treatment. It is treatment that is the foundation for construing his consent in "Good Samaritan" medicine. If we extend constructive or implied "proxy" consents beyond investigational trials related to treatment, if we also assume that the unconscious subject consents to be used for irrelevant investigations, then we adopt a violent and a false presumption.

NOTES

1. Jack Kevorkian, *Medical Research and the Death Penalty* (New York: Vantage Press, 1960); *Capital Punishment or Capital Gain?* (New York: Philosophical Library, 1962); "Capital Punishment or Capital Gain," *J. Crim. Law, Criminology and Police Science* (1959) 50: 50–51, Reprinted in Irving Ladimer and Roger W. Newman, eds., *Clinical Investigation in Medicine: Legal, Medical and Moral Aspects* (Boston University: Law-Medicine Research Institute, 1963), pp. 470–72; and in Jay Katz, et al., *Experimentation with Human Beings* (New York: Russell Sage Foundation, 1972), pp. 1027–28.
2. Kevorkian, "Capital Punishment or Capital Gain," pp. 50–51. Subsequent references are to this brief article, also in Ladimer, pp. 470–72, and Katz, pp. 1027–28.
3. Hans Jonas, "Philosophical Reflection on Human Experimentation," Ethical Aspects of Experimentation on Human Subjects, *Daedalus* (Spring 1969), 98: 241–43; reprinted in his *Philosophical Essays: From Ancient Creed to Technological Man* (Englewood Cliffs, N.J.: 1974), pp. 123–29.
4. Hans Jonas, *Philosophical Essays,* p. 126.

Fetal Research:
The State of the Question

John C. Fletcher and Joseph D. Schulman

PUBLIC policies, including policies about ethics, require a good heart (sound principles) and two good hands (sound institutional controls) to succeed. We believe that most investigators who conduct fetal research share our basic thesis: the 1975 federal regulations for fetal research "conducted by the Department of Health and Human Services (DHHS) or funded in whole or in part by a Department grant, contract, cooperative agreement or fellowship" were constructed on the soundest ethical principles: equality of protection for all research subjects; and the benefits to individuals and society that may be realized by research activities.[1]

Further, to resolve conflicts between these principles, the guidelines were set within a system of institutional controls with interaction between local and national levels. Unfortunately, since 1980 one of the hands of federal fetal research policy has been paralyzed by the lack of an Ethics Advisory Board (EAB). The other hand of policy, the local institutional review board (IRB), is now the only locus of practical control in fetal research. Consequently, fetal research in the United States is now reviewed only at the local level and receives support primarily from the private realm.

Our goal is the development of a set of public policies, ethically and institutionally coherent, to protect those toward whom research may be directed: the human embryo before and

From *Hastings Center Report*, 1985, Vol. 15. Reprinted by permission of the author and the Hastings Center.

after implantation, the pregnant woman, the developing fetus inside or outside the uterus, and the infant in the perinatal period. (The "fetus" is defined in the regulations as "the product of conception from the time of implantation . . . until a determination is made . . . that it is viable" [45 CFR 46.203 (C)]. Here we discuss mainly fetal research, although we do pay some attention to the need for research with the human embryo.

The Early Debates

Paul Ramsey,[2] Steven Maynard-Moody,[3] and others[4] have published fuller accounts of events (1967–1974) that led to Congressional debate about fetal research and creation of a National Commission for the Protection of Human Subjects of Biomedical and Behavioral Research. Between 1970 and 1972, advisory groups within the National Institute of Child Health and Development (NICHD) debated the earliest NIH policies on the review and funding of human fetal research. The NIH discussions were reported concurrently with stories of abuses by Scandinavian researchers on live, postabortion fetuses.[5]

Moral outrage over the issue resulted in the first public demonstration ever seen at the NIH.[6] Students from a local Catholic private girls' school, joined by others from a private boys' school, demonstrated in front of the normally quiet headquarters building. They protested alleged NIH funding of objectionable research in the U.S. and abroad. They were invited inside for a lengthy meeting with Charles Lowe, then scientific director of NICHD. Eunice Kennedy Shriver was the spokesperson for the demonstrators. Lowe explained that the NIH had not funded the objectionable research. However, to underscore the seriousness of the issue, NIH officials declared a moratorium on any research with the living fetus before or after abortion.

The legislation (National Research Act, P.L. 93-348, Section 213) that created the commission continued a ban on fetal research except when intended to assure the survival of a fetus, until the Commission made its recommendations. President Nixon signed this bill on July 12, 1974, and Secretary Weinberger administered the oath to the eleven-member group on December 3. Congress gave the Commission a deadline of *four months* for recommendations on fetal research, the first of several of its mandates. This short timetable reflects the emotional and polarized condition of the issue. The Commission did respond, only one month late, with recommendations[7] that became the heart and hands of the later federal regulations.

It succeeded because of its gifted, diverse membership; an irenic chairman, Kenneth Ryan; and some professional staff who advised in drafting the language of the regulations. Other factors helped too. A British working party's report was available in 1972.[8] In 1973, an NIH study group synthesized its key policy proposals to protect vulnerable human subjects, including the fetus.[9] This document contained strong language about the extension of equal protection to the fetus to be aborted, and also explained the health benefits for pregnant women and children from continued research with the nonviable human fetus. Also, many of the scientific, ethical, and legal papers prepared for the Commission were superlative.[10]

The early "bioethics" movement produced several contributors who illuminated key elements in the debate. The fledgling Kennedy Institute for the Study of Human Reproduction and Bioethics provided two whose ethical views counted strongly in a middle-ground position, between no restriction and a virtual ban of fetal research. Richard A. McCormick reasoned from an earlier defense of nontherapeutic research with children to the possibility of fetal research, premised on the proxy consent of parents and no "discernible" risk.[11] The latter term was a preface to the Commission's use of "minimal" risk, although the frame of reference was not then defined. LeRoy Walters's paper on nontherapeutic research espoused the equality principle and outlined the policy choices.[12]

Highlights of the Commission's discussions occurred during its review of fetal research for testing rubella vaccine, amniocentesis, treatment of Rh isoimmunization disease, and respiratory distress syndrome. The rubella vaccine discussion was especially important in shaping some openness toward limited research with fetuses prior to abortion. Preliminary testing of rubella vaccine in monkeys indicated that the vaccine virus did not cross the placenta. In contrast, studies on women requesting therapeutic abortion showed clearly that the vaccine virus did indeed cross the placenta and infect the fetus. At the time, it was thought that the presence of the virus transmitted by vaccine in the fetus would be teratogenic. However, many subsequent cases of infants born to women who have received rubella vaccine during early pregnancy have not shown harmful effects. This retrospective experience was not available to the Commission, whose members were impressed with a finding in the human fetus contrary to animal studies.

The Commission, with one notable dissent by David Louisell on categories (4) and (5), encouraged federal support of six categories of fetal research, conditional on IRB approval, informed consent of the mother, and the nonobjection of the father:

1. *Therapeutic research directed toward the fetus,* within appropriate medical standards;

2. *Therapeutic research directed toward the pregnant woman,* provided the research imposes minimal risk or no risk to the fetus; altered in the regulations to "fetus will be placed at risk only to the minimum extent necessary to meet" the health needs of the mother, [46.207 (a) (1)];

3. *Nontherapeutic research directed toward the pregnant woman,* if the risk to the fetus is minimal;

4. *Nontherapeutic research directed toward the fetus in utero* either: (a) not anticipating abortion, if risk to the fetus is minimal, and the knowledge is unobtainable by other means; or (b) anticipating abortion, if risk to the fetus is minimal; approval of a national ethical review body was required if such research presents "special problems related to the interpretation or application of these guidelines";

5. *Nontherapeutic research directed toward the fetus during the abortion procedure and nontherapeutic research directed toward the nonviable fetus ex utero,* provided that the fetus is less than twenty weeks gestational age, no significant changes in the interests of research alone are introduced into the abortion procedure, and no attempt is made to alter the duration of the life of the fetus; like the fourth category, only with approval by a national ethical review body, if problems arise about the interpretation of minimal or added risk.

6. *Research directed toward the possibly viable fetus,* provided that no additional risk to the infant will be imposed by the research, and that the knowledge is unobtainable by other means.

Except for the removal of the twenty weeks gestational age provision in the fifth category, and a few elisions and minor rewordings, existing federal regulations still embody these key elements, though they do not use the language of "therapeutic" and "nontherapeutic" research. Instead, they describe activities "to meet the health of the particular fetus" or "the development of important biomedical knowledge which cannot be obtained by other means." However, neither the Commission's recommendations nor the current regulations defined minimal risk *specifically* for fetal research. A specific definition for minimal risk in research with children was developed by the Commission in 1975: " 'Minimal risk' means that risks of harm anticipated in the proposed research are not greater, considering probability and magnitude, than those ordinarily encountered in daily life or during the performance of routine medical or psychological examinations or tests, of healthy children."[13] In the regulations, the last frame of reference phrase of "healthy children" was omitted, and "physical" substituted for "medical" tests [45 CFR 46.102 (g)].

What frame of reference is supposed to be used for evaluating minimal risk of research with the fetus? The logical extension of the Commission's reasoning would be healthy, wanted fetuses, and the routine tests and examinations done on them. But how does one learn to do "routine" tests, unless by research, which at first involves risks of testing the new approach? This issue has never been resolved in the fetal regulations. Regulations to protect prisoners in research include a definition of minimal risk with the frame of reference being "healthy persons" [46.303 (d)].

Understandably, the most controverted issue faced by the Commission was the meaning of equal protection in nontherapeutic research with fetuses to be aborted. A maxim was developed from the Golden Rule implications of the equality principle, that is, one ought to do or refrain from doing with a fetus to be aborted what one would likewise do or refrain from doing with a fetus to be delivered.

In the Commission discussions of this issue, most members favored a policy in which, if the research carried some risk but was acceptable to offer to fetuses to be carried to term, initial studies could be offered selectively to fetuses scheduled for abortion. However, if the research involves learning to do something new in prenatal diagnosis that carries a risk of fetal loss, should one *begin* to learn equally with both classes of fetuses or only with those to be aborted? The Commission's report (p. 67) admitted this moral dilemma, and left it unresolved with the further potential of national review:

> There is basic agreement among Commission members as to the validity of the equality principle. There is disagreement as to its application to individual fetuses and classes of fetuses. Anticipating that differences of interpretation will arise over the application of the basic principles of equality and the determination of 'minimal risk,' the Commission recommends review at the national level . . . the appropriate forum for determination of the scientific and public merit of such research. In addition, such review would facilitate public discussion of the sensitive issues surrounding the use of vulnerable nonconsenting subjects in research.

Thus the Commission intended the already intact system of independent local IRBs with the addition of one national Ethics Advisory Board as the *necessary* means to nurture and maintain the complex moral consensus they achieved.

The Ethics Advisory Board

The fetal research guidelines were adopted as federal regulations on July 29, 1975. These regulations also required that proposals involving *in vitro* fertilization (IVF) be reviewed by an EAB which, among other duties, would advise the Secretary as to their acceptability. An EAB was not chartered until 1977, and not convened until 1978, so a *de facto* moratorium continued on federal support for fetal research involving minimal risks and also on IVF.

Meanwhile, in 1977, the NIH received an application for support of IVF research, which was approved by study section. In May 1978, the EAB agreed to review the proposal and the EAB published its recommendations and forwarded them to the Secretary in May 1979. Louise Brown, the first infant born after IVF and embryo transfer (ET), was delivered in July of the same year. The EAB recommended that DHEW support research involving IVF-ET to establish the safety and efficacy of the technique when used for the treatment of infertility.[14] Conditions placed upon approval included IRB approval, informed consent, a fourteen-day limit for susbtaining embryos *in vitro,* and the use of gametes obtained only from lawfully married couples. These recommendations have yet to be approved by any of the subsequent DHHS Secretaries and no federal support of IVF research can yet be allowed.

The EAB considered only one proposal for fetal research after implantation. In 1978, investigators from the Charles R. Drew Postgraduate Medical School planned to assess the safety of fetoscopy for prenatal diagnosis of hemoglobinopathies in pregnant women who had elected abortion for reasons unrelated to the research. Working with data obtained from the earliest use of fetoscopy in the U.S., the EAB evaluated a situation in which the risk of fetal loss was estimated to be at least 5 percent but was essentially unknown. The EAB did not insist on a rigorous application of the equality maxim in this case. Because of the importance of the biomedical information, unobtainable by any other method, the EAB recommended a waiver of provisions of the regulations involving minimal risk.[15] The EAB also stipulated that the timing of the planned abortions was not to be altered by the research. Secretary Califano granted such a waiver for this single research project in September 1979, but took no action on an EAB recommendation for generic waiver for fetoscopy studies. Later in 1979, the first definitive review of the risk of fetal loss after fetoscopy showed that an initial rate of 10 percent might not be too high.[16]

A second fetoscopy proposal would have reached the EAB but did not. In 1980 NICHD's National Advisory Council approved funding for a proposal from the University of California at San Francisco to obtain fetal blood samples from controls in a study of prenatal diagnosis in three genetic disorders (severe combined immunodeficiency disease, Wiskott-Aldrich syndrome, and glycogen storage disease, Type I). Fetal blood would be obtained by fetoscopy concurrently with abortion at mid-trimester to establish the feasibility of using fetal red blood cells for prenatal diagnosis of these disorders. However, the EAB was allowed to lapse by Secretary Harris when its charter and funding expired on September 30, 1980. No national review could be done, and the research has not been able to proceed. Mitchell Golbus, the principal investigator, says that his research on prenatal diagnosis for these disorders has been "seriously restricted" by lack of access to an EAB review in the same department where approval for his project was achieved.[17]

Fetal Research Today

We recently reviewed 183 research projects on high-risk pregnancies and fetal pathophysiology supported by NICHD, the primary source of federal support for fetal research. Other than two studies that employ ultrasound and one with antibiotic therapy, we could not find an example of human fetal research that approached the threshold of minimal risk. The latter study focuses on the question of whether bacterial infections in the female genital and urinary tracts cause premature labor and whether treatment with antibiotics prevents early labor. Studies of why labor starts suggest that an enzyme, phospholipase A2, that may stimulate contractions, could also be released by bacteria that cause genitourinary infections. Subjects will be women in the sixth month of pregnancy with any of three bacterial organisms but no other symptoms. Half will be treated with an antibiotic and half with a placebo until the thirty-eighth week of pregnancy or delivery, whichever occurs first, followed by assessment of the effect of treatment on prematurity and the infant's health.

In one of the ultrasound studies, the technique is being evaluated as a predictive test for respiratory distress syndrome (RDS) following delivery. In the second, it used to study fetal heart, lung, and other functions as responses to hypoxia and the effects of smoking in pregnancy. In 1984 an NIH consensus development panel on diagnostic ultrasound imaging concluded that because some biological effects had been observed after ultrasound exposure in various experimental systems, the question of risks deserved more study than that "Data on clinical efficiency and safety do not allow a recommendation for routine screening at this time."[18] However, the panel listed twenty-seven clinically indicated uses of ultrasound, some of which parallel the uses in these two studies. By the standards set out by the panel, ultrasound examination falls well within the meaning of minimal risk applied to fetuses that may be at higher risk for RDS or for harms due to smoking. However, it would be more difficult, within current regulations, to test ultrasound for safety in studies with presumably healthy fetuses, since the examination can be challenged as a "routine" procedure for the fetus. Thus, some issues of minimal risks from questionably routine tests can only be settled by long-term studies of children who did and did not have such examinations.

All the other fetal pathophysiological studies currently funded by NICHD use animals. The high-risk pregnancy studies use only observational or health education techniques, for example, following the pregnancies of diabetic mothers for malformations or losses, and assisting the District of Columbia to identify mothers at risk for babies with low birthweight. These mothers are then given education and encouragement to stay in prenatal care.

Since 1980 some significant developments have occurred in fetal research. The single thread that runs through the story is that no initiatives in fetal research involving minimal risk have been federally conducted or supported, except for the ultrasound and antibiotic studies cited above, and one case of experimental fetal therapy cited below.

Fetal Therapy

Experimental fetal surgery has been successfully used in a few centers to correct fetal obstructive uropathy and obstructive hydrocephalus, and will likely be tried soon for diagrammatic hernia.[19] The initial plans were approved by local IRBs and financially supported by the institution or patient fees. Investigators in this new field published guidelines, including ethical considerations, for experimental fetal surgery.[20] Criteria for patient selection and a multidisciplinary team satisfied the "appropriate medical standards" required by the regulations.

Investigators in the NICHD attempted innovative steroid therapy for congenital adrenal hyperplasia in one pregnancy.[21] Their findings confirmed the feasibility of this therapy. The process for institutional review and bioethical consultation for this NIH case was also reported.[22]

Prenatal Diagnosis

The most significant advance since amniocentesis is chorionic villus sampling (CVS). With CVS, cells genetically identical to fetal cells can be obtained for study and diagnosis without puncture of the uterus and amniotic sac. CVS is usually done today between nine and eleven weeks of pregnancy.[23]

Guided by ultrasound, the physician inserts a plastic or metal cannula into the cervix and directs it to the *chorion frondosum*, a villous part of the embryonic membrane that enters the developing placenta. Small amounts of tissue are removed for direct analysis of chromosomes or subsequent tests for other genetic disorders. The early timing of CVS is a major advantage, because in most cases the negative result relieves the anxiety of parents at higher risk much sooner than is possible with amniocentesis. After a positive finding, usually followed by an elective abortion, the early timing avoids the higher physical and emotional risks of mid-trimester abortion. Emotional and moral differences between earlier and later abortion for genetic reasons also need careful study. The emotionally painful experience for mother and family of later abortions after amniocentesis has been well documented.[24]

Physicians in the U.S. brought CVS through an early research stage into the first phase of clinical practice without any federal support, although their initial studies were approved locally by IRBs. A few investigators working in states with laws banning any nontherapeutic research on the fetus to be aborted used cases of blighted ovum for the earliest studies. However, most of the initial feasibility studies obtained villi for diagnosis in the context of elective abortions. Women who had decided for first-trimester abortions were asked to participate in the research only after the procedure had been scheduled. Other than anecdotal reports, we have no record of IRB discussion of research risks to these fetuses to be aborted, or what frame of reference was used to discuss such risks. We suspect that the equality maxim could not have been applied literally in the actual choices made. The fact that CVS was already being widely used in Europe for diagnostic cases might have helped to balance the choice to allow physicians to learn to do a procedure that would eventually be beneficial to pregnant women. First-trimester diagnosis also carries a potential for earlier and more effective fetal therapy for some conditions. Presumably IRB members felt that CVS research was ethically acceptable within the intent of the regulations.

If an EAB had been available for national review of an application for early CVS research, the scientific and ethical considerations could have been shared, and perhaps improved, by many more persons. Further, the fetal regulations could have been put to another test, especially on the relevant framework for nontherapeutic research involving "minimal risk" for the human fetus. But no applications for federal support were made for three reasons. First, investigators knew an EAB review would be needed to waive "minimal risk" considerations by an EAB that did not exist. Second, they could proceed with IRB approval alone without federal support. Third, they felt a need to move promptly to evaluate a method of diagnosis already being requested by patients.

How would an EAB have evaluated the risks of CVS to the fetus to be aborted and the value of the information to be gained? Data were scanty in the U.S. at the time (1982–1983), but publications about use in diagnostic cases were out from China,[25] the Soviet Union,[26] Great Britain,[27] and available from Italy.[28] The risk of fetal loss was probably below what a previous EAB had approved in fetoscopy studies. Even without this precedent, a series of phased feasibility *and* early diagnostic studies could have been appproved in the interest of speeding delivery of a test that might benefit the health of mothers in the highest risk groups by providing early diagnosis. If an EAB took only fetal interests into account and used the equality maxim rigorously, the only feasibility study that could have been approved would have had to involve both fetuses to be aborted and fetuses at risk for genetic disorders randomly in the same study.

We believe, at the point of considering this alternative, an EAB would have considered its earlier willingness first to expose fetuses to be aborted followed by fetuses to be delivered in the same study series. In the debate, opportunities would have arisen to examine the concept of minimal risk with more specificity to fetal research. It seems to us inherently contradictory to derive a definition of minimal risk in a framework intended to apply to healthy *individuals* after birth, and to use the same definition in the context of the fetal-maternal unit. A more fitting and clearer definition is needed, based on presumably healthy mothers and fetuses, in the context of a "normal" pregnancy. However, only by constant examination of the shortcomings of the present expression of minimal risk in the light of actual research choices will the regulations be refined and improved.

What is known about the risks of fetal loss from CVS? Laird Jackson maintains a voluntary registry of fetal loss following CVS in diagnostic cases. At last report from 46 centers in Europe, Canada, and the U.S., a total of 4,054 diagnostic procedures had been done (1,609) deliveries with a maximum fetal loss rate of 4.1 percent.[29] Some fetal losses due to spontaneous abortions that would occur anyway and losses due to CVS are mixed in this figure. In the most experienced centers, like Jefferson Medical College, the loss rate is less than 2 percent (1.8 percent).

By a cooperative agreement, NICHD is now supporting the costs of data collection in a seven-center randomized trial to compare the safety and accuracy of CVS with amniocentesis.[30] Most patients to be enrolled will be women between the age of 35 and 39 whose pregnancies are at higher risk for chromosomal disorders. The patients will be randomized; those who do not agree to randomization will choose the procedure they prefer and will be included in some phases of the study. The costs of the procedures will be reimbursed by patient fees. This study, now in a stage in which patients are being admitted, will require about three years to complete.

Testing maternal serum for elevated levels of alpha-fetoprotein (AFP), an indication for higher risk of neural tube defects, began in Great Britain in the late 1970s in conjunction with analysis of AFP in amniotic fluid for a definitive fetal diagnosis. Although tests are now widely used here, no systematic study to evaluate the feasibility or safety of AFP screening in prenatal diagnosis was ever conducted in the United States. Indeed, a delay of several years took place in Food and Drug Administration action to release the test kits for commercial production. AFP-testing in maternal serum is an example of a significant step in prenatal diagnosis being introduced after exceptional delay and yet paradoxically without adequate studies of the capacity and competence of genetic centers to deliver the counseling and follow-up required.

Prevention of Birth Defects

Following encouraging but inconclusive reports in 1977 from Great Britain that vitamin supplementation around the time of conception reduces the recurrence of neural tube defects, a placebo-controlled randomized trial was begun there to answer the question conclusively.[31] One arm of the trial involved a dose of folic acid (a vitamin in the B vitamin complex) more than five times higher than the recommended daily allowance in pregnancy. Among the investigators who most favor a trial in the U.S. is Godfrey Oakley, Jr., of the Centers for Disease Control (CDC). Ethical issues in a proposed trial were extensively debated in NICHD; the agency was open to a trial that would involve only women at higher risk who had not taken vitamins and were not taking them at the time of recruitment.[32]

Oakley and others who favor a trial take the position that since current scientific evidence is not strong enough to support recommending vitamins to all women before conception, the most ethically desirable alternative is to conduct a trial. At this stage, CDC and the Spina Bifida Association of America have begun a collaborative study of the feasibility of conducting the trial. In particular, they will evaluate various recruitment mechanisms to determine how best to recruit subjects, and make a determination as to whether a full-scale trial is possible in the U.S.

Does the proposed trial, if feasible, meet the requirements of federal regulations? Two provisions apply here. First an IRB would have to determine that the fetuses on the higher dosage vitamin arm of the trial meet the requirements of 46.208 (a) (1) if that arm was seen to present greater than minimal risk: that is, would inclusion in this arm meet the health needs of the particular fetus? Second, an IRB would have to determine that the fetuses in the placebo arm met the requirements of 46.208 (a) (2), that is, that no greater than minimal risk was involved and that important biomedical knowledge was a likely outcome which could not be obtained in another way. Exact knowledge to answer these objections is unavailable. Indeed, the trial is designed to seek information about dose relationships and recurrence rates. Literally applied, the regulations appear to prevent a trial that seeks scientific information in the context of a *possibly* therapeutic trial.

In our view, the best position from which to apply the regulations to the proposed trial is one that allows some attention to early, favorable results in uncontrolled trials but includes true uncertainty as to whether vitamin-taking around the time of conception will prove to reduce the recurrence of neural tube defects or do harm to the fetus at the higher dosage when rigorously tested. On this view, since the trial is at least partly designed to "meet the health needs" of fetuses at higher risk for neural tube defects by testing the only mode of prevention other than abortion, and since the trial will distribute the risks (if any) equally to all fetuses in the trial (by random chance), each particular fetus will be placed at risk "only to the minimum extent necessary to meet such needs" [46.208 (a)]. We note, however, how difficult it is to study for the first time an important question that may involve ventures over the boundary of minimal risk.

Research with Fetuses Ex Utero, Including Nonviable Fetuses

A pressing long-range problem in fetal research is the development of methods to sustain the previable fetus (the spontaneous abortus less than twenty-four weeks) *ex utero* until it develops to the point of sufficient maturity for independent survival. These methods might be considered the development of an artificial uterine environment in the broadest sense, including the "artificial placenta" or new techniques to perfuse directly the previable fetus with nutrients or oxygen. Any work of this type, if successful, will be life-saving in cases of extreme prematurity. To *learn* to do such work and to test the technology would require research with nonviable fetuses, in our view, since it would be ethically objectionable to subject a possible viable fetus to totally unproven techniques.

To carry out this research runs counter to [42.209 (b) (1)], "no nonviable fetus may be involved as a subject . . . unless vital functions of the fetus will not be artificially maintained."

In our view, the regulations go too far in an effort to prevent recurrence of nontherapeutic research with nonviable fetuses that had no relevance to potential therapy. The nonviable fetus to be studied to "develop important biomedical knowledge which cannot be obtained by any other means" [46.209 (b) (3)] and which is clearly related to potentially life-saving therapy, should be anesthetized and the fetal experiment terminated at a specific predetermined point.

IVF

In testimony before Congress in August 1984, Gary Hodgen, Scientific Director of the Jones Institute for Reproductive Medicine in Norfolk, Va., summarized progress in IVF research. Hodgen, an expert in pregnancy and fertility research who resigned from the NIH in part because of the lack of opportunity to study human IVF, reported that the number of children born as a result of IVF-ET therapy exceeded 700 and more than 300 pregnancies were ongoing.[33] Over 200 IVF programs have been established, with perhaps fifty of these in the United States. No federal funds have been expended on research concerning the efficacy and safety of IVF-ET in its actual use. However, the first detailed follow-up study of children born after IVT-ET will be done with federal support. NICHD will soon begin such a project, through contract with a major IVF program.

Hodgen's statement about research goals with IVF included: (1) monitoring the safety and reliability of methods to freeze, store, and thaw human embryos for later transfer to infertile women, which avoids laparoscopy and prevents destruction of embryos already fertilized; (2) developing a safe method to freeze human eggs, since between five and ten can be obtained from most patients; (3) overcoming male infertility caused by oligospermia (too few living sperms) by IVF with induced fusion of egg and sperm or microsurgical placement of sperm in ooplasm; (4) developing tests predictive of the normalcy of each fertilized embryo, to avoid the risk of multiple pregnancies caused by implanting several embryos; (5) diagnosing chromosomal and/or genetic disorders in the preimplantation embryo; and (6) studying cell messengers in human embryos and their relation to normal embryonic genes, oncogenes, and development of cancer.

Officially appointed bodies were established in Great Britain[34] and Victoria, Australia,[35] to review ethical, legal, and social considerations of IVF research with preimplantation human embryos that were not to be transferred. Both recommended research that would restrict studies to a limit of fourteen days after fertilization. The EAB report of 1979 anticipated this issue in allowing for research with fertilized embryos not used for ET. "The Board believes that such research, if performed as a corollary to research designed primarily to establish safety and efficacy of IVT-ET, would also be acceptable from an ethical standpoint" (EAB Report, p. 108). The EAB report also anticipated but did not take up the issue of fertilizing human ova for the purpose of research.

Clearly, an officially appointed national body in the United States needs to consider these questions in the context of our legal, ethical, and social traditions. The ideal group would be a newly convened EAB. A decision memorandum regarding establishment of an EAB is awaiting Secretarial approval. The former Assistant Secretary for Health, Edward Brandt, prior to his recent departure from office, recommended creation of an EAB. A new EAB should be asked, as its first assignment, to establish criteria according to which the Department will support research on human embryos not to be transferred.

The Consequences of Inaction

Federal regulations on fetal research are ethically sound and widely respected by investigators. For a variety of reasons having to do with political and social conflict about the moral status of the human embryo and the fetus, federal support for an ethical review of research with virtually *any* risk to the human fetus ended in 1980 and has not resumed. The dangers of such a situation, foreseen by the framers of the guidelines, have already clearly emerged.

We close by simply listing some serious consequences of this situation and the policy choices before those who can change it.

First, a gulf has been created between local and national considerations of fetal research. The gulf is harmful to science and ethics. The NIH is being prevented, to quote Hodgen's testimony, from its "natural roles . . . in peer review of research, debate of relevant scientific, ethical and legal issues, and provision of funding for research excellence. . . ."

Second, support for fetal research has been divided. Research with risks to the fetus or mother is supported in the "private" realm. Unquestionably safe research is supported by federal sources. In no other realm of medicine and science does this situation exist. In effect, by the absence of an expert national review body for just such guidance, federal authorities cannot support research that may involve acceptable risks, as defined by federal guidelines, to achieve gains on behalf of seriously affected groups and individuals. Families at higher genetic risk, fetuses at higher risk, pregnant women, and infertile couples are being deprived of the potential benefits of research on problems that affect their life chances. The distribution of the benefits of federally supported research has become unjust in the process and, in our view, needs correction.

Third, the absence of an EAB has many unfortunate consequences. Missing is the mechanism seen by the Commission as vital for resolving conflicts of scientific opinion and ethical differences too great for any local IRB to assume. The public, broadly considered, is deprived of participation in choices of great significance. Further, if federal policies on research with human subjects are understood as a moral code, it is necessary to keep their provisions under critical evaluation. Moral codes that cannot be tested and examined in the light of actual choices usually wither and die, because they lose relevance to ever new scientific questions. A new EAB needs to be appointed to keep the specifics of the protections for human subjects under critical review. An EAB is also needed to implement the public partnership between national and local institutions that undergirded the original policy formulated in 1966 to require prior ethical review of research.[36]

Fourth, if and when an EAB is assembled, two provisions of the regulations on fetal research need careful study. A definition of minimal risk, with pregnancy, healthy mothers, and "normal" fetuses as its frame of reference, needs to be drafted and debated in an open public forum. Moreover, the fetal research guidelines need to be reexamined in the light of the potential for fetal therapy and its relation to fetal diagnosis. The Commission report was drafted in a climate of concern to protect fetuses that were to be aborted. Now that more therapeutic possibilities are available, more risks might be allowed in early therapeutically designed studies. We include in this concern the research required to learn to save and nurture babies so small and compromised that they hover between the borderline of viable and nonviable.

After a period of almost ten years since the Commission debates, the ethics of fetal research needs to be reexamined by an Ethics Advisory Board, in the context of current possibilities in research from fertilization to delivery.

NOTES

1. Title 45, Code of Federal Regulations, Part 46—Protection of Human Subjects, Subpart B-Additional Protections Pertaining to Research Development, and Related Activities Involving Fetuses, Pregnant Women, and Human In Vitro Fertilization (revised as of March 8, 1983).
2. Paul Ramsey, *The Ethics of Fetal Research* (New Haven: Yale University Press, 1975), pp. 1–20.
3. Steven Maynard-Moody, "Fetal Research Dispute," in Dorothy Nelkin (ed.), *Controversy: Politics of Technical Decisions* (Beverly Hills, CA: Sage Publications, 1979), pp. 197–211.
4. Andre E. Hellegers, "Fetal Research," in Warren T. Reich (ed). *Encyclopedia of Bioethics* (New York: The Free Press, 1978), pp. 489–93; also, Robert J. Levine, *Ethics and Regulation of Clinical Research* (Baltimore: Urban & Schwarzenberg 1981), pp. 197–206.
5. Diana Copsey and Marion Gold, "NIH Ethics Policy Near on Fetal Research," *Ob-Gyn News* (April 15, 1973), p. Al. Cases of objectionable fetal research were collected in a broad, objective review by Maurice J. Mahoney, "The Nature and Extent of Research Involving Living Human Fetuses," in *Appendix, Research on the Fetus* (Washington, D.C.: U.S. Government Printing Office, 1976), 1-1/1-48. DHEW Publication No. (OS) 76-128. The decline in the field of fetal research can be measured by the fact that a review of the excellence of Mahoney's has not since appeared.

6. Victor Cohn, "NIH Vows Not to Fund Fetus Work," *Washington Post* (April 13, 1973), p. A1.
7. National Commission for the Protection of Human Subjects of Biomedical and Behavioral Research, *Report and Recommendations. Research on the Fetus* (Washington, D.C.: ULSL Government Printing Office, 1975) DHEW Publication No. (OS) 76-127, pp. 61–88.
8. Department of Health and Social Security. *Report of the Advisory Group. The Use of Fetuses and Fetal Material for Research* (London: Her Majesty's Stationery Office 1972); the Peel Commission Report.
9. National Institutes of Health, "Protection of Human Subjects, Policies and Procedures," *Federal Register* 38 (Nov. 16, 1973), pp. 31738–49.
10. Collected in *Appendix*, cited at ref. 5.
11. Richard A. McCormick, "Experimentation on the Fetus: Policy Proposals," in *Appendix*, 8-1/8-17.
12. LeRoy Walters, "Ethical and Public Policy Issues in Fetal Research," in *Appendix*, 8-1/8-17.
13. Commission, *Research Involving Children: Report and Recommendations*, DHEW Publication No. (OS) 77-0004, 1977; the specific reference to the earliest definition of minimal risk in *Federal Register* 40:33529, 1975.
14. Ethics Advisory Board of the U.S. Department of Health, Education and Welfare, "Report and Conclusions: DHEW Support of Research Involving In Vitro Fertilization and Embryo Transfer," (May 4, 1979); also, *Federal Register* 44:35, 1979.
15. Margaret Steinfels, "At the EAB, Same Members, New Ethical Problems," *Hastings Center Report* 5 (October, 1979), p. 2.
16. R. Benzie, M.J. Mahoney, D.V.I. Fairweather, *et al.*, "Fetoscopy and Fetal Tissue Sampling," in John L. Hamerton and Nancy E. Simpson (eds.), Report of an International Workshop, *Prenatal Diagnosis* (Special Issue, December 1980), p. 32.
17. Personal Communication, December 17, 1984.
18. National Institutes of Health Consensus Development Conference, *Consensus Development Statement*, Vol. 5 (No. 1), 1984, Question 4. Available from Office of Medical Applications of Technology, Building 1, Room 216, NIH, Bethesda, MD 20205.
19. Michael R. Harrison, Mitchell S. Golbus, and Roy A. Filly, *Unborn Patient* (Orlando, FL: Grune & Stratton, 1984).

20. Michael R. Harrison, Roy A. Filly, Mitchell S. Golbus, et al., "Fetal Treatment 1982," *New England Journal of Medicine*, 307 (December 23, 1982), 1651–52.

21. Mark I. Evans, George P. Chrousos, Dean Mann, et al., "Pharmacological Suppression of the Fetal Adrenal Gland in Utero: Attempted Prevention of Abnormal External Genital Masculinization in Suspected Congenital Adrenal Hyperplasia," 253 (Feb. 15, 1985), 1015–1020 *Journal of the American Medical Association.*

22. John C. Fletcher, "Emerging Ethical Issues in Fetal Therapy," in Kare Berg and Knut Erik Tranoy, *Research Ethics* (New York: Alan R. Liss, Inc., 1983), pp. 309–11.

23. Bruno Brambati, Giuseppe Simoni, and S. Fabro (eds), *Fetal Diagnosis During the First Trimester* (1985) Marcel Dekker, Inc.

24. Three studies have appeared in the literature. The latest is the most extensively documented. B.D. Blumberg, M.S. Golbus and K.H. Hanson, "The Psychological Sequalae of Abortion Performed for a Genetic Indication," *American Journal of Obstetrics and Gynecology*, 122 (1975), 799–808; P. Donnai, N. Charles, and N. Harris, "Attitudes of Patients After 'Genetic' Termination of Pregnancy," *British Medical Journal,* 282 (1981), 621–22; N.J. Leschot, M. Verjaal and J. H. Leschot, On Prenatal Diagnosis (Doctoral Dissertation, Rodopi, University of Amsterdam, 1982), pp. 96–111.

25. Anshan Department of Obstetrics and Gynecology, "Fetal Sex Prediction by Sex Chromatin of Chorionic Villi Cells During Early Pregnancy," *Clinical Medical Journal* (1975), 117–126.

26. Z. Kazy, I.S. Rozovsky, and V. Bakharev, "Chorion Biopsy in Early Pregnancy," *Prenatal Diagnosis* 2 (1982), 39–45.

27. R.H.T. Ward, B. Modell, et al., "Method of Sampling Chorionic Villi in First Trimester of Pregnancy Under Guidance of Real Time Ultrasound," *British Medical Journal* 286 (1983), 1542.

28. G. Simoni, B. Brambati, C. Danesino, et al., "Diagnostic Application of First Trimester Trophoblast Sampling in 100 Pregnancies," *Human Genetics*, 66 (1984), 252–59.

29. Laird Jackson (ed.), "CVS Newsletter," February 5, 1985, p. 2.

30. Virginia Cowart, "NIH Considers Large-Scale Study to Evaluate Chorionic Villi Sampling," *Journal of the American Medical Association* 252 (July 6, 1984), 11–15.

31. R.W. Smithells, S. Sheppard, and C.J. Schorah, et al.,
    "Possible Prevention of Neural Tube Defects by Periconceptual
    Vitamin Supplementation," *Lancet* 1 (1980), 339–34.
32. Mortimer B. Lipsett and John C. Fletcher, "Do Vitamins
    Prevent Neural Tube Defects (And Can We Find Out Ethi-
    cally)?" *Hastings Center Report* (August 1983), pp. 5–8.
33. Gary D. Hodgen, "Testimony Before Subcommittee on
    Investigations and Oversight," Committee on Science and Tech-
    nology, U.S. House of Representatives, (August 8, 1984);
    Jeffrey L. Fox, "Scientist Quits NIH Over Fetal Rules,"
    Science 223 (March 2, 1984), 916.
34. Department of Health and Social Security, *Report on the
    Committee of Inquiry into Human Fertilization and Embryology*
    (London: Her Majesty's Stationery Office 1984), p. 84.
35. Victoria, Committee to Consider the Social, Ethical, and
    Legal Issues Arising From In Vitro Fertilization, *Report on
    the Disposition of Embryos Produced by In Vitro Fertilization*
    (Melbourne: F.D. Atkinson Government Printer, August
    1984), p. 60.
36. Surgeon General, Public Health Service, Department of
    Health, Education and Welfare, "Investigations Involving
    Human Subjects, Including Clinical Research: Requirements
    for Review to Insure the Rights and Welfare of Individuals,"
    PPO 129, Revised Policy, July 1, 1966.

Moral Obligations and the Fallacies of "Genetic Control"

Marc Lappé, Ph.D.

THE sciences of molecular biology and human genetics emerged within my own lifetime. Partly as a consequence of the development of these two sciences, my generation was the first to become swept up in what we now recognize as "The Biological Revolution." What made genetics "revolutionary" is that it was transformed from a science whose content was discernible only by inference, to one which seemingly could be known with certainty: the discovery which made the unknown knowable was made the year I was born.

Chance Events and the Myth of Genetic Certainty

In 1943, Oswald Avery wrote his brother Roy to describe his findings about a physiological principle which appeared to be able to confer the properties of virulence to a bacterium. The excited tone of his letter reflected the utter incredulity that Avery must have felt upon learning the outcome of his experiments: a *chemical* had made it possible to induce predictable and heritable changes in living cells. Genes were molecules! As

From *Theological Ethics*, Vol. 33, No. 3, Sept., 1972. Reprinted by permission of *Theological Ethics*.

such they were subject to human control and manipulation. Avery wrote: "This is something which has long been the dream of geneticists. . . . [Up until now] the mutations they induced . . . are always unpredictable and random and chance changes."[1]

Although Avery was mistaken in his assumption that this knowledge would allow us generally to control where and when mutations occur, he was correct in concluding that his discovery revolutionized our ability potentially to control what specific genetic information a cell contained or expressed. Thus, when he discovered the molecular basis for a "transforming principle," he simultaneously acquired the ability to effect genetic transformations. The phenomenon by which the acquisition of knowledge per se changes that which has become known (or affords the potential for such change) represents a subtle mechanism by which genetic information (as well as much other knowledge in science) escapes the moral scrutiny of its possessors. Hans Jonas perceptively observed:

> Effecting changes in nature as a means and as a result of knowing it are inextricably interlocked, and once this combination is at work it no longer matters whether the pragmatic destination of theory is expressly accepted . . . or not. The very process of attaining knowledge leads through manipulation of the things to be known, and this origin fits of itself the theoretical results for an application whose possibility is irresistible . . . whether or not it was contemplated in the first place.[2]

In Avery's case, he might well have foreseen that transformation could be used to confer virulence to normally nonpathogenic bacteria, but he certainly could not have anticipated that his principle, in conjunction with the later to be discovered "R" factors, would be used to make potent, antibiotic resistant biological warfare agents![3] But the prospect of nefarious application is *not* what makes genetic knowledge unique. Rather, its uniqueness lies in the manner in which "knowing" the genetics of something changes it.

For example, the simple act of acquiring prenatal genetic information about a fetus—whether or not he is carrying a particular gene, or if he will develop a genetically determined disease later in his life—automatically gets into motion a train of events which themselves change that individual's future. At the very moment you acquire a "bit" of genetic information about a fetus (or any person, for that matter), you have begun to define him in entirely novel terms. You tell him (and sometimes others) something about where he came from and who is responsible for what he is now. You project who he may or may not become in the future. You set certain limits on his potential. You say something about what his children will be like, and whether or not he will be encouraged or discouraged to think of himself as a parent. In this way the information you obtain changes both the individual who possesses it, and in turn the future of that information itself.

In addition to the potential for individual stigmatization, there is also sufficient ambiguity in genetic "facts" themselves to seriously question the judiciousness of massive operations designed to ascertain the genetic composition of whole populations. In contrast to the simplistic view of genetics in Avery's time, we now know that genetic information, by its very nature, tends to confound rational analysis. It is *redundant,* such that a flaw in replication or a mutational event need not irrevocably distort or destroy (as had previously been assumed) the information contained in the genetic material. It is *self-correcting,* containing enzymes whose sole function is to recognize damaged segments of DNA molecules, excise them, and faithfully reconstruct the whole (thereby compelling reconsideration of estimations of mutation rates and their causes). It is *heterogeneous,* with most seemingly "single" genes being in fact clusters of genes with related functions ("pleiotrophy") or products ("alleles," or "pseudalleles"), each gene having the potential property of producing different effects in different organs at different times in development (frustrating any simplistic analysis of whether or not a single gene or many is responsible for a given complex constellation of developmental defects).

These observations begin to explain why at the human level, for example, medical researchers have been at a loss to explain why some individuals who by all measurements have the defective genes for phenylketonuria[4] do *not* in fact show the physical stigmata of the condition. If, as apears likely, this genetic "defeat" (and perhaps the one responsible for the related condition galactosemia) is not an "all or none" phenomenon, but can actually be compensated for by the operation of other genes, all of our assumptions about the nature of such genes, *and* our moral decisions of what should be done in the event that an individual is discovered with them, have to be seriously reassessed. The fact that this reassessment is *not* currently going on reflects, I believe, an underlying cultural bias that affects our analyses of genetic problems. It is not just that we want simple answers to complex questions; it is that we would like to be able to *control* a material whose nature eludes our dominion.

Intolerance for Uncertainty and the Quest for Genetic Control

If genetic systems are so inherently difficult to understand, why do we feel impelled to seek to control them? The problem appears to be rooted in our Western psyche and philosophical assumptions about the use of knowledge. Avery's letter gives us a sense of the deep-seated aversion most Western scientists (and philosophers) feel towards the chance events that appear to govern genetic systems. (Recall Avery's mistaken assumption that he had discovered the means to *control* the class of events we call "random mutations," when in fact he had merely discovered an analogue for one specific mutational event.)

Joseph Fletcher, an ethicist, echoes this profound disquiet towards uncertainty in genetic systems when he states: "We cannot accept the 'invisible hand' of blind chance or random nature in genetics."[5] An implicit assumption in Fletcher's remarks is that the reduction of uncertainty is equivalent to progress, a view widely held in the West.[6] In genetic systems, the paradox is that progress (in this sense evolutionary progress) is accomplished *because* of genetic instability and susceptibility to chance events, not in spite of it.

James Crow, a renowned population geneticist, has described the operation of chance in sexual reproduction by pointing out that "In a sexual population, genotypes are formed and broken up by recombination every generation, and a particular genotype

is therefore evanescent: what is transmitted to the next generation is a sample of genes, not a [whole] genotype."[7] It is
difficult to reconcile evolutionary progress with this image alone,
since Crow omits (by intention, I am sure) discussion of the
mechanisms by which variation is introduced into sexual populations. Faced with the reality of incessant fluctuation and change
of genetic systems, the Nobel laureate geneticist Joshua Lederberg
asked at one point: "If a superior individual . . . is identified,
why not copy it directly, rather than suffer all the risks of
recombinational disruption, including those of sex? . . . Leave
sexual reproduction for experimental purposes; when a suitable
type is ascertained, take care to maintain it by clonal propagation."[8]

If from Avery's day scientists believed they had discovered
the means to control the transmission of hereditary information, why does Joshua Lederberg believe that the only real
means of control for man would be to clone him? The answer in
part is that the kinds of control which were possible in bacteria
thirty years ago remain an illusive quest for human organisms
today. Not only is cloning a distant and limited prospect for
man, but so is the much-vaunted genetic engineering which
would precede it. Mammalian cells, unlike bacterial ones, appear to be extraordinarily resistant to the introduction of most
forms of genetic information. Although reports have appeared
indicating that bacterial viral genes will function after being
introduced into human cells in tissue culture[9] (a feat proving
difficult to replicate), enormous difficulties remain in attempting to use the same techniques actually to treat individuals with
the genetic defect that the virus appears to correct. Another
technique for correcting "defective genes" also appears to pose
currently insuperable problems for human application. It entails
fusing or "hybridizing" a cell lacking a particular gene with one
containing the active equivalent.[10] This technique may prove to
be limited to tissue-culture studies, since the number of cells
needed to correct the same defect in a person would be astronomically large and the problem of immunologic acceptance of
the cells a thorny one.

While tantalizing in the control that such techniques appear
to promise for the future, there is a danger in their seductiveness
in the present. In the first place, they obfuscate the need for
solving current problems which do not need novel technical
solutions, such as general health care. Secondly, they pose the

threat of dehumanization that Jacques Ellul identifies with technique per se. Ellul observes that "When technique enters into every area of life, including the human, it ceases to be external to man and becomes his very substance. It is no longer face to face with man but is integrated with him, and it progressively absorbs him."[11] In the context of the above examples, Ellul would envision man's existence becoming dependent upon and inevitably indistinguishable from the vast array of artificially engineered genes and tissue-culture support systems needed to sustain him. More importantly, such techniques do not offer permanent solutions to human problems but merely transiently replace one technique (e.g., insulin for treating diabetes) with another (genetic engineering of Islets of Langerhans cells in the pancreas) for coping with man's medico-genetic dilemmas. Since none of these projected genetic techniques offer the prospect of the permanent change that can only be accomplished by changing the germ plasm itself, they offer only the illusion of changing man.

The "New" Eugenics and the "Old"

In presenting a scenario of genetically "engineering" man,[12] Lederberg and Fletcher believe that current knowledge of genetics mandates a new eugenics to meet pressing human needs. There are two points to be made about any such proposal: (1) Concern about effecting widespread genetic changes in a population is unwarranted, given existing demographic trends; but (2) the general *motivation* for proposing cloning or other engineering of man must be taken seriously, because it reveals a tacit approval by some of the best minds of the country for both the legitimacy and the need for introducing genetic controls.

To some geneticists, the recrudescence of a social concern for applied human genetics is mandated by an assumed or projected deterioration of the genetic quality of the species. They frankly admit that this concern must be properly construed as a "eugenic" one, but insist that it is based on hard facts. They maintain their concern is not tainted with the racial connotation that irrational eugenicists had applied in the past. Nevertheless,

both the basis for this concern—a progressive "genetic deterioration" of man—and the proposed remedy—a humane form of
"genetic counseling" or at an extreme "negative eugenics"—
actually are synonymous with the analyses of a hundred years
ago.

While Galton is the name usually associated with the "eugenics" movement of the late 1800's, it is actually Darwin whose
ideas have endured. Galton described the aim of eugenics[13] (a
word he coined) in blatantly racist, class-society terms. Its purpose was "to give the more suitable races or strains of blood a
better chance of prevailing speedily over the less suitable [races]
than they otherwise would have had."[14] Darwin, not Galton,
represented the more representative and "morally enlightened"
tone of the eugenics movement:

> With savages, the weak in body or mind are soon
> eliminated; and those that survive commonly exhibit a
> vigorous state of health. We civilized men, on the
> other hand, do our utmost to check the process of
> elimination; we build asylums for the imbecile, the
> maimed, and the sick; we institute poor-laws; and our
> medical men exert their utmost skill to save the life of
> everyone to the last moment. There is reason to be-
> lieve that vaccination has preserved thousands, who
> from a weak constitution would formerly have suc-
> cumbed to small pox. Thus the weak members of
> civilized society propagate their kind. No one who has
> attended to the breeding of domestic animals will doubt
> that this must be highly injurious to the race of man. It
> is surprising how soon want of care, or care wrongly
> directed leads to the degeneration of a domesticated
> race; but excepting in the case of man himself, hardly
> anyone is so ignorant as to allow his worst animals to
> breed. . . .
> The aid which we feel impelled to give to the help-
> less is mainly an incidental result of the instinct of
> sympathy, which was originally acquired as part of the
> social instincts, but subsequently rendered, in the man-
> ner previously indicated, more tender and more widely
> diffused. Nor could we check our sympathy, even at
> the urging of hard reason, without deterioration in the
> noblest part of our nature . . . if we were to neglect

the weak and helpless, it could only be for a contingent benefit, with an overwhelming present evil. *We must therefore bear the undoubtedly bad effects of the weak surviving and propagating their kind; but there appears to be at least one check in steady action, namely that the weaker and inferior members of society do not marry so freely as the sound; and this check might be infinitely increased by the weak in body or mind refraining from marriage, though this is more to be hoped for than expected.*[15]

"Expecting" the weak to refrain from marriage may strike us as a quaint nineteenth-century idea; but it faithfully echoes some contemporary statements of the value of "quasi-coercive" genetic counseling. There are some today who no longer "hope" but "expect" the weak in body and mind to refrain from marriage or its genetic equivalent, childbearing. A growing number of people use moral arguments to urge those who are genetically "handicapped" (and this may only mean individuals who *carry* but do not express aberrant genes) to fulfil their social responsibility by refraining from procreation.[16] This moral suasion is mistakenly based on the assumption that genetic deterioration of the species will be the inevitable consequence of the "unbridled" procreation of the unfit.

Moral Obligations in the Face of Genetic Realities

Darwin's focus on the moral dilemmas facing those who think they recognize a genetic basis for human suffering and feel impelled to act on this assumption has a contemporary ring. Theodosius Dobzhansky assessed the eugenic situation in 1961 in this Darwinian tradition: "We are then faced with a dilemma —if we enable the weak and the deformed to live and to propagate their kind, we face the prospect of a genetic twilight; but if we let them die or suffer when we can save them, we face the certainty of a moral twilight. How to escape this dilemma?"[17] Thus ten years ago, the moral problems were not posed in terms of the need for genetic improvement, but rather in terms of the need for societal protection against genetic deterioration. The genetic information which made such an analysis valid thirty or even ten years ago has been substantially amended today.

In the recent past, the chief proponent of the need for eugenic practice was Hermann Muller. In 1959 he stated: "If we fail to act now to eradicate genetic defects, the job of ministering to infirmities would come to consume all the energy that society could muster for it, leaving no surplus for general, cultural purposes."[18] Other, more contemporary authors have voiced similarly concerned if not alarmist views.[19]

While no one can conclusively refute the contention that *sometime* in the future we may have to come to grips with an increased incidence of genetically disabling disorders, it would have been extremely difficult to have made the case, even in 1959, for our moral obligations to act to anticipate them. As Martin Golding, in a review of genetic responsibility to future generations, concluded: "We are thus raising a question about our moral obligation to the community of the remote future. I submit that this relationship is far from clear, certainly less clear than our moral obligations to communities of the present. . . ."[20]

What actually is the "threat" posed to future generations (or, for that matter, to our very own children) by the specter of genetic deterioration? Golding and others appear to believe that current trends in medical treatment and protection of the "genetically unfit" condemn the future to suffer the weight of our omissions. He states, for example, that "the tragedy of the situation may be that we will have to reckon with the fact that the amelioration of short-term evils . . . and the promotion of good for the remote future are mutually exclusive alternatives."[21]

Part of the fallacy of this form of pessimism is the assumption that genes and genes alone are the only means by which we project ourselves into the future. Certainly, most anthropologists, when faced with the question of the most important way in which we influence the future, would emphasize the primacy of *cultural* factors in establishing human societies through time, because purely genetic trends are highly uncertain in fluctuating and migrating human populations.

The Fallacy of a Genetic Apocalypse

The other part of the fallacy is the assumption that we actually do face a genetically deteriorating situation. In the ten years since Dobzhansky originally posed the dilemma of a "genetic twilight," we have acquired enough information to enable us to draw back from the vision of a genetic apocalypse. Imminent "genetic deterioration" of the species is, for all intents and purposes, a red herring. The officers of the American Eugenics Society acknowledged this in a six-year report ending in 1970. In spite of the fact that they reaffirmed the long-range objective of the society to pursue the goal of maintaining or improving genetic potentialities of the human species, they stated that "neither present scientific knowledge, current genetic trends, nor social value justify coercive measures as applied to human reproduction." In fact, the officers wrote, "at this stage the need is for better identification of present and potential directions of changes rather than action to alter these trends in any major way."[22]

Our contemporary population is in a unique situation. The "gene pool" is in fact undergoing a period of stabilization, not change. In an analysis of the demographic trends characterizing the current population in the United States, Dudley Kirk observed that while the tremendous relaxation in the intensity of selection accomplished by modern medical achievements may be inexorably increasing the load of mutations the population carries, the over-all demographic trends are such as to reduce the number of children born with serious congenital abnormalities. He summarized his paper in the following way:

> A relaxation of selection intensity of the degree and durability now existing among Western and American peoples has surely never before been experienced by man. . . . In the short run, demographic trends (in and of themselves) are reducing the incidence of serious congenital anomalies. . . . In the foreseeable future, the possibility of medical and environmental correction of genetic defects will far outrun the effects of the growing genetic load.[23]

Demographic trends such as lowered average age of childbearing, smaller number of children, and the reduction of consanguineous marriages *themselves* effect dramatic changes in the quality of life experienced by the next generation. In the thirteen years between 1947 and 1960 when Japan instituted a revolutionary (if misleadingly termed) "Eugenic Protection Law," there was a ⅓ reduction in the number of children born with Mongolism and a ⅒ reduction in aggregate of all of the other major congenital abnormalities. This startling statistic was accomplished simply as a result of introducing legal abortion and encouraging smaller and earlier families.[24] A similar trend may well be expected in Western countries if we act to encourage the same *non*-genetic changes in our population. The data on the close relationship between higher maternal ages at birth, number of previous offspring, and the high incidence of such devastating congenital defects as anencephaly[25] and Mongolism make the moral imperative of recommending basic changes in childbearing patterns obvious. It is important to note that this kind of recommendation (for example, proscribing childbearing in women over thirty-five) has a universal basis, unlike proscriptions on individual childbearing for genetic reasons.

Societal vs. Individual Costs of Genetic Disease

Statistics such as these do not, however, tell us what specific moral questions are at stake for the future childbearing of individuals who themselves are born with a genetically determined disorder. Society's interest in this question acquires legitimacy only if it is true that society is paying an increasing social (not just monetary) cost for the offspring of the genetically unfit.

The origin of the notion of "social cost" is rooted in the assumption that the care extended by society to the "unfit," while morally desirable, cannot be accomplished without heavy burden. It is widely accepted, for example, that medical advances have contributed to our genetic load by permitting individuals who are born with genetically determined disorders to survive to childbearing age. Is this in fact the case? The answer appears to be that *some* advances in medicine may have this effect, but that on the whole medical practice is neither generating a race of Orwellian invalids requiring daily injections of insulin, enzymes, and other crucial but absent substances *nor* is it permitting a critical number of the truly "unfit" to procreate.[26] A key but unique case in point would be retinoblastoma, a treatable eye tumor which until recently was fatal. "Treatment" here is understood to entail enucleation of the eye, with an increasing residual risk of cancer elsewhere in the body even if initial surgery is successful. It is undeniable that the survival of individuals who can transmit the dominant mutant gene to their children poses grave moral problems to both the parents and society as a whole. Between 1930 and 1960 in the Netherlands, for example, the frequency of this dread cancer *doubled*, probably as a result of the procreation of survivors carrying the gene.[27] Another cogent example would be the legitimate societal interest in counseling or even in regulating childbearing in mothers with phenylketonuria, where there is grave danger of fetal damage and retardation. The moral issue becomes whether or not such statistics establish society's right to intervene in childbearing decisions by parents known to carry genes directly or indirectly causing grave disability in offspring.

With rare exception there is, in my opinion, no compelling case for societal restrictions on childbearing. I am profoundly disturbed by the advocacy of societal intervention in childbearing decisions for genetic reasons, denial of medical care to the congenitally damaged, or sterilization of those identified as likely to pass on the genetic basis for a constitutional disability. Such an advocacy is implicit in the tone of the following excerpt from a letter in *Science*: "Even elementary biology tells us that hereditary disease or susceptibility to disease which leads to death or diminished reproduction rids a population of genes which perpetuate these maladies. Yet modern medical practice is leading to the accumulation of such genes in the most highly advanced society of man."[28]

This statement, like the one of Darwin's one hundred years ago, miscasts the facts of natural selection in human populations. *The consensus of the best medical and genetic opinion is that whatever genetic deterioration is occurring as a result of decreased natural selection is so slow as to be insignificant when contrasted to "environmental" changes, including those produced by medical innovation.*[29] Even where we have identified a disease in which medical advances can be *shown* to have increased the over-all population incidence, as in schizophrenia,[30] few if any competent geneticists would advocate reducing the number of offspring schizophrenic individuals would be permitted to bear. The principal reason is ignorance. We simply do not know what (if any) intellectually desirable attributes are also transmitted with the complex of genes responsible for schizophrenia. Bodmer notes that the conditions which have led to an increase in the frequency of schizophrenia "may also conceivably increase the frequency of some desirable genetic attributes in other individuals."[31]

The variability that we (and geneticists with considerably more perceptivity) "see" in people represents the top of an iceberg of genetic diversity in human populations. Most of the variability which can be found at the genetic level is the result of spontaneous mutations which become fixed in the population. The traditional attitude of geneticists was that these mutations were in the main "undesirable," and the number of mutations and the extent to which a population as a whole was subjected to them constituted society's genetic load. Dobzhansky has been diligent in pointing out that the original definitions of "genetic load" tended to be spurious because they hypothesized a single "best" genotype, specifically one which was "homozygous" (i.e., having the same genes on each chromosome pair) for all of its genes. In Dobzhansky's estimation, this notion was inconsistent with the fact that the nature of human populations is to have a tremendous proportion of their genomes (perhaps as much as 30%) made up of "heterzygous" genes, and thus, to be consistent, geneticists would have to regard genetic uniformity beneficial and genetic heterogeneity inimical to the fitness of the population.[32]

It now appears that the term "genetic load" must be considered as almost synonymous with "genetic variability" and to be similarly bereft of utility. An appreciable portion of the expressed and even greater portion of the concealed variability that we can recognize in man consists of variants that—in most environments—are to some degree unfavorable to the organism.[33] In spite of the tendency to term this unfavorable, deleterious, ostensibly unadaptive part the genetic "load" or "burden" of the population, there is little evidence that it is deleterious to the population as a whole to carry so many variant genes. In fact, the opposite appears true. To be consistent, those who favor this definition must regard genetic uniformity as the *summum bonum*, an attitude incompatible with the adaptive value of genetic diversity in nature. (A sophisticated analysis of the concept of genetic load is available.)[34]

While many would concur that the "load" imposed by novel or recurrent mutations should be minimized, the natural load of variant genes carried by a population is the result of forces exerted by natural selection. The "burden" of variant genes is a "load," according to Dobzhansky, only in the sense in which the expenditures a community makes to bring up and to educate its younger members are a "load" on that community. Genetic diversity is in one sense capital for investment in future adaptations. Since genetic variability represents evolutionary capability, it is a load we should be ready and willing to bear.

It is indeed ironic that just as man is coming to realize the value of the immense genetic diversity of his species,[35] he has embarked in a direction which threatens to restrict or curtail that diversity. For example, it would be unfortunate if the move to reduce the frequencies of specific "deleterious" genes through identification of heterozygotes by carrier detection screening resulted in broad sanctions on the very mating combinations (heterozygous x normal) which tend to perpetuate genetic diversity. Even where the deleteriousness of a *specific* gene is unquestionable, as in the case of the Hemoglobin S gene responsible for sickle-cell anemia, and the "diversity value" of maintaining high frequencies of the gene largely unsubstantiated, I believe that it would *still* be morally unacceptable to restrict childbearing by those heterzygotes married to normals. Part of the conceptual problem underlying the focus on heterozygous individuals as those responsible for ladening us with our "genetic load" is the false assumption that this load is in fact imposed on society only by a select few individuals. Hermann Muller professed this view when he stated:

> A conscience that is socially oriented in regard to reproduction will lead many of the persons who are loaded with more than the average share of defects

. . . to refrain voluntarily from engaging in reproduction to the average extent, while vice versa it will be
considered a social service for those more fortunately
endowed to reproduce to more than the average extent.[36]

Such a statement raises but fails to answer the profound
moral question of how one identifies the "unfortunately" or
"fortunately" genetically endowed. Today we realize that *each*
individual bears a small but statistically significant number
(variously estimated at 3–8) of deleterious genes. The moral
attitude best fitted by our knowledge is that *a genetic burden is
not something that a population is laden with, it is what a family
is laden with.*

We now know that the very definition of the phrase "genetic
load" is fraught with difficulty. As an alternative, Muller would
ultimately have preferred to evaluate genetic load in man, as
Sewall Wright did, in terms of the balance between the contribution that a carrier of a particular genotype makes to society
and his "social cost."[37] Yet even this seemingly enlightened
view suffers from the assumption that the worth of man lies
exclusively in his social utility. One quickly gets into the moral
dilemma that Robert Gorney proposes when he attempts to
assess the relative social worth of mentally defective people on
the basis of their mother instincts, or dwarfs on the basis of their
"court jestering."[38] Do not individuals have value unto themselves and their own families?

Protecting the Gene Pool
or Supporting General Well-Being?

What then are the positions of geneticists themselves on the
issue of how genetic knowledge should be used to guide human
actions? Virtually all geneticists agree with James Crow that the
principal hazard facing the human population stems from the
introduction of new mutations through environmental agencies.
Thus both James Neel and Joshua Lederberg feel that it is the
geneticists' primary obligation to "protect the gene pool against

damage." (Presumably, this would mean principally reducing the background levels of radiation and population exposure to mutagens.) However, they differ dramatically in their secondary concerns. Neel emphasizes the importance of stabilizing the gene pool through population control, realizing the genetic potential of the individual, and improving the quality of life through parental choice based on genetic counseling and prenatal diagnosis.[39] In contrast, Lederberg speaks of the crucial need for the detection and "humane containment" of the DNA lesions (*sic*, mutations) once they are introduced into the gene pool.[40]

There is a profound danger in discussing the need for "containment" or "quarantine," for purportedly genetically "hygienic" reasons, of individuals who by no fault of their own carry genes which place their offspring in jeopardy.[41] The case for society's concern for the genetic welfare of the population and its rights in opposing sanctions on individuals hinges on the demonstration of a clear and present danger of genetic deterioration, which, as I have indicated, is still forthcoming. Yet, a letter I received from a government official rhetorically equated the potential societal threat of genetic disease with that of a highly contagious bacterial one. An individual carrying a deleterious gene was, according to this analysis, analogous to a "Typhoid Mary." Such an attitude is at best naive, and at worst ominously coercive. To equate a genetic disease with one which can be transmitted from person to person is to fail to recognize the salient difference between the two: Genetic diseases are transmissible only to offspring of the same family. Contagious diseases not only enjoy a much wider and rapid currency, but also an often fateful degree of anonymity, as in the faceless patrons of Typhoid Mary's restaurant. Only in the case of *genetic* disease do affected siblings and relatives serve as constant reminders of the fate of a subsequent affected child. Those who would argue that legal sanctions are necessary to protect society against genetic disease fail to recognize the basic reality of the deep and enduring bonds that draw a parent to his child. As Montaigne put it, "I have never seen a father who has failed to claim his child, however mangy or hunchbacked he might be. Not that he does not perceive his defect . . . but the fact remains the child is his."[42] A father bearing a heritable disorder himself or having experienced a lifetime of suffering in the genetic disability of his child would be the best judge to make the decision to deny life to his subsequent offspring. I know of no such situation (including retinoblastoma) where the decision to procreate or bear children should be the choice of other than the parents. The moral obligations of parents faced with genetic disease are to conscientiously weigh and act based on the prospects for their *children*, not for society at large. Genetic knowledge does not now justify enjoining any family with the societal obligation to refrain from procreation.

The Peril of a Genetic Imperative

In spite of the weight of evidence which shows that we do not have sufficient information to predict any but the grossest genetic changes following individual or population shifts in child-bearing habits, the latent fear remains that to do *nothing* will itself lead to an increase in detrimental genes and thereby compound the genetic problem for future generations.[43] Joshua Lederberg has argued that we are so locked into a genetic double blind that we *should* in fact do nothing. He states:

> Our problem is compounded by every humanitarian effort to compensate for a genetic defect, insofar as this shelters the carrier [of the defective gene] from natural selection. So it must be accepted that medicine, even prenatal care which may permit the fragile fetus to survive, already intrudes on the questions of "Who shall live." . . .
>
> It is so difficult to do only good in such matters that we are best off putting our strongest efforts in the prevention of mutation, so as to minimize the heavy moral and other burdens of decision making once the gene pool has been seeded with them.[44]

Certainly, any decision to act or not to act in the face of the dilemmas posed by human genetics is a moral choice. But one does not escape the moral burden of choosing by rationalizing that intrinsic contradictions in relative goods freeze one into inaction.

As Lederberg rightfully observes, the moral contradictions in choices of this sort are never more clearly visible than in the protection of the "fragile" and by inference damaged fetus. In fact, developments in prenatal and postnatal care now make it possible to ensure the survival of infants burdened with spina bifida and meningomyelocoele, spinal abnormalities which were life-limiting before this decade. To the extent that such abnormalities (like cleft palate or harelip) are heritable, there is an ethical question in encouraging the survival and successful procreation of the affected individuals. What is too often ignored in simplistic analyses of this sort is that the increased survival of the defective and deformed is *not* the result of special and sometimes "precious" care of the weak, but rather is usually accomplished as an indirect result of dramatic improvements in health care to *all* infants. As a recent editorial in the *British Medical Journal* observed, "Indiscriminate lowering of early mortality may impose terrible burdens on the survivors. But for the overwhelming majority of infants, the normal and healthy, there is hope and increasing evidence that the measures which lower mortality tend to produce a corresponding improvement in the quality of life offered them."[45]

Lederberg's course of nonaction is effectively a course of action, and one which is as morally unacceptable today as bringing newborns to the *Lesch* for sorting and disposal in ancient Sparta. Improvement in prenatal and postnatal care may well encourage the survival of more of those "fragile" and presumably genetically defective fetuses and newborns who would normally succumb, but, as the experience in Britain shows, the cost of that type of action may well be worth paying. Would not mothers in a society which offered the promise of nondiscriminative prenatal and postnatal care feel more secure than one (as in ancient Sparta) in which they knew that their children would be subjected to a test of normalcy? If selective care of only the genetically fit leads to a decrease in the survival of the specific few who are congenitally handicapped, it will be at the cost of a general *increase* in the damage wrought by uterine and early environmental deprivation (e.g., cerebral palsy and mental retardation). That would seem a high price for society to pay for its genetic well-being.

Summary

Our knowledge of genes and genetic systems in man shows them to be too complex to readily lend themselves to controlled manipulation. Deep-seated psychologic needs to reduce uncertainty appear to drive our search for genetic control in spite of this complexity. The need for genetic intervention is today justified on the basis of the same unsubstantiated analysis of "genetic deterioration" that characterized the eugenics movement in the late nineteenth century. The notion of a genetic "burden" imposed on society by individuals carrying deleterious variant genes is a misleading concept: the "burden" of deleterious genes is borne by families, not society. Decisions to have or not have children are best made by parents who have experienced genetic disease in their own families, not by society. Society's obligation is to provide universal maternal and postnatal care, even at the cost of survival of the congenitally handicapped. To do less is both to deprive the healthy of the optimum conditions for their development and to jeopardize the moral tone of society itself.

NOTES

1. Letter from Oswald Avery to Roy Avery, May 17, 1943, in *Readings in Heredity*, ed. John A. Moore (New York: Oxford Univ. Press, 1972) pp. 249–51.
2. Hans Jonas, *The Phenomenon of Life* (New York: Harper & Row, 1966) p. 205.
3. See Marc Lappé, "Biological Warfare," in *Social Responsibility of the Scientist*, ed. Martin Brown (Berkeley: Free Press, 1970).
4. A condition resulting from an enzymatic defect in the ability to metabolize phenylalanine which is usually associated with mental retardation.
5. Joseph Fletcher, "Ethical Aspects of Genetic Controls," *New England Journal of Medicine* 285 (1971) 776–83.
6. See the discussion by Carl Jung in the Introduction to the *I Ching*, tr. Richard Wilhelm (Princeton: Bollingen Series XIX, 1967) p. xix, where he begins: "An incalculable amount of human effort is directed to combating the nuisance and danger represented by chance. . . ."

7. J. F. Crow, "Rates of Genetic Changes under Selection," *Proc. National Academy of Sciences* 59 (1968) 655–61.

8. J. Lederberg, "Experimental Genetics and Human Evolution," *American Naturalist* 100 (1966) 519–26. (Clonal propagation means using the nucleus of a single cell to propagate a whole organism genetically identical with it.)

9. Carl R. Merril, Mark R. Geier, and John Petricciani, "Bacterial Virus Gene Expression in a Human Cell," *Nature* 233 (1971) 398–400.

10. A. G. Schwartz, P. R. Cook, and Henry Harris, "Correction of a Genetic Defect in a Mammalian Cell," *Nature New Biology* 230 (1971) 5–7.

11. Jacques Ellul, *The Technological Society* (New York: Vintage, 1964) p. 11.

12. See J. Lederberg, "Unpredictable Variety Still Rules Human Reproduction," *Washington Post,* Sept. 30, 1967.

13. Eugenics is defined as "an applied science that seeks to maintain or improve the genetic potentialities of the human species" (Gordon Allen, in *International Encyclopedia of the Social Sciences* 5 [1968] 193).

14. Francis Galton, *Hereditary Genius* (London, 1870).

15. Charles Darwin, *The Descent of Man and Selection in Relation to Sex* (1871; New York: Random House Modern Library Edition) pp. 501–2 (italics mine).

16. See in particular Fletcher, *art. cit.*, and Bentley Glass's letter in reply to Leon R. Kass, *Science,* Jan. 8, 1971, p. 23.

17. Theodosius Dobzhansky, "Man and Natural Selection," *American Scientist* 49 (1961) 285–99.

18. H. J. Miller, "The Guidance of Human Evolution," *Perspectives in Biology and Medicine* 1 (1959) 590.

19. W. T. Vukovich, "The Dawning of the Brave New World—Legal, Ethical and Social Issues of Eugenics," *Univ. of Illinois Law Forum* 2 (1971) 189–231; B. Glass, "Human Heredity and Ethical Problems," *Perspectives in Biology and Medicine* 15 (1972) 237–53; R. Gorney, "The New Biology and the Future of Man," *UCLA Law Review* 15 (1968) 273–356.

20. M. Golding, "Our Obligations to Future Generations," *UCLA Law Review* 15 (1968) 443–79.

21. Golding, *ibid.*, p. 463.

22. T. Dobzhansky, D. Kirk, O. D. Duncan, and C. Bajema, *The American Eugenics Society, Inc. Six Year Report, 1965–1970* (published by the Society, New York).

23. Dudley Kirk, "Patterns of Survival and Reproduction in the United States," *Proc. Nat. Acad. Sci.* 59 (1968) 662–70.

24. *Ibid.*

25. Jean Fredrick, "Anencephalus: Variation with Maternal Age, Parity, Social Class and Region in England, Scotland, and Wales," *Ann. Human Genetics* (London) 34 (1970) 31–38.

26. Peter Brian Medawar, "Do Advances in Medicine Lead to Genetic Deterioration?" *Mayo Clinic Proceedings* 40 (1965) 23–33.

27. Anonymous, "The Changing Pattern of Retinoblastoma," *Lancet* 2 (1971) 1016–17.

28. "Biological Unsoundness of Modern Medical Practice," *Science* 165 (1969) 1313.

29. James V. Neel, "Lessons from a 'Primitive' People," *Science* 170 (1970) 815–22. See also John R. G. Turner, "How Does Treating Congenital Disease Affect the Genetic Load?" *Eugenics Quarterly*, 1968, pp. 191–96.

30. Walter F. Bodmer, "Demographic Approaches to the Measurement of Differential Selection in Human Populations," *Proc. Nat. Acad. Sci.* 59 (1968) 690–99.

31. Bodmer, *ibid.*, p. 699.

32. T. Dobzhansky, *Genetics and the Evolutionary Process* (New York: Columbia Univ. Press, 1970) p. 191.

33. Heterozygotes carrying a single dose of a recessive variant gene which is deleterious in the homozygous form are—contrary to popular belief—on the average *less* fit than the person who has both "normal" genes. The sickle-cell heterozygote, for example, is *only* at an advantage in malarial regions, having statistically less fitness than the normal in nonmalarial regions.

34. Bruce Wallace, *Genetic Load: Its Biological and Conceptual Aspects* (Englewood Cliffs, N.J.: Prentice-Hall, 1970).

35. L. C. Dunn, "The Study of Genetics in Man—Retrospect and Prospect," *Birth Defects Original Article Series* (The National Foundation, 1965).

36. H. J. Muller, "The Guidance of Human Evolution," *Perspectives in Biology and Medicine*, 1959, p. 590.

37. Dobzhansky, *Genetics and the Evolutionary Process*, p. 191.

38. Gorney, *art. cit.*, pp. 308–9.

39. Neel, *art. cit.*

40. Joshua Lederberg, "The Amelioration of Genetic Defect—A Case Study in the Application of Biological Technology," *Dimensions* 5 (1971) 13–51.

41. Margery Shaw, "*De jure* and *de facto* Restrictions on Genetic Counseling," *Proceedings of the Airlie House Conference* on "Ethical Issues in the Application of Human Genetic Knowledge," Oct. 10–14, 1971 (Plenum Press).
42. Michel de Montaigne, "On the Education of Children," *Selected Essays*, tr. D. M. Frame (New York: Van Nostrand, 1943) chap. 26, p. 5.
43. Bentley Glass, *art. cit.*
44. Lederberg, "The Amelioration of Genetic Defect," p. 15.
45. Anonymous, "Early Deaths," *British Medical Journal*, 1971, pp. 315–16.

SECTION V

ISSUES IN URBAN PRIMARY CARE

Long-Term Care for the Elderly and Disabled: A New Health Priority

Anne R. Somers

O F all the difficult health-care issues facing the nation today, none is more complex or urgent than the formulation of a viable policy of long-term care for the elderly and the chronically ill and disabled. The tragic irony of the existing neglect is clearly evident in the plight of millions of frail and dependent elders, rejected by both Medicare and Medicaid as well as by most private carriers of health insurance, even as the costs of these programs soar.

Although many of the current remedial proposals recognize the importance of long-term care, they appear to be prepared to settle for a second-class program, separate in both organization and financing from the mainstream of acute care. Given the dominance of chronic disease in the American health picture today and the importance of professional continuity in its management, such separation is inappropriate. Some way must be found to integrate long-term and acute care under a single financing program, with similar quality and cost controls. One practical approach would be to incorporate a basic schedule of long-term-care benefits into Medicare—our major program for financing acute care for both the elderly and the seriously disabled—while providing for supplementary, community-based case management, perhaps under a separate Title XXI of the Social Security Act.

From *New England Journal of Medicine*, July 22, 1982, Vol. 307, No. 4.

The Failure of Current Policy

As of 1979, Medicare enrollees numbered about 28 million. Ninety percent were 65 or over, 2.9 million were disabled, and about 60,000 had end-stage renal disease.[1] (Although the program for end-stage renal disease provides some useful lessons for any long-term-care program, the problems are sufficiently different to call for lengthier treatment than is possible in this paper.) With the exception of patients with end-stage renal disease, however, Medicare eligibility at present means virtually nothing with respect to long-term care. The Medicare message to the average patient is clear: "Get well fast or get lost." It specifically prohibits payment for most long-term or custodial care (Social Security Act, Section 1862). The meaning of "custodial" is spelled out in the official *Medicare Handbook* as follows:

> Care is considered custodial when it is primarily for the purpose of meeting personal needs and could be provided by persons without professional skills or training; for example, help in walking, getting in and out of bed, bathing, dressing, eating and taking medicine.

Anyone familiar with long-term care of the patient who has had a stroke, for example, will appreciate that these are precisely the skills that constitute the heart of effective rehabilitation. To denigrate such skills, to consign such patients to custodial care outside the responsibility of either public policy or the health professions, is not only morally unconscionable but economically and politically unfeasible.

The private health-insurance industry has also looked the other way. Although redundant policies for the hospitalized are promoted ad nauseam, it is extremely difficult to find any insurance for long-term benefits. Even major medical insurance usually excludes nursing-home and home care, or limits the latter category to full-time private-duty nursing. In 1980, private insurance accounted for only 0.7 percent of nursing-home expenditures[2]; it accounted for even a smaller fraction of home care.

Medicaid does cover long-term care, but only for the very poor, including some who have deliberately impoverished themselves for this purpose. A 1974 survey by the Congressional Budget Office found that nearly half of Medicaid nursing-home patients were not initially poor by state definitions but were forced to deplete their resources in order to qualify as "medically needy."[3] The financial burden is especially great for patients' spouses. In 1976, spouses contributed an average of $2,025 a year for the cost of nursing-home care, although their average income was only $7,890.[4]

A 1980 study by the former Assistant Commissioner of Health of New Jersey notes:

> Children are not financially responsible for the care of parents . . . but spouses are; hence the phenomenon of couples married 50 years divorcing to enable one of them to get nursing home subsidy without totally impoverishing the other.
>
> The spend-down for nursing home care presents many middle-class families with an excruciating dilemma. Either they violate the law by covertly attempting to transfer the parent's assets before admission to the nursing home . . . or they can watch passively an inheritance go up in smoke. For those families unable or unwilling to transfer assets covertly, nursing home services have thus become the most effective barrier to intergenerational transfer of income ever seen in this country.[5]

Some nursing homes require large down payments, sometimes representing charges for a year or more. Once paid, such payments can result in making the patient a virtual hostage; alternatively, the patient may be forced out when all private funds are consumed and Medicaid status becomes inevitable.

Despite numerous supposedly cost-saving limits, the costs of Medicare and Medicaid have increased astronomically. By 1980, expenditures reached $63 billion, up 19 percent from 1979.[2] They now consume nearly 10 percent of the federal budget.[6] The costs of long-term care in 1980 are estimated at $32 billion (exclusive of income maintenance, housing assistance, or any imputed value of informal care by the patient's family or friends).[7]

About two thirds of this—$21 billion—went for nursing-home care, now the fastest growing segment of the health-care industry. Nursing-home costs are projected to reach $42 billion by 1985 and $76 billion by 1990.[8] The Medicaid portion of these vast sums has grown steadily and is now about 50 per cent,[2] creating a serious distortion in the original purpose of this program.

Altogether, despite the lack of a positive long-term-care policy—or more probably because of this lack—public funds accounted for nearly $12 billion of national nursing-home costs in 1980. This includes about $10.4 billion from Medicaid, $0.4 billion from Medicare, and $1.1 billion from the Veterans Administration and other federal and state government programs.[2] At current rates and under current arrangements, that figure will rise to about $24 billion by 1985 and $43 billion by 1990. It is not surprising that those responsible for the federal budget feel desperate and are preparing to advance some desperate proposals in the effort to control these costs. However, the gradual dismantling of Medicare—through the introduction of "pro-competition" policies, vouchers, exorbitant cost sharing, and similar measures—bears about the same relation to the underlying problems as rearranging the chairs on the Titanic bears to the problem of icebergs in the North Atlantic.

Factors Behind the Growing Need For Long-Term Care

Three basic demographic factors underlie the growing need for long-term care: increasing life expectancy for the elderly, the dominance of chronic disease as the major cause of morbidity in the United States, and the "shrinking" American family.

Paradoxically, the more successful we are in conquering acute disease and postponing death, the more we aggravate the problem of long-term disability. Between 1950 and 1978, for example, 2.4 years were added to the life expectancy of the average 65-year-old American—more than were gained in the 50 years from 1900 to 1950.[9] In 1978, the average woman of 65 could look forward to over 18 more years of life, and the average man to more than 14 years. But most of those whose lives were saved from acute heart attacks, strokes, early death from cancer, complications of diabetes or other chronic diseases, and accidents were added to the millions who require lifetime medical surveillance and often some form of long-term care. Chronic disease has become the dominant pattern of illness, and by definition chronic disease is never cured. According to the National Center for Health Statistics, for those 65 and over, 83 percent of all "restricted-activity days" in 1980 and 87 percent of all deaths in 1978 were due to chronic conditions (Rice DP; personal communication).

As for the shrinking family, all the major trends—more working women, later marriage, more divorces, fewer children, and greater geographic mobility—mean less available direct family care.[10] Sixty percent of all persons over 65 are women.[11] Of these, over 60 percent are unmarried—widowed, divorced, or never married—and 43 percent live alone or with people who are not relatives. There is often no one at home to care for the elderly widow recovering from a broken hip or the widower with paralysis after a stroke. An increasing number are asking why they should be kept alive only to be condemned to years of disability, poverty, loneliness, and misery.

Essential Elements of a New Long-Term-Care Policy

Basically, the problem results from trying to fit the new needs onto the Procrustean bed of outmoded policy. What is needed is a new policy that takes changes in both health needs and family structure into account, acknowledges that the quality of life in the later years is at least as important as the quantity, and recognizes that costs can be contained only through appropriate controls applied consistently and fairly to both long-term and acute care.

Such reorientation cannot be achieved overnight. But there is a growing consensus on some basic guidelines: *(1)* Focus on functional independence for the patient rather than on "cure."[12-16] *(2)* Emphasize prevention at all ages.[17] *(3)* Do not expect the impossible of families; help them to cope. *(4)* Ensure neutrality of public financing between acute and long-term care, and between institutional and home-based care, as opposed to the current bias toward acute institutional illness. *(5)* Involve not only physicians but nurses, social workers, aides, and others, and provide incentives for these workers to master geriatric skills. *(6)* Encourage continuity of professional surveillance. *(7)* Provide adequate quality and cost controls, including fixed payment schedules for all covered benefits. *(8)* Ensure equal access to publicly funded benefits, regardless of economic status. *(9)* Encourage some transfer of resources from acute care to primary and long-term care.

These are not revolutionary measures. They do not involve repudiation of the Medicare commitment to first-rate acute care. On the contrary, such a new policy would constitute a tribute to the remarkable effectiveness of Medicare in extending the life expectancy of millions of frail or dependent elderly persons and in helping to save lives that would otherwise have been lost to acute illness or trauma. What is now needed is a synthesis of the past and present—a policy that will preserve Medicare's original commitment but will balance it and link it with the best possible long-term services, at a price that the nation can afford.

Portions of the recommended policy are already being implemented in a number of long-term-care demonstration projects.[18-25] Some have already made notable contributions in this area. Unfortunately, however, there is a frequent tendency to accept, and even strengthen, the existing barriers—both professional and financial—between acute and long-term care. On the contrary, there should be no financial barriers between the two areas, and professional distinctions should involve not acute versus long-term care but primary versus specialized care.

The case for a separate long-term-care system is frequently supported by both those who believe it to be very important and those who do not. The former stress the recent neglect on the part of many physicians and other leaders of the medical establishment, as well as their fear of the "medical model" or "physician domination" if adequate third-party payment should become available. At the same time, some supporters of the acute-care system fear that the extension of third-party coverage to long-term care could seriously dilute the funds now available for acute care.

Despite these understandable concerns and others that could be advanced, the case for programmatic integration (or at least close coordination) is compelling. Among the many reasons, two are of special concern. In the first place, even a well-funded long-term-care program, if separate from the mainstream of acute care, will never achieve the same level of quality; it will remain a stepchild, as Medicaid has been from the beginning. "Separate but equal" will not be equal in this area any more than in education. Secondly, good long-term care is achieved through a blending of medical and socioeconomic concerns and activities. It cannot operate exclusively on a social model any more than on a medical model. The long-term-care team must involve social workers and case managers, but it must also include nurses, therapists, and other health personnel, and ideally it should be headed by a primary physician who can best deal with the underlying health problems, command the respect of all parties, and assume legal responsibility.

A New Proposal

The following proposal is similar but not identical to that submitted to the White House Conference on Aging by its Technical Committee on Health Services.[12] It is presented here simply as my own, first suggested to the National Council on Aging on April 1, 1981.[26] It is outlined in very general terms, as it should be at this early stage. What we need now is not a technical debate over administrative or financial details but agreements on broad goals and objectives. The proposal is in two parts.

Part I: Medicare Payment for Appropriate Long-Term Care

The Medicare definition of eligibility, though ultraconservative with respect to disability—coverage cannot begin until the 30th month after the first full month of disablement—does provide a practical initial framework for identifying and reaching the elderly and the most seriously disabled. Section 1862 of the Social Security Act should be amended to eliminate the prohibition against "custodial care." The need for continuity between acute and long-term care should be explicitly recognized, and a defined schedule of benefits for long-term care—both institutional and home-based—should be included. Medicare (rather than Medicaid) reimbursement for such services would be provided.

The Secretary of Health and Human Services should review (and, when appropriate, revise) the conditions of Medicare participation for providers of long-term care. To help pay for the new benefits, several measures should be undertaken: First of all, funds currently budgeted for long-term care of the elderly and the disabled, under Medicaid, Title XX, and possibly other public programs, or funds that would have been budgeted were it not for the new program, should be transferred to Medicare for the same purpose. Secondly, all Medicare providers—those providing acute care as well as those providing long-term care—should be paid on the basis of fixed (prospective) rates, to be negotiated periodically between Medicare or its intermediaries and the major provider associations. Thirdly, cost-sharing formulas for the various long-term benefits should be developed by the Secretary and applied as appropriate. Finally, the feasibility of additional cost sharing for very expensive care, whether acute or long-term (e.g., expenditures over $100,000 in any one year) should be at least studied.

Part II: Community Long-Term-Care Coordinating Services

A new federal, state, and community program to coordinate long-term care for Medicare beneficiaries should be established, either as an amendment to Title XVIII or possibly as a new

Title XXI. It would be under the Department of Health and Human Services at the federal level but would be financed by a combination of federal, state, local, and possibly private funds. Actual administration should be at the community or county level, by an appropriate public or private body, within guidelines established by the federal and state governments. It would have three principal functions: to ensure maximum feasible coordination among health-care institutions, agencies, and programs involved in care of the elderly and disabled; to help allocate long-term-care resources in the most equitable and effective manner and ensure adequate facilities and personnel; and to provide comprehensive assessment, appropriate placement, and cost-effective case management of individual long-term Medicare patients, under the general supervision of a responsible primary physician or group and through some appropriate interdisciplinary mechanism, with guaranteed opportunity for patient and family input.

The proposal is a compromise between those who would simply extend Medicare to include long-term care and those who would prefer a completely separate program with different methods of financing, standards of eligibility, and administration. It aims to retain the proved strengths of Medicare, including its nearly universal entitlement for the elderly and seriously disabled, its requirement for physician responsibility, its quasi-insurance type of financing, its tremendous resources, and its high standards of quality, while suggesting new restraints on provider payments for all types of benefits. It builds on the momentum started by the 1980 expansion of Medicare home-care benefits (removal of the requirement for prior hospitalization under Part A and the 100-visit limit under both Parts A and B). President Reagan's proposal (delivered in his 1982 State of the Union address) to federalize Medicaid in return for state assumption of several other social-welfare programs, if enacted, might also facilitate this joining of acute and long-term care for the elderly.

At the same time, the proposal recognizes the special complexities inherent in good long-term care—complexities relating both to the interdisciplinary nature of such care and to the length of time over which it may have to be sustained. For these and other reasons, a supplementary community-based coordinating and monitoring service is proposed, but medical and legal responsibility for the individual patient remains in the hands of the patient's primary physician or a legally defined surrogate, and eligibility for benefits is based on the same general Medicare criteria used for acute-care patients. This does not mean that issues of eligibility for a specific service—e.g., whether a certain patient requires a skilled-nursing-facility or intermediate-care-facility level of care—would not differ. But it does mean that age, the definition of disability, and other basic eligibility criteria would be standardized between acute and long-term care. Financial resources would probably have a role in determining the degree of cost-sharing, but not in defining basic eligibility.

With respect to costs, the proposal primarily envisions a transfer of existing expenditures, personnel, and other resources, rather than any large additions. By transferring the responsibility for long-term care of the elderly and disabled from Medicaid to Medicare, it should cut Medicaid expenditures by nearly half and contribute substantially to solving the state "Medicaid problem." The over $12 billion currently being spent by Medicaid and other public programs for nursing-home services—a figure that will double by 1985 under the existing arrangements—would constitute the basic financial underpinning for the expanded benefits.

Although the total costs will inevitably rise with the increase in the number of elderly persons, continuing progress in acute care, and inflation, the rise should be substantially moderated by the change in methods of provider payment, the appropriate use of cost-sharing provisions (possibly involving children as well as the spouse), and continuous professional monitoring, with an emphasis, insofar as possible, on noninstitutional care.

As an intermediate and immediate step, I urge the states to take advantage of the greater flexibility now available under the Budget Reconciliation Act of 1981 to strengthen health-care services under Medicaid and thus help to reverse the traditional bias toward institutional care in that program as well as Medicare.[27]

It may be helpful at this point to compare this proposal with another, Local Area Management Organizations (LAMOs), recently presented in the *Journal.*[20] There are, in fact, several points of similarity. Both proposals are concerned with long-term care for the elderly and the disabled. Both call for the integration of acute and long-term care for the populations they propose to cover. Both call for local or community agencies to carry out the actual case management of individual patients.

However, the differences are more important than the similarities. The LAMO proposal is limited to the severely disabled and the "vulnerable elderly," who would be expected to pull out of Medicare even for their acute care and to enroll in the new organizations. Unlike Medicare, LAMOs would be financed by federal and state block grants, would be paid on a capitation basis, would be "at risk," and would thus be expected to do everything possible to cut costs. The opportunity for reform of Medicare payment procedures would be lost, whereas the prospect of perpetuating and even deepening the present qualitative differences between Medicare and Medicaid would be strengthened. Physician involvement in the LAMO appears minimal.

In brief, whereas the LAMO proposal extends the present two-class system of long-term care to acute care for the "vulnerable elderly" and the disabled, the proposal that I suggest seeks to extend the Medicare one-class acute-care system to long-term care for all Medicare beneficiaries: just the reverse.

The LAMO proposal is strongly anti-government. For example, the authors state, "Reliance on public funding imparts a de facto aura of charity or welfare to an activity that should be a person's own responsibility. Concomitantly, it creates an environment in which concern for quality is not deemed a priority."[20] Such a sweeping generalization is simply inaccurate. Some public programs are very poor, and some very good. Medicare is clearly one of the most popular programs in the country—with both beneficiaries and providers. And there is no doubt that it has contributed substantially to the quality of care available to older Americans, as well as to their access to such care. Despite its shortcomings, which have been stressed in this article, the main thrust of my proposal is not to destroy or even weaken Medicare but to reform and strengthen it by incorporating some essential long-term-care benefits and simultaneously introducing some badly needed cost controls.

The most frequent criticism of this proposal involves its alleged political unrealism. Obviously, it will not be popular with those whose sole concern is budget cutting, especially at the federal level. On the contrary, it involves the transfer of a substantial portion of current state-funded Medicaid costs to

Medicare—i.e., to the federal government—as well as the allocation of some new money for new programs, at least for the first few years. However, for those concerned with the long-run efficiency and economy of the health-care system, as well as the health of the American people, it could be an important step in the right direction.

Already, there are signs that the epidemic of anti-government feeling that gripped the country in 1980 is waning in favor of a more balanced blend of public and private responsibilities. And unless the American people are prepared to repeal their 1966 commitment "to assure comprehensive health services of high quality for every person" (P.L. 89-749), they will have to come to grips with the problem of long-term care for the elderly and chronically disabled. This, in turn, will inevitably involve not only a blend of public and private initiatives but also some trade-off between acute and long-term care, or more precisely between primary care (defined to include long-term care) and specialty care.

Moreover, the proposal contains many elements of a viable political solution, even in the current polarized atmosphere. To the elderly themselves, traditional liberals, and others committed to the Medicare tradition, it offers an extension of benefits to recipients of long-term care in return for some limits on acute care. To the federal government and others primarily concerned with economy, it offers fixed fees for all health-care providers, reasonable cost sharing, and some limits on acute care in return for coverage for long-term care. To the medical profession, it offers continued primacy in the management of both acute and chronic illness, professional independence, and freedom from inappropriate competitive pressures in return for fixed fees and the assumption of responsibility for long-term care.

To private health-insurance carriers, it offers a new market for supplementary coverage for long-term care, even more extensive than the "Medigap" market opened up in 1965, because more cost sharing will inevitably be required. To social workers and others who may fear the "medical model," it offers a piece of the action in the mainstream rather than an illusory independence in a peripheral program. No group will be totally happy, but neither will any be badly hurt. In short, it is a design that all the major interested parties can live with, at least for several decades, and this is the essence of progress in our pragmatic democracy.

NOTES

1. Muse DN, Sawyer D. Medicare and Medicaid data book, 1981. Washington, D.C.: United States Department of Health and Human Services, 1982. (DHHS publication no. (HCFA) 82-03128).
2. Gibson RM, Waldo DR. National health expenditures, 1980. Health Care Financ Rev. 1981; 3(1):1–54.
3. United States Congress, Congressional Budget Office. Long-term care for the elderly and disabled. Washington, D.C.: Government Printing Office, 1977.
4. Callahan JJ, Jr, Diamond LD, Giele JZ, Morris R. Responsibility of families for their severely disabled elders. Health Care Financ Rev. 1980; 1(3):29–48.
5. Vladeck BC. Unloving care: the nursing home tragedy. New York: Basic Books, 1980:24.
6. Congress Q Weekly Rep. February 13, 1982; 40:231,243.
7. Home Health Line. January 8, 1982; 7:1–2.
8. Freeland M, Calat C, Schendler CE. Projections of national health expenditures, 1980, 1985, and 1990. Health Care Financ Rev. 1980; 1(3):1–27.
9. Allan C, Brotman H. Chartbook on aging in America. Washington, D.C.: 1981 White House Conference on Aging, 1981:8–9.
10. Somers AR. Marital status, health, and the use of health services: an old relationship revisited. JAMA. 1979; 241:1818–22.
11. Department of Health and Human Services, Administration on Aging. Facts about older Americans 1979. Washington, D.C.: Government Printing Office, 1980. (DHHS publication no. 80-20006).
12. Beck JC. White House Conference on Aging: report on Technical Committee on Health Services. Washington, D.C.: Government Printing Office, 1981 (720-019/6963).
13. Fahey SJ. 1981 White House Conference on Aging: report of Technical Committee on Social and Health Aspects of Long-Term Care. Washington, D.C.: Government Printing Office, 1981 (720-019/6889).
14. Cluff LE. Chronic disease, function, and the quality of care. J Chronic Dis. 1981; 34:299–304.
15. Somers AR, Fabian DR, eds. The geriatric imperative: an introduction to gerontology and clinical geriatrics. New York: Appleton-Century-Crofts, 1981.

16. Long-term care: in search of solutions. Washington, D.C.: National Conference on Social Welfare, 1981.

17. Fries JF. Aging, natural death, and the compression of morbidity. N Engl J Med. 1980; 303:130–5.

18. Brickner PW. Nine years of long-term home health care, 1973–1981. New York: St. Vincent's Hospital & Medical Center, 1982.

19. Hicks B, Raisz H, Segal J, Doherty N. The Triage experiment in coordinated care for the elderly. Am J Public Health. 1981; 71:991–1002.

20. Ruchlin HS, Morris JN, Eggert GM. Management and financing of long-term-care services: a new approach to a chronic problem. N Engl J Med. 1982; 306:101–6.

21. New York State Department of Social Services & Health Care Financing Administration. Third year evaluation of the Monroe County long-term-care program. Silver Spring, Md.: Macro Systems, 1980.

22. Program for the health-impaired elderly. Princeton, N.J.: Robert Wood Johnson Foundation, 1979.

23. United States Department of Health, Education, and Welfare, Office of the Secretary. National long-term care channeling demonstration request for proposal. (RFP-74-80-HEW-PS, April 25, 1980.

24. Diamond LD, Berman D. The social HMO: a single entry prepaid long-term-care system. In: Callahan JS, Wallack SE, eds. Reforming the long-term-health care system. Lexington, Mass.: Lexington Books, 1980:185–213.

25. Kleinman L, Snope FC, Somers AR, Kane WS. Are you ready for the graying of America? Patient Care. 1981; 15:227–91.

26. Somers AR. Long-term care for the elderly: toward a positive policy. Perspect Aging. 1981; 10(4):5–10.

27. PL 97-35 (The omnibus budget reconciliation act of 1981). Section 217b 97th Congress. 1st Session.

Homelessness, Health and Human Needs: Summary and Recommendations

National Academy of Science Report

Origin of This Study

Among congressional actions taken in recent years to address both the broader aspects of homelessness and the more narrow issues relating to the health of homeless people was the Health Professions Training Act of 1985 (P.L. 99-129). This mandated that the secretary of the Department of Health and Human Services ask the Institute of Medicine of the National Academy of Sciences to study the delivery of health care services to homeless people. This report is the result of that study.

The study committee was composed of experts in fields such as medicine, nursing, and social sciences; two public officials who administer statewide health and human services programs also served on the committee.

The charge to the committee and its staff was stated in P.L. 99-129:

The members of the study committee endorse the analyses and conclusions of the report but unanimously wish to express their strong feeling that the recommendations are too limited in addressing the broader issues of homelessness—especially the supply of low-income housing, income maintenance, the availability of support services, and access to health care for the poor and uninsured.

1. evaluate whether existing eligibility requirements for health care services actually prevent homeless people from receiving those services;
2. evaluate the efficiency of health care services to homeless people; and
3. make recommendations as to what should be done by the federal, state, and local governments as well as private organizations to improve the availability and delivery of health care services to homeless people.

At the request of the study's funding agency in the Department of Health and Human Services, the Health Resources and Services Administration, the committee took a broad view of health care and of needs for health care-related services, including matters such as nutrition, mental health, alcohol and drug abuse problems, and dental care.

Study Process

The study committee met five times during a 10-month period (December 1986 to September 1987); individual committee members participated in site visits to 11 cities and to rural areas of four states to observe the problems of the homeless firsthand. The committee also commissioned 10 papers on specific areas of concern, such as the legal aspects of access to health care and the problems of providing health care for homeless people in the rural areas of America. Committee members, assisted by a study staff of two professionals, reviewed what is known about the health of homeless people, as evidenced in the scholarly literature, reports of public and private organizations, and—in particular—the ongoing evaluation of work of the 19 Health Care for the Homeless projects funded by the Robert Wood Johnson Foundation and the Pew Memorial Trust.

In the course of this study, the committee encountered several major methodological problems. For example, the lack of a uniform definition of homelessness results in substantial disagreement about the size of the homeless population. Some people define the homeless as only those who are on the streets or in shelters; others include those who are temporarily living with family or friends because they cannot afford housing. For its working definition, the committee adopted the one contained in the Stewart B. McKinney Homeless Assistance Act of 1987 (P.L. 100-77), which defines a homeless person as one who lacks a fixed, permanent nighttime residence or whose nighttime residence is a temporary shelter, welfare hotel, transitional housing for the mentally ill, or any public or private place not designed as sleeping accommodations for human beings (U.S. Congress, House, 1987).

The committee commissioned a study of the methodology of counting the homeless, but refrained from providing its own quantitative estimate of the number of homeless people. One recent estimate of the number of homeless people in the United States, published in June 1988 by the National Alliance to End Homelessness (Alliance Housing Council, 1988), calculates that currently, on any given night, there are 735,000 homeless people in the United States; that during the course of 1988, 1.3 million to 2.0 million people will be homeless for one night or more; and that these people are among the approximately 6 million Americans who, because of their disproportionately high expenditures for housing costs, are at extreme risk of becoming homeless.

What Was Learned

Who Are the Homeless?

Contrary to the traditional stereotypes of homeless people, the homeless of the 1980s are not all single, middle-aged, male alcoholics. Neither are they all mentally ill people made homeless as a by-product of the policy of deinstitutionalization of mental health care.

The homeless are younger, more ethnically diverse, and increasingly are more likely to be members of families than is generally believed by the public. In most cities around the country, minorities—especially blacks and Hispanics—are represented disproportionately among the homeless as compared with their percentage of the overall population of those cities.

Children under the age of 18, usually as part of a family headed by a mother, are the fastest-growing group among the many subpopulations of the homeless. On the other hand, the elderly are underrepresented among the homeless in comparison with their percentage in the general population. There are a substantial number of veterans among the homeless, especially from the Vietnam era.

Homeless people tend to be long-term residents of the city in which they live. The homeless in rural areas, as well as homeless urban families, usually have gone through several stages of doubling up with family and friends before becoming visibly homeless.

Although the old stereotype of the public inebriate does not reflect the diversity of homelessness in the 1980s, alcohol abuse and alcoholism are still the most frequently diagnosed medical problems among homeless men (more than 40 percent). Substance abuse with drugs other than alcohol also appears to be more prevalent among homeless adults than among the general population, as is "comorbidity"—that is, multiple problems in the same individual such as alcoholism and mental illness.

The homeless have also been stereotyped as uniformly mentally ill, in part because *severe* disorders such as schizophrenia are conspicuously overrepresented among homeless individuals on the street. Most studies of mental illness among the homeless reveal that 30 to 40 percent of the adults show evidence of some type of major mental disorder; 15 to 25 percent acknowledge having been hospitalized for psychiatric care in the past. These rates are several times higher than those of the general population.

Why Do People Become Homeless?

The answer to this seemingly simple question is quite complex. Among the many causes of homelessness, the committee identified three major, interrelated factors that, in the face of a relatively strong economy, have contributed to the increased number of homeless people in this decade:

1. *Housing*—the supply of housing units for people with low incomes has decreased considerably, while the number of people needing such housing has increased.

2. *Income and employment*—There has been a tightening of the eligibility criteria for public assistance programs (especially locally funded general relief), as well as a decline in the purchasing power of such benefits for those who do establish eligibility. This reduction in benefits comes at a time when the number of people living in poverty has increased.

3. *Deinstitutionalization*—The policy of deinstitutionalization, which characterizes the way state mental health systems have been administered since the early 1960s, is clearly a contributing factor; in addition, a policy of noninstitutional— that is, not admitting people for psychiatric care except for very brief periods of time—has further exacerbated the problems of mentally ill homeless adults. Both policies were based upon the assumption that treatment, rehabilitation, and appropriate residential placement would be provided in the community. This has not happened anywhere near the extent originally envisioned. Similar attitudes regarding extended confinement have come to characterize policy toward general hospitals and correctional, rehabilitation, and mental retardation facilities.

One result of these factors is that the system for providing temporary shelter for people who are homeless has been burdened beyond its capacity, despite enormous expansion in the last few years; people are staying in these emergency facilities for many months, not only a few days or weeks.

What Are the Health Problems of the Homeless?

Homeless people experience illnesses and injuries to a much greater extent than does the population as a whole. The committee identified three sets of health problems that specifically relate to homelessness:

1. Some health problems can cause a person to become homeless, for example, injury on the job resulting in the loss of employment and income, severe mental illness, alcoholism, drug abuse, and, more recently, AIDS (acquired immune deficiency syndrome).

2. Other health problems result from homelessness, for example, problems resulting from exposure, such as hypothermia; problems resulting from not being able to lie down, such as vascular and skin disorders of the legs and feet; and problems resulting from specific hazards of the homeless life-style, such as trauma from being mugged or raped on the streets.

3. Many health problems require treatment that is made more complicated or impossible by the fact that the patient is homeless. Almost all illnesses and injuries fall within this category, and the difficulty encountered in attempting to treat even minor ailments when the patient is homeless is one of the major issues facing health care providers. One example would be the dietary limitations and the medication regimen that are part of the routine care of hypertension, a problem of particular significance among those past middle age and among blacks. Medication can rarely be taken as prescribed, and the sodium content of food derived from soup kitchens cannot be controlled. A simpler example would be the frequent order to "rest in bed"; this is virtually impossible if one does not have a bed, and very difficult at best if one must give up one's bed in a shelter every morning and wait until evening to be reassigned a bed.

What Other Problems Do Homeless People Have with Health Care?

The primary problem that homeless people have with health care is access, both financial and physical. With regard to financial access, homeless people generally face the same problems as do other poor and near-poor people: eligibility requirements for financial assistance, benefit levels well below the current market price for health care, and a reluctance of health care providers to supply low-cost treatment (especially in specialties like obstetrics, for which malpractice premiums are extremely high). Recent legislation has begun to eliminate one of the most serious obstacles to financial access for homeless people, that is, the requirement for a fixed address as a prerequisite for determining eligibility for public health care benefits.

Depending on the state and the city, however, many homeless people—especially single, nondisabled adult individuals—are simply not eligible for such benefits.

With regard to physical access, those obstacles that often prevent the domiciled poor from obtaining health care prove to be still more difficult for the homeless. Hospitals, clinics, and mental health centers often are located far from the districts of cities where homeless people congregate. The primary means of getting to health care programs is public transportation, which homeless people often cannot afford. In addition, if they do get to such programs, the long wait for services may mean that they miss the deadline when they must be back at the shelter to sign up for a bed for the night. Given a forced choice between treatment and a shelter for the night, shelter invariably becomes a first priority.

Responding to the health care needs of the homeless is more difficult than serving the medically indigent population generally. Personnel need special training and support for working with people who are often very distrustful, lack a network of social supports, and have a multiplicity of medical and social needs.

What is Being Done About the Health Problems of Homeless People?

During the course of the study, members of the committee and the staff observed many commendable, well-utilized (and often overextended) health care and health care-related programs for homeless people throughout the country. Meetings were held with local officials, service providers, volunteers, and advocates for the homeless; numerous reports of other programs were evaluated. Of particular interest were the efforts of the 19 Robert Wood Johnson Foundation-Pew Memorial Trust Health Care for the Homeless projects, because they represented a particular targeted approach to providing health care services to homeless people. Moreover, while this study was in progress, Congress passed and the President signed into law the Stewart B. McKinney Homeless Assistance Act (P.L. 100-77), which provides new funding for a range of services, including general health and mental health care, in an effort to help the homeless (U.S. Congress, House, 1987).

However, even the most energetic health care worker is repeatedly confronted with the reality that poor and homeless people have trouble separating a specific need, such as health and mental health care, from the other activities needed for survival, such as securing housing and food. The committee concluded that even if the health care services that are clearly needed by so many of the homeless were widely available and accessible, the impact of such services would be severely restricted as long as the patients remained on the streets or in emergency shelters.

Conclusions and Recommendations

Five Critical Observations

The fundamental problem encountered by homeless people—lack of a stable residence—has a direct and deleterious impact on health. Not only does homelessness cause health problems, it perpetuates and exacerbates poor health by seriously impeding efforts to treat disease and reduce disability.

Although the urgent need for focused health care and other prompt interventions is readily recognized, the committee found that the health problems of the homeless are inextricably intertwined with broad social and economic problems that require multifaceted, long-term approaches for their resolution. In spite of the limitations brought about by the committee's charge and the limitations of the committee's resources in its ability to formulate detailed recommendations to deal with the root causes of homelessness, the committee believes that those who seek solutions to the homelessness problem itself and to its attendant health-related problems must take into consideration the five critical observations described below.

1. **More than anything else, homeless people need stable residences.**

   The health problems of homeless people that differ from those of other poor people are directly related to their homeless state. Homelessness is a risk factor that predisposes people to a variety of health problems and complicates treatment. The committee considers that decent housing is not only socially desirable but is necessary for the prevention of disease and the promotion of health. Yet the number of housing units for people with low incomes has been steadily decreasing since 1981, while the number of people needing such housing has been increasing during that same period.

2. **People need income levels that make housing affordable, both to reduce and to prevent homelessness.**

   The issue of affordable housing has two sides; On one side is the supply of housing at a given price; on the other is the amount of money an individual or family has with which to pay rent. The committee observed that in many communities neither employment at the current minimum wage nor welfare benefits for those who are eligible provide enough income for them to acquire adequate housing. Given the irreducible economic cost of housing in those communities, income adequacy must also be addressed if homelessness and its attendant health problems are to be prevented or remedied.

3. **Supportive services are necessary for some homeless people who require assistance in establishing and maintaining a stable residence.**

   Although the main issue is housing, for some homeless people, such as the chronically ill, the mentally retarded, the physically disabled, those with histories of alcohol and drug abuse, the very young, and the very old, housing alone may not be sufficient. They need the kind of social support systems and appropriate health care that would allow them to maintain themselves in the community. Effective discharge planning, outreach services, and casework are necessary to identify needs and to ensure that these needs are met. With the proper support systems, many will outgrow their need for therapeutic milieus and specialized housing and will eventually become self-reliant. For some, however, the need may be lifelong.

4. **Ensuring access to health care for the homeless should be part of a broad initiative to ensure access to health care for all those who are unable to pay.**

In its deliberations, the committee examined ways to increase and to try to ensure access to health care for the homeless as a special group. It concluded, on both ethical and practical grounds, that a targeted approach was inappropriate in the long run. The committee found that, as a practical matter, those who provide health care services to homeless people also encounter other poor, uninsured people seeking access to health care. Moreover, the boundary between the homeless and the nonhomeless is thin and permeable. Although there are some chronically homeless people, many poor people slip in and out of homelessness. Extending health care services to the homeless while continuing to deny them to the domiciled poor is, thus, not only administratively impractical and bureaucratically cumbersome but also ethically difficult for those who provide or finance health care services. The committee agrees with the President's Commission for the Study of Ethical Problems in Medicine and Biomedical and Behavioral Research (1983) that the federal government has an obligation regarding access to needed health care:

When equity occurs through the operation of private forces, there is no need for government involvement, but the ultimate responsibilty for ensuring that society's obligation is met, through a combination of public and private sector arrangements, rests with the federal government.

5. **Short-term solutions will not resolve what has clearly become a long-term problem.**

The immediate and desperate need for shelter and food has overridden attempts to design and implement policies that might provide some long-term solutions. In the committee's view, what is needed now is planning and action at the federal, state, and local levels to coordinate and ensure the continuity of appropriate services and housing for homeless people. Although short-term, problem-specific approaches provide essential and sometimes lifesaving services, the committee does not believe that they will result in major enduring change.

Keeping these five observations in mind, the committee

offers some recommendations about preventing and reducing homelessness before turning to recommendations focused on the immediate health care and other service needs of homeless people.

Preventing and Reducing Homelessness and Its Related Health Problems

As expressed throughout this report, health care and other services, including temporary shelters, can only help relieve some of the symptoms and consequences of homelessness. Coordinated efforts to address housing, income maintenance, and discharge planning are needed to prevent and reduce homelessness.

Housing The problem of homelessness will persist and grow in the United States until the diminution and deterioration of housing units for people with low incomes are reversed and affordable housing is made more widely available. Because of recent media attention to the refusal of certain homeless people to reside in institutional domiciles, there may be a misconception that homeless people will reject offers of decent and appropriate housing. There are no known studies that prove that if affordable housing were provided to homeless people they would use it, but several reports of the U.S. Conference of Mayors (1986a,b; 1987) regarding shelter utilization in excess of capacity support the belief that if such housing were available, the great majority of homeless people would surely accept it.

This is not a report on housing, nor was this committee made up of housing experts.* However, in light of the frequency with which the subject of housing arose during the course of this study, the committee makes the following observations:

1. For nearly five decades, beginning with the National Housing Act of 1938, the federal government has acknowledged, as a matter of explicit policy, its obligation to help ensure that every American family has access to decent housing. Because of the retreat from that commitment over the last several years, there has been a dramatic

---

*For a thoughtful analysis of this very complicated set of issues, see Alliance Housing Council (1988).

increase in the number of homeless people. The committee believes that if the health problems caused by homelessness are to be prevented, this commitment to housing should be reaffirmed.

2. Increasing the number of housing units for low-income people obviously requires major budgetary commitments. The lack of funds, however, is only one of several impediments to augmenting the housing supply. Among the nonfiscal issues that must be addressed are the impact of zoning regulations, real estate tax exemptions as incentives or disincentives to construct low-cost housing, local building construction standards, and the need for greater communication and coordination between the public agencies responsible for the disposition of abandoned housing and the public and private agencies that seek to help the homeless and ensure an adequate supply of affordable housing.

3. Many individuals and families only require a stable place to live, but some, especially the mentally ill, alcohol and drug abusers, the physically handicapped, and those with chronic and debilitating diseases, need housing and an array of professionally supervised supportive services in order to remain in the community—and, in many cases, to enable a transition to independent living. The committee believes that supportive housing programs for homeless people with disabilities are likely to be cost-effective and may lead to a reduction in future public expenditures; eventually, they may also enable these individuals to become economically productive citizens. Although there has long been a commitment to provide specialized housing (in the Community Mental Health Centers Act of 1962 [P.L. 88-164], for example, and implicitly in state governments' deinstitutionalization policies), the federal and state governments have not lived up to this commitment.

4. The Emergency Assistance program plays an important role in the provision of housing, especially as it relates to homeless families. In the committee's opinion, major aspects of this program that need to be reassessed include voluntary versus mandatory participation by the states, the use of Emergency Assistance funds to prevent—rather than simply to alleviate—homelessness, and the period of

time and type of facilities (hotel rooms versus apartments) for which Emergency Assistance funds can be used. This reassessment is especially urgent in light of the present high prevalence of homelessness and the widespread expectation that the problem will get worse before it gets better.

Income and Benefits Throughout its deliberations, the committee was impressed by the fact that improvements in income maintenance and other benefit programs for people in poverty would help appreciably in preventing and reducing homelessness and its related health problems. In this section the committee offers some observations and conclusions, urges the implementation of existing legislation, and recommends that some new legislation be considered.

The committee observes that a growing number of people with full-time jobs are becoming homeless. During its site visits around the country, the committee heard numerous references to people who are working but who cannot afford the most basic form of housing, not even a single room. This suggests that the relation of the minimum wage level to housing costs should be reexamined.

The committee also observed that many homeless people do not qualify for federally supported entitlement programs such as Medicaid and food stamps. Moreover, for those who do qualify, the benefit levels are so low as to make it impossible for them to obtain adequate housing or services. The committee did not find that there is any substantial justification for major geographic variations in eligibility standards. There may be a basis for some differences in benefit levels because of regional variations in the cost of living, but the dramatic differences in benefit levels from state to state do not appear to be justified.

Therefore, we recommend **that the federal government should review all federally funded entitlement programs in order to create rational eligibility standards and establish benefit levels based upon the actual cost of living in a specific region.** The committee commends state courts, such as those in Massachusetts and New York, for their recent decisions holding that entitlement benefits should be great enough to enable the recipients to afford that for which the benefits are intended, whether it be housing, food, or health care and recommends that this approach be adopted by other states and the federal government in establishing benefit levels.

In terms of eligibility for benefits, the committee found that the 1986 federal legislation requiring the development of procedures to ensure that the absence of a permanent address does not constitute a barrier to receipt of cash assistance, food stamps, Medicaid, and other benefits has yet to be fully implemented. **The committee urges prompt, uniform implementation of these procedures. Furthermore, the committee recommends that state and local governments reexamine their documentation requirements for public benefit programs** to ensure that they, too, do not impose unrealistic requirements on homeless people.

The committee observed that some homeless people who are eligible for income and other benefits are unaware of their eligibility or are unable to secure them. Augmented outreach efforts to identify and assist the homeless and those at risk of becoming homeless (especially those about to be discharged from institutions) could reduce and prevent homelessness (see the section Health Care and Related Services in this chapter for a more complete discussion of outreach). The committee recommends the following:

- **The effects of extending the presumptive eligibility guidelines for Supplemental Security Income (SSI) to include disabled homeless people (especially homeless people who have been discharged from a mental hospital within the preceding 90 days) should be evaluated in order to assess the costs and impact on the rates of homelessness.**
- **The effects of the current federal regulation that mandates a 33.3 percent cash reduction in benefits for SSI recipients who live with other people should be carefully assessed.** Questions such as the following need to be addressed: To what extent is the regulation contributing to homelessness by deterring people from sharing housing? Given the high cost of even the most basic forms of shelter services, would there be savings that would result from removing this regulation and, if so, what would the magnitude of the savings be?

Finally, the committee recommends that **serious consideration** be given to the following two changes in the Medicaid system:

- **Medicaid eligibility should be decoupled from eligibility for other benefits, and a national minimum eligibility standard should be established for Medicaid.** These changes would enhance access to health care for certain vulnerable groups— such as families whose Medicaid eligibility is lost if they lose Aid to Families with Dependent Children (AFDC) benefits.
- **Medicaid regulations should be amended to provide reimbursement for community-based services (e.g., day treatment and case management) for homeless people with psychiatric or physical disabilities in order to assist them in community integration and reduce current incentives for institutionalization.**

Discharge Planning Inadequate discharge planning coupled with inadequate community-based support and housing can cause homelessness. State, local, and private mental hospitals; inpatient substance abuse facilities; facilities for mentally retarded and developmentally disabled people; general hospitals; nursing homes; and correctional facilities all share a common responsibility to help arrange access for their clients or patients to appropriate and affordable postinstitutional living arrangements, including supportive services when necessary. Three sets of variables appear to affect the likelihood of postinstitutional placement most frequently:

1. Whether a person was homeless at the time of admission or became homeless during his or her institutional stay.
2. Whether there is a supply of affordable housing and supportive services or whether such housing or services are virtually nonexistent.
3. Whether even a basic minimum effort to locate housing and services is expended by the institution or whether that task is inappropriately delegated to shelters.

Some people become homeless because the institutions that are responsible for their care fail to ensure that they can maintain themselves in the community after they are discharged. Although the committee recognizes that there is a shortage of affordable housing, it believes that more effective discharge planning will help homeless people have greater access to that which is available. (On the related issue of the need for additional services for those who require posthospital nursing care, see the section Convalescent Services later in this chapter.) Just as it is inappropriate for a person who is not sick to remain in a hospital, so is it inappropriate for institutions simply to discharge people to shelters or to the streets without having made even the most basic efforts to find alternative living arrangements.

The committee recommends that public and private institutions adopt and observe discharge planning processes that ensure in advance of discharge—to the extent possible—that clients have suitable living arrangements and necessary supportive services. To help increase the availability of adequate postdischarge arrangements, such institutions must work to improve communications and coordination with organizations that provide postdischarge ambulatory care, home health care services, and other relevant community agencies and organizations.

Moreover, **federal and state agencies that provide financing to hospitals and other relevant institutions should extend to all beneficiaries of public programs the standards for discharge planning that now apply to Medicare patients.**

Health Care and Related Services

The committee found that the most effective health care and other services for homeless people are those that recognize the special needs and characteristics of the homeless. With this in mind, the committee recommends that the following general strategies be adopted:

- **services should be provided on a voluntary basis,** respectful of individual privacy and dignity;
- **intensive efforts should be made to engage homeless people by reaching out to them at the places where they congregate;** this requires appropriately skilled and trained health care professionals who can link clients to and provide continuity of services in community-based health care centers, freestanding clinics, hospital outpatient departments, and other existing providers of services;
- **health care providers should be trained in the special problems of patient engagement and communication;**

- health care providers should be trained in the diagnosis, treatment, and follow-up of those conditions that are especially prevalent among homeless people;
- techniques should be developed to address the particular difficulties homeless people have in maintaining medication or dietary regimens; and
- ways should be developed for homeless patients to obtain needed medicines, medical supplies, or equipment.

In many respects, homeless people have the same health care needs as other poor people. A high prevalence of acute and chronic diseases is found among the homeless, so health care needs to be available and accessible. **The committee recommends that serious efforts be made to identify those in need of treatment and to encourage intervention at the earliest appropriate time in order to avoid unnecessary deterioration in their health status. Such health care should include, for example, either by direct provision or by contractual agreement, primary health care services such as pediatric care (including well-baby care and immunizations), prenatal care, dental care, testing and treatment for sexually transmitted diseases, birth control, screening and treatment for hypertension, podiatric care, and mental health services.**

Outreach As discussed throughout this report, homeless people have multiple service needs. The provision of such services is complicated by the state of being homeless. Although there have been occasional reports of homeless people refusing services, data from the 19 Johnson-Pew projects indicate that, when properly approached, the homeless welcome services. In fact, demand for services has exceeded earlier projections for the utilization of both health care services and shelter space (U.S. Conference of Mayors, 1986a; Wright and Weber, 1987).

Aggressive outreach efforts and coordinated case management are crucial to successful service provision to homeless people. Intensive efforts to identify homeless people who are in need of health care and other services, to determine eligibility for benefits, to encourage acceptance of appropriate treatment, and to facilitate receipt of services are needed.

The committee recommends that the Social Security Administration substantially expand its outreach efforts, already man-

dated by statute, to include sites at which homeless people congregate. Special efforts should be made to expedite the assessment of eligibility for disability benefits of chronically mentally ill people about to be discharged from institutions. For example, consideration should be given to:

- developing descriptive materials on the current prerelease program for use by the Social Security Administration's (SSA) local offices;
- requiring a specific period within which state agencies must file and act upon disability applications received as part of the prerelease program;
- amending SSI regulations to permit applications for SSI to be completed and processed (either granted or denied) before a person's discharge;
- requiring local SSA personnel to routinely seek, accept, and process disability applications from patients in state mental hospitals; SSA workers should be trained to become effective liaisons with institutions in their area; and
- establishing a system for collecting national, regional, and local data on approval or denial of SSI disability claims of individuals in institutions.

Given the apparent effectiveness of the Veterans Administration's (VA) pilot project to reach homeless veterans suffering from mental illness, the committee recommends the following:

- **Additional funding should be appropriated to allow the expansion of the outreach program to those facilities that did not receive outreach staff under the original pilot project and, when necessary, to allow additional staffing for those facilities serving geographic areas with a high prevalence of homeless people. Furthermore, ways should be found to expand the VA's outreach effort to include homeless veterans who are not chronically mentally ill.**
- Because the VA has already shown itself to be willing to assist in preventing homelessness by serving those "at serious risk" of becoming homeless, **the VA should consider expanding its efforts to include outreach to such institutional settings as mental hospitals, acute-care hospitals, and**

prisons so that assessment and placement can be arranged before people are released from such facilities.

• The VA has given recognition to the possibility that some homeless veterans are "wary about coming to a hospital" (Rosenheck et al., 1987). **It is recommended that the VA consider alternatives to having psychiatric and medical assessments done at a medical facility and to determine whether changes will increase the number of veterans for whom follow-up care and placement is actually accomplished.**

• **The VA should increase its efforts to publicize its outreach program to providers of non-health care-related services to the homeless; as the outreach program becomes more fully established, the VA should pursue more formal means of linkage with other providers of services.**

• During several of its site visits, including a site visit to the community placement program at the VA Medical Center in Lexington, Kentucky, committee members heard frequent reference to a lack of appropriate supportive residential programs for veterans from the Vietnam era. Programs such as the community placement program, although rendering excellent service to the older veterans from World War II and the Korean conflict, were not seen as appropriate for the younger, more active Vietnam veterans. Because the initial outreach effort has determined that a majority of the homeless veterans whom they have seen were from the Vietnam era, **the VA should place a greater priority on developing programs that are more appropriate for meeting the needs of younger veterans.**

Casework After food and shelter, effective social casework is the fundamental service needed for nearly every homeless person. Such an approach, under appropriate professional supervision, is essential because of the multiple problems homeless people encounter in the complex interactions among employment, personal behavior, and public and private benefit and service programs. A coordinated local effort that enables public and private agencies to improve their communications would increase the likelihood that homeless people would use the programs and services to which they are entitled. In many communities, the creation of such a network will take time.

Therefore, in the interim, the committee recommends the following:

- **Ways should be found for providers of services to the homeless, including, for example, shelters, soup kitchens, and drop-in centers, to make casework services available to all clients willing to accept them.** Such intensive case management should focus on enrollment for benefits, services management, health care management, services coordination, and vocational assistance. These efforts should be aimed at ending the client's homelessness and facilitating his or her reintegration into the community.
- **Casework services must be adequately funded.** Federal, state, local, and voluntary agencies that fund services to the homeless should be encouraged to provide adequate resources. For example:
  1. For AFDC families, Federal Financial Participation for the administrative costs of casework should be increased as an incentive to states to increase their support.
  2. The Protection and Advocacy for Mentally Ill Individuals Act (P.L. 99-319), which currently applies only to mentally ill people in residential settings, should be amended to support protection and advocacy services for homeless people who are mentally ill, irrespective of their location.

Nutrition Nutrition is of particular concern to the health and well-being of the homeless, who are usually too poor to purchase adequate food and who have no place to prepare it. For those who receive food in soup kitchens and shelters, they get what is available without regard for special dietary needs. Homeless infants, children, and chronically ill adults are especially vulnerable to nutritional problems. Therefore, the committee recommends the following:

- **Providers of food to the homeless, such as operators of shelters, soup kitchens, and food pantries, should be educated in and encouraged to follow principles of sound nutrition and the special nutritional needs of the homeless.**
- **The recently established practice of permitting food stamps to be used at soup kitchens and other feeding sites should**

be extended to permit the use of food stamps to purchase prepared foods from restaurants and elsewhere.

- Because even the most prudent and imaginative parents in homeless families cannot provide adequate nutrition for young children at existing levels of food stamp benefits, such benefits should be recalculated to reflect realistic expenses to meet nutritional requirements.

- The Special Supplemental Food Program for Women, Infants, and Children (WIC) provides food assistance and nutritional screening to women and children below 185 percent of the poverty level; however, funding for this program is not adequate to provide such benefits to all those who are eligible (U.S. Congress, House, Committee on Ways and Means, 1987). Because many homeless women are pregnant and a growing number of homeless people are children, it is especially important that **the WIC Program be strengthened in order to address comprehensively the nutritional needs of pregnant women and young children.**

Mental Health, Alcoholism, and Drug Abuse Alcohol-related problems and mental disorders are the two most prevalent health problems among homeless adult individuals, and drug abuse appears to be on the increase. Since the early 1980s the National Institute of Mental Health, the National Institute on Alcohol Abuse and Alcoholism, and the National Institute on Drug Abuse have each funded programmatic and basic research in these areas as they relate to homelessness. More recent programs, such as the community mental health services demonstration projects for homeless individuals who are chronically mentally ill and the community demonstration projects for the treatment of homeless individuals who abuse alcohol and drugs (as mandated by Sections 612 and 613 of the Stewart B. McKinney Homeless Assistance Act), have significant potential for combating the major problems of these populations. Increased efforts to aid other homeless people, whether they are individuals or families, should not be at the expense of these existing programs.

In recent years, the trend has been to separate programs that serve the mentally ill, alcoholics, and drug abusers. However, because there is growing evidence of dual and multiple diagnoses among these populations and because there are certain basic similarities in efforts to provide treatment, those recommendations that address elements common to programs that treat individuals with all three diagnoses are identified before those recommendations relating to individuals with a specific diagnosis. In seeking to resolve the very complicated interrelationships among homelessness and mental illness, alcoholism, and drug abuse, the following services should be included:

- **targeted outreach services** directed at homeless individuals suffering from mental illness, alcoholism, or drug abuse;
- **supportive living environments** encompassing programs ranging from the most structured to the least structured; this is necessary so that as the individual improves, progress can be made through several stages of decreasing support and on to independent living, when possible (some will need various support services throughout their lifetimes);
- **treatment and rehabilitation services** appropriate to the individual's diagnosis and functional level; this must be a range of such services so that, again, the individual who improves can become less dependent on such programs while moving to self-sufficiency; and
- **specialized case management** provided by professionals who not only understand the complexities of these illnesses as they relate to homelessness but who also understand the complexities of systems that seek to provide mental health, alcoholism, and drug abuse services.

In addressing the issues of the mentally ill, alcoholic, or drug-abusing homeless, the committee saw repeated reference in the literature and heard from those actively engaged with these populations that **greater communication, consultation, and continuing liaison** between providers of services are needed. This is especially true for homeless adult individuals who suffer from more than one of these diagnoses, who suffer from one such diagnosis along with some other disabling condition (e.g., a physical disability), or who suffer from one form of substance abuse while using other substances as "enhancers." It is critical that **people suffering from dual or multiple diagnoses (physical illnesses, mental disorders, and addictions) not be left unserved or underserved because of overspecialization of treatment programs.** It is far more cost-effective to coordinate existing services than it would be to create new treatment programs directed at each possible combination of diagnoses.

With regard to specific problem areas, the committee offers the following conclusions and recommendations.

Mental Health The institutional mental health system appears to be an inappropriate place to focus policymakers' attention in trying to resolve the broad problems of homelessness. Proposals purporting to resolve the problem of homelessness by changing commitment laws or by substantially relaxing standards for admission to mental hospitals are misguided and lead to an erroneous belief that the mental health system alone can correct a problem for which all systems bear a responsibility. The central issue in mental health care is the lack of an adequate supply of appropriate and high-quality services throughout the mental health care system, including state psychiatric centers and psychiatric units in acute-care hospitals and in the community. **The committee recommends that the first priority in addressing the problems of the mentally ill homeless must be to ensure the adequate availability of clinical services (including professionally supervised supportive housing arrangements) at all levels.** Of these, the most serious deficiency between supply and demand—and that which is most directly linked to homelessness—is at the community level.

Alcoholism and Alcohol Abuse In addition to an inadequate supply of those services cited earlier (outreach, supportive living, treatment, and case management) as they relate to homeless individuals suffering from alcoholism, the committee notes a serious shortage of services directed toward the specific relationship between alcoholism and homelessness. In light of the fact that studies have shown that homeless alcoholics are at significantly greater risk of certain health problems (e.g, tuberculosis and hypothermia) than nonalcoholic homeless individuals and that alcoholism may become an integral part of the life-style of homelessness, the treatment of alcoholism among the homeless in the same manner and at the same locations as those for the domiciled alcoholic may not be the most effective. **The committee recommends that both public and private agencies and organizations treating alcoholism develop programs specifically for the homeless and those alcoholics at high risk of**

becoming homeless. The committee notes that recent developments such as alcohol-free living environments (e.g., "sober hotels") and programs that combine both medical and social approaches to the treatment of alcoholism appear to be especially promising.

Drug Abuse While not yet as prevalent as mental illness or alcoholism among the homeless single adult population, drug abuse, especially among younger adult men, is increasing. In particular, because of its close correlation with AIDS, the issue of intravenous drug abuse has come to greater public awareness, as has the inability of the existing drug abuse treatment system to respond to the increased demand for treatment services. **The committee joins with others in recommending that treatment services for intravenous drug abusers be increased to the extent that anyone desiring such services can be accommodated.** The cost of such services is relatively minor when compared with the costs of treatment and care for those physical diseases associated with intravenous drug abuse, such as AIDS and hepatitis.

The prevalence rates for mental illness, alcoholism, and drug abuse are much lower among adults who are members of homeless families than among homeless adults who are not, but the fact remains that such health problems are more prevalent among homeless parents than among the general population. Furthermore, the long-term impact on treatment programs and social service systems resulting from the effect of the parents' problems on the children could become very costly in the future. Both in terms of their value as a preventive measure and as the more cost-effective approach to contain the need for such services years from now, the committee recommends that **the relevant federal, state, and local agencies, as well as the relevant private not-for-profit agencies, should begin to examine alternate ways to treat mental illness, alcoholism, and drug abuse among homeless parents, giving due consideration to the limitations of time and mobility inherent in a parent's role.** In addition, **Congress should consider extending the provisions of the Stewart B. McKinney Homeless Assistance Act of 1987 that currently deal with mental illness and the treatment of alcoholism and drug abuse in individual adults to cover homeless parents, children, and adolescents as well.**

Convalescent Services **The committee recommends that Federal Emergency Management Administration funds and other funds be made available, in every community, to support the development and operation of facilities in which homeless people can safely convalesce from subacute illness or transient exacerbations of chronic illness, or to which they can safely and appropriately be discharged form acute-care facilities.** Adequate health care for homeless people is often made impossible by the simple absence of a secure place for them to convalesce. There is a clear need for facilities that provide appropriate rest and nutrition as well as limited personal care for periods generally not in excess of 30 days.

Other Services The Stewart B. McKinney Homeless Assistance Act of 1987 (P.L. 100-77) creates a federal Interagency Council on the Homeless and charges it to "review all federal activities and programs to assist homeless individuals." This study committee, in the course of its many site visits, observed several programs that are partially federally funded. For example, the Cardinal Medeiros Center in Boston receives some of its funding under the Older Americans Act (P.L. 89-73), and the Larkin Street Youth Center in San Francisco receives some of its support under the Runaway and Homeless Youth Act (P.L. 98-473). Often, these programs are not targeted directly toward, or identified with, the homeless. In some cases, such funding is due to expire along with the enabling legislation.

The committee recommends that the interagency council mandated by P.L. 100-77 give high priority to its review of all programs that might be of assistance in helping subpopulations among the homeless, irrespective of whether such programs are specifically directed toward helping homeless people. The council should:

- conduct an extensive review of such support programs, primarily to identify programs that are providing or that could provide help to subpopulations among the homeless;
- review joint federal-state efforts, such as state veterans homes with partial federal funding, that, although not targeted directly to the homeless, might help many homeless people;

- publicize successful efforts to help the homeless as a means of encouraging other groups to develop similar programs in their communities; and
- consider ways and means of extending or enhancing the funding for programs that are deemed effective in relieving or preventing homelessness until the current prevalence of homelessness is substantially reduced.

Special Needs of Homeless Children and Their Parents

The committee feels strongly that the growing phenomenon of homeless children is nothing short of a national disgrace that must be treated with the urgency that such a situation demands. The committee has chosen to offer a number of recommendations relating to services for homeless children, only because it believes that the fundamental reforms to income maintenance programs, the child welfare system, and foster care programs, will take a number of years to implement and that, in the interim, the tens of thousands of homeless children are in urgent need of a broad range of services.

Recent studies have documented that the majority of homeless children of various ages manifest delayed development, serious symptoms of depression and anxiety, or learning problems (Bassuk and Rubin, 1987; Bassuk and Rosenberg, 1988). These are early signs that vulnerability is turning into disability for these youngsters; efforts by human service professionals may be able to reverse these liabilities and to prevent further damage. There is now a considerable body of evidence demonstrating the benefits to disadvantaged and disorganized families of intensive family-oriented services; such approaches are characterized by flexibility in meeting families' multiple needs and by specific aids such as developmental day care, infant stimulation programs, parental counseling, and Head Start. Such intensive intervention efforts—even if expensive to begin with —have proved to be cost-effective in the long run (Schorr, 1988). Because the homeless are an especially vulnerable subpopulation of poor people, the committee believes that such programs would be of similar benefit to this group. It recognizes that because the population of homeless families includes some of the most hopeless and alienated among the poor—and because they are more likely to move from place to place—there may be obstacles to participation in such programs; therefore, the committee recommends the following:

- **Federal support for enriched day care and Head Start programs should be expanded and coupled with the development of outreach efforts to encourage homeless parents to take advantage of enrichment programs for themselves, their infants, and their young children.**
- **Local and state agencies that receive federal Head Start funds should be mandated to develop plans to identify and evaluate homeless children of preschool age and to provide them with appropriate services.**
- **Federal support for local and state education agencies should be conditional on the adoption of plans for identifying, evaluating, and serving homeless children of school age, including needed transportation services. These plans should include specific mechanisms for liaison and service coordination among educational, shelter, and social service agencies.**
- **Apart from any mandates that may accompany federal support, community agencies—acting in concert with school boards, local philanthropies, and other organizations—should be encouraged to develop programs of family-oriented services for homeless children and their parents. Such services need to be both intensive and comprehensive.**

Shelters

In the committee's view, **shelters should not become a permanent network of new institutions or substandard human service organizations.** As desirable housing is developed, the shelter system should be substantially reduced in size and returned to its original intent to provide short-term crisis intervention. In the interim, the committee recommends that action be taken to reduce the hazards to the health of homeless people that may be created or exacerbated by shelters.

- **The federal government should convene a panel of appropriate experts to develop model standards for life and fire** safety, sanitation, and disease prevention in shelters and other facilities in which 10 or more homeless people are domiciled. This code should be predicated on the recognition that shelters, welfare hotels, and the like should provide short-term, emergency housing and are not satisfactory longer term substitutes for housing and other services.

- Once a model code is developed and after a reasonable amount of time has passed for compliance to be obtained, **the federal government should adopt the standards as a condition for receipt of Emergency Assistance payments or other federal assistance, including Federal Emergency Management Agency funds.** However, Federal Emergency Management Agency funds should be made available to assist existing shelters to achieve compliance with the standards.

- **The federal government should disseminate the model code to encourage voluntary compliance.** State and local governments should be encouraged to adopt it on a mandatory basis for shelters that do not receive federal funds but that do receive funds from state and local governments.

- **Adequate provision must be made to shelter families as a unit.** The consequences of homelessness are serious enough without being worsened by family disruption.

- **In light of the increasing prevalence of sexually transmitted diseases, including AIDS, and unplanned pregnancies among the homeless, the committee recommends that shelters, particularly those used by younger single men, women, and adolescents, provide birth control counseling and services, including free condoms, to reduce the risks of these conditions.** It is recognized that data on the effectiveness of these recommendations in shelter populations do not exist and that many individuals, including some providers of services, may have ethical or philosophical objections, but it is the consensus of the committee that this recommendation represents sound public health practice.

Volunteer Efforts

The provision of services to homeless people depends heavily on the efforts of volunteers. Even with the recommended expansion of federal, state, and local government support, volunteers will be needed. The committee believes that the extraordinary contributions of services to homeless people by volunteer professionals and laymen must be better recognized, encouraged, and rewarded. **Federal, state, and local governments and local United Way and other charitable agencies should work with service-providing organizations to improve their capacity to recruit, train, use, and recognize volunteers.** Universities should play a major role in providing support by using programs for the homeless as part of their training curricula, especially in social work, law, medicine, dentistry, nursing, optometry, and the allied health professions. Not only would this improve the quantity and quality of volunteer efforts, but it would also provide students with extraordinary learning experiences and make them more sympathetic to those whom they will serve during their careers. Hospitals and other health care facilities should be encouraged to provide in-kind support (including clinic space and medications) for volunteers in their communities who help the homeless. Health professionals and lawyers should be encouraged to provide *pro bono* services, and professional organizations on the national, state, and local levels should establish formal programs in support of such efforts and provide recognition of those who provide such services.

State insurance commissioners should take measures to prevent carriers of medical, professional, or institutional liability insurance from charging additional, excessive, or discriminatory premiums or refusing to provide coverage for health care providers who serve the homeless without adequate documented actuarial experience to justify such action. This is especially critical in regard to malpractice and liability insurance because it is already difficult to recruit volunteers and to create university affiliations for training in the settings in which homeless people are served; these programs can ill afford to bear the additional burden of excessive insurance premiums or the potential loss of coverage.

Research

Many questions about the health of the homeless remain unanswered. Research is needed to elucidate the health and mental health disorders of the homeless, the methods of providing health care, and the factors that affect accessibility.

The Johnson-Pew Health Care for the Homeless projects provide the only extensive data base on the general health condition of homeless people (Wright and Weber, 1987). The shortcomings of these data are that they document health problems in individuals seeking help at clinics and are based on presenting complaints rather than systematic health evaluations; therefore, hidden health problems are not included.

There are no longitudinal data that document the fate of homeless people. For example, it is a frequent observation that there are relatively few homeless people over the age of 50, but the reasons for this are unknown. Though there have been calls from many quarters for additional resources to meet the needs of homeless people, there is still a paucity of information as to the ways in which resources should be allocated.

Various subgroups of the homeless have different health service needs; to consider the homeless as a homogeneous population is to be mistaken. Research is needed to identify the various subgroups of homeless people and their particular problems and health service requirements. Regional variations are also important; the problems of displaced workers in rural areas or small towns of the South or Midwest can be very different from those of displaced factory workers in the eastern industrial cities, which have more diversified economies.

Specific disorders deserve particular attention by researchers in epidemiology and health care services. These include tuberculosis and AIDS. Alcoholism has traditionally been and continues to be the most prevalent single medical condition of homeless people; improved methods of outreach, detoxification, rehabilitation, and long-term maintenance should be developed and evaluated. Abuse of other drugs also needs further research. The National Institute of Mental Health and the Robert Wood Johnson Foundation are to be especially commended for the initiatives that they have taken in encouraging and supporting research in the financing, organization, and delivery of services to the severely mentally ill.

Public and private research funding organizations should encourage research into the dynamics of homelessness, the health problems of homeless people, and effective service provision strategies. Specifically, the following research is most critically needed:

- longitudinal studies of the natural history of homelessness;
- studies of the prevalence of acute and chronic diseases in homeless populations;
- the role of illness as a precipitant of homelessness and the ability of health care and social service systems to prevent this outcome;
- studies of the homeless population and the prevalence of infectious diseases (e.g., tuberculosis, hepatitis, and AIDS) and chronic disorders or disabilities (e.g., mental retardation and epilepsy);
- studies of effective treatment programs for homeless alcoholics;
- development and evaluation of programs for homeless people who are mentally ill; and
- studies of the effects of homelessness on the health and development of children and evaluation of strategies to prevent homelessness in families and to give additional support to homeless families.

NOTES

Alliance Housing Council. 1988. Housing and Homelessness. Washington, D.C.: National Alliance to End Homelessness.

Bassuk, E. L., and L. Rosenberg. 1988. Why does family homelessness occur? A case-control study. American Journal of Public Health 78(7):783–788.

Bassuk, E. L., and L. Rubin. 1987. Homeless children: A neglected population. American Journal of Orthopsychiatry 5(2):1–9.

President's Commission for the Study of Ethical Problems in Medicine and Biomedical and Behavioral Research. 1983. Securing Access to Health Care: The Ethical Implications of Differences in the Availability of Health Services, Volume 1. Washington, D.C.: U.S. Government Printing Office.

Rosenheck, R., P. Gallup, C. Leda, P. Leaf, R. Milstein, I. Voynick, P. Errera, L. Lehman, G. Koerber, and R. Murphy. 1987. Progress Report on the Veterans Administration Program for Homeless Chronically Mentally Ill Veterans. Washington, D.C.: Veterans Administration.

Schorr, L. B. 1988. Within Our Reach: Breaking the Cycle of Disadvantage. New York: Doubleday.

U.S. Conference of Mayors. 1986a. The Growth of Hunger, Homelessness, and Poverty in America's Cities in 1985: A 25-City Survey. Washington, D.C.: U.S. Conference of Mayors.

U.S. Conference of Mayors. 1986b. The Continued Growth of Hunger, Homelessness and Poverty in America's Cities: 1986. A 25-City Survey. Washington, D.C.: U.S. Conference of Mayors.

U.S. Conference of Mayors. 1987. Status Report on Homeless Families in America's Cities: A 29-City Survey. Washington, D.C., U.S. Conference of Mayors.

U.S. Congress, House, 1987. Stewart B. McKinney Homeless Assistance Act, Conference Report to accompany. H. R. 558. Report 100-174. 100th Cong., 1st sess.

U.S. Congress, House, Committee on Ways and Means. 1987. Background material and data on programs within the jurisdiction of the Committee on Ways and Means. 100th Cong., 1st sess. March 6, 1987.

Wright, J. D., and E. Weber. 1987. Homelessness and Health. New York: McGraw-Hill.

Supplementary Statement on Health Care for Homeless People

THIS supplementary statement was prepared by nine members of the Committee on Health Care for Homeless Persons, not in opposition to the Committee's report, but from concern that the report is too limited in its discussion of the broader aspects of the issues it addresses. We endorse the report and its recommendations. We especially feel that the fact-finding efforts it embodies were thorough and thoughtful. But the report fails to capture our sense of shame and anger about homelessness, and it incompletely addresses the context in which all discussions regarding the health of homeless persons should be placed.

Any IOM (Institute of Medicine) report necessarily must undergo a process of negotiation among Committee members, and then between the Committee and external reviewers: such a process assures the objectivity, credibility, and defensibility of the report and its principal findings. This is just as it should be in order for the IOM and the National Academy of Sciences to fulfill the critical role of providing objective expert advice. There are invariably frustrations in such a process, but they too are an expected part of a committee's and the Institute's work. Another frustration, however, affected the work of this Com-

Ellen L. Bassuk, William R. Breakey, A. Alan Fischer, Charles R. Halpern, Gloria Smith, Louisa Stark, Nathan Stark, Bruce Vladeck, Phyllis Wolfe wrote this statement in response to the National Academy of Sciences report on *Health and Homelessness*. The supplement was not published with the NAS report.

From National Academy of Science Report, 1988. Reprinted by Permission of the United Hospital Fund.

mittee, and while the Committee's staff did an excellent job of managing this frustration within the Academy's ground rules, we feel the need to articulate our feelings in a supplementary statement.

The frustration we all experienced working on this report arises from the nature of the problem we were charged to address. Contemporary American homelessness is an outrage, a national scandal. Its character requires a careful, sophisticated, and dispassionate analysis—which this report provides—but its tragedy demands something more direct and human, less qualified and detached. We have tried to present the facts and figures of homelessness, but we were unable to capture the extent of our anger and dismay. We have summarized available studies on homeless children, but we had no means to paint the pathos and tragedy of these displaced, damaged, innocent lives. We have reviewed the demographic and clinical data and then, walking home, passed men asleep on heating grates or displaced people energetically searching in garbage piles for a few cents' income from aluminum cans. We analyzed mortality data for the homeless but lacked any platform from which to shout that our neighbors are dying needlessly because we are incapable of providing the most basic services.

As the Committee's deliberations progressed, we became increasingly aware that homelessness causes some illnesses and exacerbates and perpetuates others by seriously complicating efforts to treat disease and reduce disability. Therefore, only a comprehensive long-term strategy for eliminating homelessness will permanently improve the health status of homeless persons. Because of its charge and its limited resources, however, the Committee was unfortunately constrained in its ability to formulate essential long-term recommendations that dealt with the root causes of homelessness.

The most basic health problem of homeless people is the lack of a home; to condemn someone to homelessness is to visit him or her with a host of other evils. Ignoring the causes of homelessness leads to treating only symptoms and turns medical programs into costly but necessary stopgap measures. Attempts to address the health problems of homeless persons separately from their systemic causes is largely palliative.

A broad long-term strategy is needed to solve the health care problems of homeless people. Such a strategy must emphasize the context of homelessness. It must focus on gross inadequacies in four areas; supply of low-income housing, income maintenance, support services, and access to health care for the poor and uninsured.

1. *Housing.* As the Committee observed in its report, the health problems of homeless people that differ from the health problems of other poor people relate directly to their homeless state. We agree with the World Health Organization's statement (1987) on the International Year of Shelter for the Homeless: "Shelter to protect against the elements and to serve as a locus of family life is a basic human need. . . . At its best, appropriate shelter promotes emotional and social health."

   We support the principle that decent, affordable housing is every American's right. This view reaffirms the Federal Housing Act of 1948, which describes the Federal Government's obligation to assure that every household has access to decent, affordable housing. To this end, we strongly recommend that the Federal Government work to substantially increase the supply and availability of low-income housing. More specifically, we recommend that, as a start, funding for federal housing programs be restored to 1981 levels.

2. *Income and Benefits.* As the committee also observed, people must have income levels that make housing affordable, both to prevent and to end existing homelessness. We were grieved to encounter ever-growing numbers of homeless people with full-time jobs, who were unable to afford any kind of housing because they were being paid the minimum wage. It is our judgment that the minimum wage should be set at a level that makes decent housing affordable.

   Many people must rely on entitlements for their income and financial support. Not only have these benefits become more difficult to obtain, but today's federal entitlements are not sufficient to support housing for the elderly, the disabled, or those on welfare. If homelessness and its resultant health problems are to be eliminated, those benefits must be significantly augmented.

3. *Supportive Services*. Many homeless persons are disconnected from supportive relationships and caretaking institutions, as the report notes. Some, such as chronically mentally ill individuals, substance abusers, those with physical disabilities, and the very young and the very old, have very special needs. Many homeless people urgently require a wide array of support services, including job training, psychosocial rehabilitation, outreach, and case management.

For the most chronically disabled among the homeless population, psychosocial rehabilitation services must be offered, but for those who cannot be rehabilitated the goal is to provide decent and humane asylum in the community. Disabled people must not be consigned to lives of degradation.

4. *Access to Medical Care*. While homeless people encounter many obstacles obtaining access to health care, the single greatest problem is one shared by many other Americans; they are unable to pay for health care and therefore often do not receive it. While the Constitution does not promise citizens health care, neither does it guarantee universal free education or old age pensions, but these rights have long been recognized by policy makers. Additionally, the President's Commission for the Study of Ethical Problems in Medicine and Biomedical and Behavioral Research in their 1983 report *Securing Access to Health Care* concluded that:

. . . society has an ethical obligation to ensure equitable access to health care for all.

The societal obligation is balanced by individual obligations.

Equitable access to health care requires that all citizens be able to secure an adequate level of care without excessive burdens. When equity occurs through the operation of private forces, there is no need for government involvement, but the ultimate responsibility for ensuring that society's obligation is met, through a combination of public and private sector arrangements, rests with the Federal Government.

The cost of achieving equitable access to health care ought to be shared fairly.

Efforts to contain rising health care costs are important but should not focus on limiting the attainment of equitable access for the least well served portion of the public.

Approximately 37 million Americans, including many of the homeless, are without any form of public or private health insurance. Medicaid has tended to some needs of one large constituency, but we believe the time has come to move towards establishing universal access to health care.

The Committee tried to make its report as dispassionate as the IOM/NAS process requires, but the reality cries out for immediate action. As we witnessed the suffering of America's poorest citizens, we came to understand that the individual health problems of homeless people combine to form a major public health crisis. We can no longer sit as spectators to the elderly homeless dying of hypothermia, to the children with blighted futures poisoned by lead in rat-infested, dilapidated welfare hotels, to women raped, to old men beaten and robbed of their few possessions, and to people dying on the streets with catastrophic illnesses such as AIDS. Without eliminating homelessness, the health risks and concomitant health problems, the desperate plight of homeless children, the suffering, and the needless deaths of homeless Americans will continue. We agree with the recommendations set forth in the committee report, but we felt continuously uneasy because of our inability to state the most basic recommendation: Homelessness in the United States is an inexcusable disgrace and must be eliminated.

Deinstitutionalization and the Homeless Mentally Ill

H. Richard Lamb, M.D.

Is deinstitutionalization the cause of homelessness? Some would say yes and send the chronically mentally ill back to the hospitals. A main thesis of this paper, however, is that problems such as homelessness are not the result of deinstitutionalization per se but rather of the way deinstitutionalization has been implemented. It is the purpose of this paper to describe these problems of implementation and the related problems of the lack of clear understanding of the needs of the chronically mentally ill in the community. The discussion then turns to some additional unintended results of these problems, such as the criminalization of the mentally ill that usually accompanies homelessness. The paper concludes with some ways of resolving these problems.

To see and experience the appalling conditions under which the homeless mentally ill exist has a profound impact upon us; our natural reaction is to want to rectify the horrors of what we see with a quick, bold stroke. But for the chronically mentally ill, homelessness is a complex problem with multiple causative factors; in our analysis of this problem we need to guard against settling for simplistic explanations and solutions.

For instance, homelessness is closely linked with deinstitutionalization in the sense that three decades ago most of the chronically mentally ill had a home—in the state hospital. Without deinstitutionalization it is unlikely there would be large

From *Hospital and Community Psychiatry*. 35:899–907, 1984. Reprinted by permission of the author and of *Hospital and Community Psychiatry*.

numbers of homeless mentally ill. Thus in countries such as Israel, where deinstitutionalization has barely begun, homelessness of the chronically mentally ill is not a significant problem. But that does not mean we can simply explain homelessness as a result of deinstitutionalization; we have to look at what conditions these persons must face in the community, what needed resources are lacking, and the nature of mental illness itself.

With the mass exodus into the community that deinstitutionalization brought, we are faced with the need to understand the reactions and tolerance of the chronically mentally ill to the stresses of the community. And we must determine what has become of them without the state hospitals, and why. There is now evidence that nationwide very substantial numbers of the severely mentally ill are homeless at any given time.[1,2,3] Some are homeless continuously and some intermittently. We need to understand what characteristics of society and the mentally ill themselves have interacted to produce such an unforeseen and grave problem as homelessness. Without that understanding, we will not be able to conceptualize and then implement what needs to be done to resolve the problems of homelessness.

With the advantage of hindsight, we can see that the era of deinstitutionalization was ushered in with much naivete and many simplistic notions about what would become of the chronically and severely mentally ill. The importance of psychoactive medication and a stable source of financial support was perceived, but the importance of developing such fundamental resources as supportive living arrangements was often not clearly seen, or at least not implemented. "Community treatment" was much discussed, but there was no clear ideas as to what it should consist of, and the resistance of community mental health centers to providing services to the chronically mentally ill was not anticipated. Nor was it foreseen how reluctant many states would be to allocate funds for community-based services.

It had been observed that persons who spend long periods in hospitals develop what has come to be known as institutionalism —a syndrome characterized by lack of initiative, apathy, withdrawal, submissiveness to authority, and excessive dependence on the institution.[4] It had also been observed, however, that this syndrome may not be entirely the outcome of living in dehumanizing institutions; at least in part, it may be characteristic of the schizophrenic process itself.[5] Many patients who are liable to institutionalism and vulnerable to external stimulation may develop dependence on any other way of life outside hospitals that provides minimal social stimulation and allows them to be socially inactive.[6] These aspects of institutionalism were often not recognized or were overlooked in the early enthusiasm about deinstitutionalization.

In the midst of very valid concerns about the shortcomings and antitherapeutic aspects of state hospitals, it was not appreciated that the state hospitals fulfilled some very crucial functions for the ill. The term "asylum" was in many ways an appropriate one, for these imperfect institutions did provide asylum and sanctuary from the pressures of the world with which, in varying degrees, most of these patients were unable to cope.[7] Further, these institutions provided such services as medical care, patient monitoring, respite for the patient's family, and a social network for the patient as well as food, shelter, and needed support and structure.[8]

Fernandez,[9] working in Dublin, recognizes these needs that used to be met, though not well, by state hospitals. He warns about the tendency to "equate the concept of homelessness exclusively with the lack of a permanent roof over one's head. This deflects attention from what is believed to be the essential deficit of homelessness, namely, the absence of a stable base of caring or supportive individuals whose concern and support help buffer the homeless against the vicissitudes of life. In this context, it is felt that the absence of such a base, or the inability to establish or to approximate such a base, is the essential deficit of patients with 'no-fixed-abode.' "

In the state hospitals what treatment and services that did exist were in one place and under one administration. In the community the situation is very different. Services and treatment are under various administrative jurisdictions and in various locations. Even the mentally healthy have difficulty dealing with a number of bureaucracies, both governmental and private, and getting their needs met. Further, patients can easily get lost in the community as compared to a hospital, where they may have been neglected but at least their whereabouts were known. It is these problems that have led to the recognition of the importance of case management. It is probable that many of the homeless mentally ill would not be on the streets if they were on the caseload of a professional or paraprofessional trained to deal with the problems of the chronically mentally ill, monitor them (with considerable persistence when necessary), and facilitate their receiving services.

In my experience [10] and that of others,[11] the survival of long-term patients, let alone their rehabilitation, begins with an appropriately supportive and structured living arrangement. Other treatment and rehabilitation are of little avail until patients feel secure and are stabilized in their living situation. Deinstitutionalization means granting asylum in the community to a large marginal population, many of whom can cope to only a limited extent with the ordinary demands of life, have strong dependency needs, and are unable to live independently.

Moreover, that some patients might need to reside in a long-term, locked, intensively supervised community facility was a foreign thought to most who advocated return to the community in the early years of emptying the state hospitals. "Patients who need a secure environment can remain in the state hospital" was the rationale. But in those early years most people seemed to think that such patients were few, and that community treatment and modern psychoactive medications would take care of most problems.

Most people are now recognizing that a number of severely disabled patients present major problems in management, and can survive and have their basic needs met outside of state hospitals only if they have a sufficiently structured community facility or other mechanism that provides support and controls.[12] Some of the homeless appear to be in this group. A function of the old state hospitals often given too little weight is that of providing structure. Without this structure, many of the chronically mentally ill feel lost and cast adrift in the community, however much they may deny it.

There is currently much emphasis on providing emergency shelter to the homeless, and certainly this must be done. However, it is important to put the "shelter approach" into perspective; it is a necessary stopgap, symptomatic measure, but does not address the basic causes of homelessness. Too much emphasis on shelters can only delay our coming to grips with the underlying problems that result in homelessness. We must keep these problems in mind even as we sharpen our techniques for working with mentally ill persons who are already homeless.

Most mental health professionals are disinclined to treat "street people" or "transients."[13] Moreover, in the case of the homeless, we are working with persons whose lack of trust and desire for autonomy cause them to not give their real names, to refuse our services, and to move along because of their fear of closeness, of losing their autonomy, or of acquiring a mentally ill identity. Providing food and shelter with no strings attached, especially in a facility that has a close involvement with mental health professionals, a clear conception of the needs of the mentally ill, and the ready availability of other services, can be an opening wedge that ultimately will give us the opportunity to treat a few of this population.

At the same time we have learned that we must beware of simple solutions and recognize that this shelter approach is not a definitive solution to the basic problems of the homeless mentally ill. It does not substitute for the array of measures that will be effective in both significantly reducing and preventing homelessness: a full range of residential placements, aggressive case management, changes in the legal system that will facilitate involuntary treatment, a stable source of income for each patient, and access to acute hospitalization and other vitally needed community services.

Still another problem with the shelter approach is that many of the homeless mentally ill will accept shelter but nothing more, and eventually return to the wretched and dangerous life on the streets. A case example will illustrate.

A 28-year-old man was brought to a California state hospital with a diagnosis of acute paranoid schizophrenia. He had been living under a freeway overpass for the past six weeks. There was no prior record of his hospitalization in the state. After a month in the hospital he had gone into partial remission and was transferred to a community residential program. There he was assigned to a skilled, low-key, sensitive clinician. Over a period of several weeks he gradually improved and returned to what was probably his normal state of being guarded and suspicious but not overtly psychotic.

Though he isolated himself much of the time, he appeared quite comfortable with the program and with the staff and indicated that he would, if allowed, stay indefinitely. He denied possessing a birth certificate, baptismal certificate, driver's license, or any other proof of identity. He steadfastly refused to give the whereabouts of his family or reveal his place of birth or anything else about his identity, even though he realized such information was necessary to qualify him for any type of financial or housing assistance. Clearly his autonomy was precious to him. And in an unguarded moment he said, "I couldn't bear to have my family know what a failure I have been." At the end of the three months, the maximum length of stay allowed by the community program's contract, he had to be discharged to a mission.

What was not foreseen in the midst of the early optimism about returning the mentally ill to the community and restoring and rehabilitating them so they could take their places in the mainstream of society was what was actually to befall them. Certainly it was not anticipated that criminalization and homelessness would be the lot for many. But first let us briefly look at how deinstitutionalization came about.

A Brief History
of Deinstitutionalization

For more than half of this century, the state hospitals fulfilled the function for society of keeping the mentally ill out of sight and thus out of mind. Moreover, the controls and structure provided by the state hospitals, as well as the granting of almost total asylum, may have been necessary for many of the long-term mentally ill before the advent of modern psychoactive medications. Unfortunately the ways in which state hospitals achieved this structure and asylum led to everyday abuses that have left scars on the mental health professions as well as on the patients.

The stage was set for deinstitutionalization by the periodic public outcries about these deplorable conditions, documented by journalists such as Albert Deutsch;[14] mental health professionals and their organizational leaders also expressed growing concern. These concerns led ultimately to the formation of the Joint Commission on Mental Illness and Health in 1955 and its recommendations for community alternatives to state hospitals, published in 1961 as a widely read book, *Action for Mental Health*.[15]

When the new psychoactive medications appeared,[16,17] along with a new philosophy of social treatment,[18] the great majority of the chronic psychotic population was left in a state hospital environment that was now clearly unnecessary and even inappropriate for them, though, as noted above, it met many needs. Still other factors came into play. First was a conviction that mental patients receive better and more humanitarian treatment in the community than in state hospitals far removed from home. This belief was a philosophical keystone in the origins of the community mental health movement. Another powerful motivating force was concern about the civil rights of psychiatric patients; the systems then employed of commitment and institutionalization in many ways deprived them of their civil rights. Not the least of the motivating factor was financial. State governments wished to shift some of the fiscal burden for these patients to federal and local governments—that is, to federal Supplemental Security Income(SSI) and Medicaid and local law enforcement agencies and emergency health and mental health services.[19,20]

The process of deinstitutionalization was considerably accelerated by two significant federal developments in 1963. First, categorical Aid to the Disabled (ATD) became available to the mentally ill, which made them eligible for the first time for federal financial support in the community. Second, the community mental health centers legislation was passed.

With ATD, psychiatric patients and mental health professionals acting on their behalf now had access to federal grants-in-aid, in some states supplements by state funds, which enabled patients to support themselves or to be supported either at home or in such facilities as board-and-care homes or old hotels at comparatively little cost to the state. Although the amount of money available to patients under ATD was not a princely sum, it was sufficient to maintain a low standard of living in the community. Thus the states, even those that provided generous ATD supplements, found it cost far less to maintain patients in the community than in the hospital. (ATD is now called Supplemental Security Income, or SSI, and is administered by the Social Security Administration.)

The second significant federal development of 1963 was the passage of the Mental Retardation Facilities and Community Mental Health Centers Construction Act, amended in 1965 to

provide grants for the initial costs of staffing the newly constructed centers. This legislation was a strong incentive to the
development of community programs with the potential to treat
people whose main resource previously had been the state
hospital. It is important to note, however, that although rehabilitative services and precare and aftercare services were among
the services eligible for funding, an agency did not have to offer
them in order to qualify for funding as a comprehensive community mental health center.

Also contributing to deinstitutionalization were sweeping
changes in the commitment laws of the various states. In California, for instance, the Lanterman-Petris-Short Act of 1968
provided further impetus for the movement of patients out of
hospitals. Behind this legislation was a concern for the civil
rights of the psychiatric patient, much of it from civil rights
groups and individuals outside the mental health professions.
The act made the involuntary commitment of psychiatric patients a much more complex process, and it became difficult to
hold psychiatric patients indefinitely against their will in mental
hospitals. Thus the initial stage of what had formerly been the
career of the long-term hospitalized patient—namely, an involuntary, indefinite commitment—became a thing of the past.[21]

Some clearly recognized that while many abuses needed to be
corrected, this legislation went too far in the other direction
and no longer safeguarded the welfare of the patients. (For
instance, Richard Levy, M.D., of San Mateo, California, argued this point long and vigorously.) But these were voices in
the wilderness. We still have not found a way to help some
mental health lawyers and patients' rights advocates see that
they have contributed heavily to the problem of homelessness—
that patients' rights to freedom are not synonymous with releas-
ing them to the streets where they cannot take care of themselves,
are too disorganized or fearful to avail themselves of what help
is available, and are easy prey for every predator.

The dimensions of the phenomenon of deinstitutionalization
are revealed by the numbers. In 1955 there were 559,000 patients
in state hospitals in the United States; today at any given time
there are approximately 132,000.[22]

What Happened to the Patients

What happened to the chronically and severely mentally ill as a result of deinstitutionalization? In the initial years approximately two-thirds of discharged mental patients returned to their families.[23] The figure is probably closer to 50 percent in states such as California, which has a high number of persons who are without families.[24] This discussion is limited to those aged 18 to 65, for those over 65 are a very different population with a very different set of problems.

In most recent years, there has been a growing number of mentally disabled persons in the community who have never been or have only briefly been in hospitals. Problems in identifying and locating them make it difficult to generalize about them. But we do know they tend to be younger and often manifest less institutional passivity than the previous generation, who had spent many years in state hospitals.

A large proportion of the chronically mentally ill—in some communities as many as a third or more of those aged 18 to 65—live in facilities such as board-and-care homes.[24] These products of the private sector are not the result of careful planning and well-conceived social policy. On the contrary, they sprang up to fill the vacuum created by the rapid and usually haphazard depopulation of our state hospitals. Suddenly many thousands of former state hospital patients needed a place to live, and private entrepreneurs, both large and small, rushed to provide it.

"Board-and-care home" is used in California to describe a variety of facilities, many of which house large numbers of psychiatric patients. These patients include both the deinstitutionalized and the new generations of chronically mentally ill. The number of residents ranges from one to more than a hundred. Board-and-care homes are unlocked and provide a shared room, three meals a day, dispensing of medications, and minimal staff supervision; for a large proportion of long-term psychiatric patients, the board-and-care home has taken over the functions of the state hospitals. And for many, the alternative to the board-and-care home would be homelessness.

There is a great deal of variability in facilities such as board-

and-care homes. Generally they could and should provide a higher quality of life than they do, and services should be made more available to their residents. Services should include social and vocational rehabilitation, recreational activities, and mental health treatment. But considering the funding available, these facilities are for the most part not bad in the sense that there is no life-threatening physical neglect or other gross abuses.[25]

What does stand out is the significantly higher funding for similar resources for the developmentally disabled and the resulting increased quality in terms of location of the facility, condition of repair, general atmosphere, and staffing. For instance, as of 1984 the rate paid to operators of board-and-care facilities for the developmentally disabled in California varies from a minimum of $525 a month for easily manageable residents to $840 a month for "intensive treatment." For the mentally ill there is only one rate of $476 per month, regardless of the severity of the problem and the need for intensive supervision and care; many of the better board-and-care home operators have stopped serving the mentally ill in order to take advantage of the higher rates for the developmentally disabled. Clearly this is a gross inequity.

But facilities such as board-and-care homes and single-room-occupancy (SRO) hotels, even when adequate, often do not attract and keep the homeless.[1] If they do enter one of these facilities, their stay may be brief—they drift in and out, to and from the streets. Further, these facilities are not prepared to provide the structure needed by some of the chronically mentally ill, as discussed below.

This paper is, of course, concerned with the undomiciled chronically mentally ill, those who live neither with family nor in board-and-bare homes nor in SRO hotels nor in nursing homes nor in their own homes or apartments. Some are homeless continuously, and some intermittently. While estimates of the extent of the problem are highly variable and there are no reliable data, it seems reasonable to conclude that nationwide the homeless mentally ill number in the tens of thousands, and perhaps the many tens of thousands. They live on the streets, the beaches, under bridges, in doorways. So many frequent the shelters of our cities that there is concern that the shelters are becoming mini-institutions for the chronically mentally ill, an ironic alternative to the state mental hospitals.[26]

The Tendency to Drift

Drifter is a word that strikes a chord in all those who have contact with the chronically mentally ill—mental health professionals, families, and the patients themselves. It is especially important to examine the phenomenon of drifting in the homeless mentally ill. The tendency is probably more pronounced in the young (aged 18 to 35), though it is by no means uncommon in the older age groups. Some drifters wander from community to community seeking a geographic solution to their problems; hoping to leave their problems behind, they find they have simply brought them to a new location. Others, who drift in the same community from one living situation to another, can best be described as drifting through life: they lead lives without goals, direction, or ties other than perhaps an intermittent hostile-dependent relationship with relatives or other caretakers.[27]

Why do they drift? Apart from their desire to outrun their problems, their symptoms, and their failures, many have great difficulty achieving closeness and intimacy. A fantasy of finding closeness elsewhere encourages them to move on. Yet all too often, if they do stumble into an intimate relationship or find themselves in a residence where there is caring and closeness and sharing, the increased anxiety they experience creates a need to run.

They drift also in search of autonomy, as a way of denying their dependency, and out of a desire for an isolated life-style. Lack of money often makes them unwelcome, and they may be evicted by family and friends. And they drift because of a reluctance to become involved in a mental health treatment program or a supportive out-of-home environment, such as a halfway house or board-and-care home, that would give them a mental patient identity and make them part of the mental health system: they do not want to see themselves as ill.

Those who move out of board-and-care homes tend to be young; they may be trying to escape the pull of dependency and may not be ready to come to terms with living in a sheltered, segregated, low-pressure environment.[28] If they still have goals, they may find life there extremely depressing. Or they may want more freedom to drink or to use street drugs. Those who move on are more apt to have been hospitalized during the preceding year. Some may regard leaving their comparatively static milieu as a necessary part of the process of realizing their goals—but a process that exacts its price in terms of homelessness, crisis, decompensation, and hospitalizations.

Once out on their own, they will more than likely stop taking their medications and after a while lose touch with Social Security and no longer be able to receive their SSI checks. They may now be too disorganized to extricate themselves from living on the streets—except by exhibiting blatantly bizarre or disruptive behavior that leads to their being taken to a hospital or to jail.

The Question of Liberty

Perhaps one of the brightest spots of the effects of deinstitutionalization is that the mentally ill have gained a greatly increased measure of liberty. There is often a tendency to underestimate the value and humanizing effects for former hospital patients of simply having their liberty to the extent that they can handle it (even aside from the fact that it is their right) and of being able to move freely in the community. It is important to clarify that, even if these patients are unable to provide for their basic needs through employment or to live independently, these are separate issues from that of having one's freedom. Even if they live in mini-institutions in the community, such as board-and-care homes, the homes are not locked, and the patients generally have access to community resources.

However, the advocacy of liberty needs to be qualified. A small proportion of long-term, severely disabled psychiatric patients lack sufficient impulse control to handle living in an open setting such as a board-and-care home or with relatives.[12] They need varying degrees of external structure and control to compensate for the inadequacy of their internal controls. They are usually reluctant to take psychotropic medications and often have problems with drugs and alcohol in addition to their mental illness. They tend not to remain in supportive living situations, and often join the ranks of the homeless. The total number of such patients may not be great when compared to the total population of severely disabled patients. However, if placed in community living arrangements without sufficient structure, this group may require a large proportion of the time of mental health professionals, not to mention others such as the police. More important, they may be impulsively self-destructive or sometimes present a physical danger to others.

Furthermore, many of this group refuse treatment services of any kind. For them, simple freedom can result in a life filled with intense anxiety, depression, and deprivation, and often a chaotic life on the streets. Thus they are frequently found among the homeless when not in hospitals and jails. These persons often need ongoing involuntary treatment, sometimes in 24-hour settings such as locked skilled-nursing facilities or, when more structure is needed, in hospitals. It should be emphasized that structure is more than just a locked door; other vital components are high staff-patient ratios and enough high-quality activities to structure most of the patient's day.

In my opinion, a large proportion of those in need of increased structure and control can be relocated from the streets to live in open community settings, such as with family or in board-and-care homes, if they receive assistance from legal mechanisms like conservatorship, as is provided in California. But even those who live in a legally structured status in the community, such as under conservatorship or guardianship, have varying degrees of freedom and an identity as a community member.

Some professionals now talk about sending the entire population of chronically and severely mentally ill patients back to the state hospitals, exaggerating and romanticizing the activities and care the patients are said to have received there. To some, reinstitutionalization seems like a simple solution to the problems of deinstitutionalization such as homelessness.[19,29] But activity and treatment programs geared to the needs of long-term patients can easily be set up in the community, and living conditions, structured or unstructured, can be raised to any level we choose—if adequate funds are made available.

The provision of such community resources, adequate in quantity and quality, would go a long way toward resolving the problems of homelessness. In the debate over which is the better treatment setting—the hospital or the community—we must not overlook the patients' feelings of mastery and heightened self-esteem when they are allowed their freedom.

Criminalization

Deinstitutionalization has led to large numbers of mentally ill persons in the community. At the same time, there are a limited amount of community psychiatric resources, including hospital beds. Society has a limited tolerance of mentally disordered behavior, and the result is pressure to institutionalize persons needing 24-hour care wherever there is room, including jail. Indeed, several studies describe a criminalization of mentally disordered behavior—that is, a shunting of mentally ill persons in need of treatment into the criminal justice system instead of the mental health system. [30,31,32,33,34] Rather than hospitalization and psychiatric treatment, the mentally ill often tend to be subject to inappropriate arrest and incarceration. Legal restrictions placed on involuntary hospitalization also probably result in a diversion of some patients to the criminal justice system.

Studies of 203 county jail inmates, 102 men and 101 women, referred for psychiatric evaluation[32,35] shed some light on the issues of both criminalization and homelessness. This population had extensive experience with both the criminal justice and the mental health systems, was characterized by severe acute and chronic mental illness, and generally functioned at a low level. Homelessness was common; 39 percent had been living, at the time of arrest, on the streets, on the beach, in missions, or in cheap, transit skid row hotels. Clearly the problems of homelessness and criminalization were interrelated.

Almost half of the men and women charged with misdemeanors had been living on the streets or the beach, in missions, or in cheap transient hotels, compared with a fourth of those charged with felonies (p<.01 by chi-square analysis). One can speculate on some possible explanations. Persons living in such places obviously have a minimum of community supports; committing a misdemeanor may frequently be a way of asking for help. It is also possible that many are being treated for minor criminal acts that are really manifestations of their illness, their lack of treatment, and the lack of structure in their lives. Certainly these were the clinical impressions of the investigators as they talked to these inmates and their families and read the police reports.

The studies also found that a significantly larger percentage of inmates aged 35 or older had a history of residence in a board-and-care home, compared with those under age 35 ($p<.02$, chi-square analysis). Obviously the older one is, the more opportunity one has had to live in different situations, including board-and-care homes. However, in talking with these men and women, other factors emerged: the tendencies of the younger mentally ill person to hold out for autonomy rather than living in a protected, supervised setting, and to resist both entering the mental health system and being labeled as a psychiatric patient, even to the extent of living in a board-and-care home. Board-and-care homes had been repeatedly recommended to a large number of the younger persons as part of their hospital discharge plans, but they had consistently refused to go. It appeared that eventually many gave up the struggle, at least temporarily, and accepted a board-and-care placement. However, most left the homes after relatively brief periods, many to return to the streets.

In some cases the board-and-care situation did not appear to be structured enough for them. In other cases, they seemed to want to regain their autonomy, their isolated life-style, and their freedom to engage in antisocial activities. Despite the fact that a high proportion of the study population had serious psychiatric problems, only eight men (out of 102) and five women (out of 101) were living in board-and-care homes at the time of arrest.

Clearly the system of voluntary mental health outpatient treatment is inadequate for this population, who are extremely resistant to it. If they do agree to accept treatment, they tend not to keep their appointments and not to take their medications, and to be unwelcome at outpatient facilities.[36] This is confirmed by our findings, which showed that only 10 percent of the inmates were receiving any form of outpatient treatment, such as medication, at the time of arrest, and that only 24 percent ever received outpatient treatment.

The need for mental health services in jails is apparent.[37] Even so, many mentally ill inmates will not participate in release planning and will not accept referral for housing or treatment. As a result they are released to the streets to begin anew their chaotic existences characterized by homelessness, dysphoria, and deprivation. To work with this population of mentally ill in jail is to be impressed by their need for ongoing involuntary treatment.

Conclusions

The majority of chronically mentally ill persons live with their families or in sheltered living situations such as board-and-care homes. Some live in situations such as single-room-occupancy hotels or otherwise alone. Many are in and out of hospitals. Some are continuously homeless, and some intermittently so. While a minority of the total population of chronically mentally ill are homeless at any given time, very substantial numbers of persons are involved, and homelessness of the chronically mentally ill is a critical nationwide problem.

What have we learned from our experience with more than two decades of deinstitutionalization? First of all, it has become clear that what is needed is a vast expansion of community housing and other services and a whole revamping of the mental health system to meet the needs of the chronically mentally ill. Markedly increased funding is needed to increase the quality, quantity, and range of housing and other services, improve the quality of life for this population, and meet their needs for support and stability. The availability of suitable services should make it possible to attract many of the homeless to stable living arrangements and retain them there.

Many of the chronically mentally ill are not able to find or retain such community resources as housing, a stable source of income, and treatment and rehabilitation services. The need for monitoring and treating these patients by means of aggressive case management has become increasingly apparent. Aggressive case management for all of the chronically mentally ill, given the availability of adequate housing and other resources, would probably minimize homelessness.

It is one of the injustices of deinstitutionalization that, compared with the developmentally disabled, the chronically mentally ill in the community do not fare well in terms of funding, housing, and services. Surely the needs of the mentally ill should be given equal priority. The success of deinstitutionalization for the developmentally disabled, however, does demonstrate what can be accomplished when there is determined advocacy and adequate funding and community resources.

We have learned in this era of deinstitutionalization that many of the homeless mentally ill feel alienated from both society and the mental health system, that they are fearful and suspicious, and that they do not want to give up what they see as their autonomy, living on the streets where they have to answer to no one. They may be too acutely and chronically mentally ill and disorganized to respond to our offers of help. Their tolerance for closeness and intimacy is very low, and they fear they will be forced into relationships they cannot handle. They may not want a mentally ill identity, may not wish to or are not able to give up their isolated life-style and their anonymity, and may not wish to acknowledge their dependency. Thus we are dealing with an extremely difficult and challenging population.

As with most problems, we have learned that there are no simple and universal solutions to the problems of homelessness. Let us take the shelter approach as an example. Some of the chronically mentally ill will accept food and shelter, but nothing else, and sooner or later return to the streets, despite the efforts of our most sensitive clinicians. A few will not accept simple shelter, even with no conditions attached.

Certainly we must provide emergency shelter, but also we need to be aware that this is a symptomatic approach. Instead our primary focus should be on the underlying causes of homelessness, and we should work to provide a full range of residential placements, aggressive case management, changes in the legal system, a ready availability of crisis intervention including acute hospitalization, and other crucial community treatment and rehabilitation services.

We have also learned that some of the chronically mentally ill, because of their personality problems, their lack of internal controls, and their resort to drugs and alcohol, will not be manageable, or welcome, in open settings, such as with family or in board-and-care homes, or even in shelters. Some will need more structure and control; they may need involuntary treatment in a secure intermediate or long-term residential setting or in the community, facilitated by mechanisms such as conservatorship or mandatory aftercare. Such intervention should not be limited to those who can be proven to be "dangerous," but should be extended to gravely disabled individuals who do not respond to aggressive case management and are too mentally incompetent to make a rational judgment about their needs for care and treatment. In this way we can help those homeless mentally ill who are unwilling to accept our assistance and whose self-destructive tendencies, personality disorganization, and inability to care for themselves result in lives lived alternately in jails, in hospitals, and on the streets. In some cases such intervention is the only act of mercy left open to us.

We have learned that we must accept patients' dependency when dealing with the chronically mentally ill. And we must accept the total extent of patients' dependency needs, not simply the extent to which *we* wish to gratify these needs. We have learned, or should have learned, to abandon our unrealistic expectations and redefine our notions of what constitutes success with these patients. Sometimes it is returning them to the mainstream of life; sometimes it is raising their level of functioning just a little so they can work in a sheltered workshop. But oftentimes success is simply engaging patients, stabilizing their living situations, and helping them lead more satisfying, more dignified, and less oppressive lives.

The reluctance of mental health professionals and society to fully accept the dependency of this vulnerable group, inadequate case management systems, the preference of many mental health professionals to work with more "healthy" and "savory" patients, and an ideology that "coercive" measures should be used only in cases of "extreme danger" leave the homeless mentally ill in extreme jeopardy. If deinstitutionalization has taught us anything, it is that flexibility is all important. We must look objectively at the clinical and survival needs of the patients and meet those needs without being hindered by rigid ideology or a distaste for dependency.

NOTES

1. Arce AA, Tadlock M, Vergare MJ, et al: A psychiatric profile of street people admitted to an emergency shelter. Hospital and Community Psychiatry 34:812–817, 1983
2. Baxter E, Hopper K: Troubled on the streets: the mentally disabled homeless poor, in The Chronic Mental Patient: Five Years Later. Edited by Talbott JA. New York, Grune & Stratton, 1985
3. Lipton FR, Sabatini A, Katz SE: Down and out in the city: the homeless mentally ill. Hospital and Community Psychiatry 34:817–821, 1983
4. Wing JK, Brown GW: Institutionalism and Schizophrenia. New York, Cambridge University Press, 1970
5. Johnstone EC, Owens DGC, Gold A, et al: Institutionalization and the defects of schizophrenia. British Journal of Psychiatry 139:195–203, 1981
6. Brown GW, Bone M, Dalison B, et al: Schizophrenia and Social Care. London, Oxford University Press, 1966
7. Lamb HR, Peele R: The need for continuing asylum and sanctuary. Hospital and Community Psychiatry 35:798–802, 1984
8. Bachrach LL: Asylum and chronically ill psychiatric patients. American Journal of Psychiatry 141:975–978, 1984
9. Fernandez J: "In Dublin's fair city": the mentally ill of "no-fixed-abode." Lecture at Conference on Homelessness, Dublin, Sept 1983.
10. Lamb HR: What did we really expect from deinstitutionalization? Hospital and Community Psychiatry 32:105–109, 1981.
11. Baxter E, Hopper K: The new mendicancy: homeless in New York City. American Journal of Orthopsychiatry 52:393–408, 1982
12. Lamb HR: Structure: the neglected ingredient of community treatment. Archives of General Psychiatry 37:1224–1228, 1980
13. Larew BI: Strange strangers: serving transients. Social Casework 63:107–113, 1980

14. Deutsch A: The Shame of the States. New York, Harcourt Brace, 1948.

15. Joint Commission on Mental Illness and Health: Action for Mental Health: Final Report of the Commission. New York, Basic Books, 1961.

16. Brill H, Patton RE: Analysis of 1955–56 population fall in New York State mental hospitals in the first year of large-scale use of tranquilizing drugs. American Journal of Psychiatry 114:509–514, 1957

17. Kris EB: The role of drugs in after-care, home-care, and maintenance, in Modern Problems of Pharmacopsychiatry: The Role of Drugs in Community Psychiatry, vol. 6. Edited by Shagass C. Basel, Karger, 1971

18. Greenblatt M: The third revolution defined: it is sociopolitical. Psychiatric Annals 7:506–509, 1977

19. Borus JF: Deinstitutionalization of the chronically mentally ill. New England Journal of Medicine 305:339–342, 1981

20. Goldman HH, Adams NH, Taube A: Deinstitutionalization: the data demythologized. Hospital and Community Psychiatry 34:129–134, 1983

21. Lamb HR, Sorkin AP, Zusman J: Legislating social control of the mentally ill in California. American Journal of Psychiatry 138:334–339, 1981

22. Redick RW, Witkin MJ: State and County Mental Hospitals, United States, 1970–80 and 1980–81. Mental Health Statistical Note 165. Rockville, Md, National Institute of Mental Health, Aug 1983

23. Minkoff K: A map of chronic mental patients, in The Chronic Mental Patient. Edited by Talbott JA. Washington, DC, American Psychiatric Association, 1978

24. Lamb HR, Goertzel V: The long-term patient in the era of community treatment. Archives of General Psychiatry 34:679–682, 1977

25. Dittmar ND, Smith GP: Evaluation of board and care homes: summary of survey procedures and findings. Special briefing for Department of Health and Human Services, Denver Research Institute, 1983

26. Bassuk L, Rubin L, Lauriat A: Is Homelessness a Mental Health Problem? American Journal of Psychiatry, V141:12, 1546–1550, 1984

27. Lamb HR: Young adult chronic patients: the new drifters. Hospital and Community Psychiatry 33:465–468, 1982

28. Lamb HR: Board and care home wanderers. Archives of General Psychiatry 37:136–137, 1980

29. Feldman S: Out of the hospital, onto the streets: the over-selling of benevolence. Hastings Center Report 13:5–7, 1983

30. Abramson MF: The criminalization of mentally disordered behavior. Hospital and Community Psychiatry 23:101–105, 1972

31. Grunberg F, Klinger BI, Grument BR: Homicide and the deinstitutionalization of the mentally ill. American Journal of Psychiatry 134:685–687, 1977

32. Lamb HR, Grant RW: The mentally ill in an urban country jail. Archives of General Psychiatry 39:17–22, 1982

33. Sosowsky L: Crime and violence among mental patients reconsidered in view of the new legal relationship between the state and the mentally ill. American Journal of Psychiatry 135:33–42, 1978

34. Urmer A: A study of California's new mental health law. Chatsworth, Calif, ENKI Research Institute, 1971

35. Lamb HR, Grant RW: Mentally ill women in a county jail. Archives of General Psychiatry 40:363–368, 1983

36. Whitmer GE: From hospitals to jails: the fate of California's deinstitutionalized mentally ill. American Journal of Orthopsychiatry 50: 65–75, 1980

37. Lamb HR, Schock R, Chen PW, et al: Psychiatric needs in local jails: emergency issues. American Journal of Psychiatry 141:774–777, 1984

Providing Health Care for Low-income Children: Reconciling Child Health Goals with Child Health Financing Realities

Sara Rosenbaum and Kay Johnson

E VERY child needs access to health care, including assessment and diagnostic services, preventive treatment, and medical care for episodic and chronic illnesses and conditions. We provide children with health care because it is both an ethical and moral social obligation (President's Commission for the Study of Ethical Problems in Medicine and Biomedical and Behavioral Research 1983). We also provide health care for children because many pediatric health interventions are known to be both effective and cost-effective (Starfield 1982), and because when we invest in children we invest in our own futures.

Unfortunately, however, the goal of equitable access to health care for children has always been an elusive one in the United States. In recent years, it has grown more so, as rising poverty, changing employment patterns, and cutbacks in public health programs have left 35 million Americans—33 percent of whom are children and two-thirds of whom have family incomes below 200 percent of the federal poverty level—uninsured (Swartz 1985).

The purpose of this article is to examine health care financing for low-income children. Specifically, we will consider the Medicaid program and its special preventive health benefit for chil-

From *The Milbank Quarterly*, Vol. 64, No. 3, 1986. Reprinted by permission of *The Milbank Quarterly*, Milbank Memorial Fund.

dren, known as the Early and Periodic Screening Diagnosis and Treatment program (EPSDT), in order to assess how well major child health goals are being served for low-income children.

Medicaid is the single most important public health program for low-income children, accounting for over 55 percent of all public health expenditures for children, compared to only 25 percent of public health expenditures for the elderly (Budetti, Butler, and McManus 1982). Medicaid has played a crucial role in reducing the disparity in access to health care between poor and nonpoor children (Davis and Schoen 1978).

The EPSDT program, added to the Medicaid program in 1967, ensures that all Medicaid-eligible children are covered not only for health care for acute and chronic medical problems but also for a wide range of preventive benefits, including health assessments, immunizations, vision, hearing and dental care, and medical treatment for episodic or chronic conditions disclosed during the screening process. Thus, the Medicaid program, in both its diagnosis-related and preventive health aspects, contains enormous potential for helping poor children secure access to the full range of health care they need.

However, Medicaid has substantially shortchanged the children it was meant to serve. Even prior to the dramatic 1981 reductions in federal eligibility standards, Medicaid provided only one out of three poor children with full-year coverage and left another one-third of all poor children completely uninsured (Butler et al. 1985). Despite the broad range of preventive and primary health services available to Medicaid-eligible children through the EPSDT program, over half of all black preschool children were inadequately immunized against various preventable childhood diseases in 1982 (Children's Defense Fund 1985b). Poor children continue to be at increased risk of death from all causes, including preventable factors, and are more likely to suffer greater and more severe and prolonged levels of many childhood illnesses (Egbuanu and Starfield 1982). Finally, when adjusted for health status, poor children have less access to medical care than their nonpoor counterparts (Kleinman 1981).

This article examines two separate but highly related issues. First, it analyzes Medicaid as a current source of health care financing for children. Second, it evaluates key structural decisions that states have made in implementing their EPSDT programs in order to determine whether the states' approach to

EPSDT administration is compatible both with the limitations of Medicaid and the needs of low-income children.

We focus particularly on EPSDT in this article because, as the component of Medicaid devoted exclusively to children, it provides insight into how adequately states finance a range of pediatric medical services for low-income children. Since EPSDT covers both assessment and medical treatment services, examination of EPSDT can identify how a variety of low-income children's health care service needs are met.

Finally, we conclude this article by exploring a series of possibilities for improving health care financing and service delivery arrangements for poor children.

Children and Medicaid: An Uneasy Relationship

Despite the fact that poor children have a disproportionately large stake in Medicaid, their relationship with the program has never been an easy one. Furthermore, children's link to Medicaid has deteriorated significantly over the last several years as a direct result of major federal restrictions imposed on the program by the Reagan administration and Congress.

Medicaid is a federal grant-in-aid program that entitles certain categories of poor individuals to coverage for a range of medical benefits (Rosenbaum 1983b). States are granted sizeable flexibility in fashioning their Medicaid plans. However, as a condition of participation in the program, states must cover certain groups of persons and must provide certain benefits to enrollees.

Payments for covered services are made directly by state Medicaid agencies to providers participating in the program for care furnished to enrollees. States maintain considerable flexibility in developing provider-participation standards, and establishing reimbursement rates, particularly in the case of outpatient services.

The federal government reimburses states for a certain percentage of the costs Medicaid agencies incur. The federal reimbursement level is based on a formula tied to a state's per capita income level.[1] While federal funding for Medicaid is open-ended, as a practical matter a state will budget a set amount for a Medicaid program of a certain size and will control amounts expended by limiting the categories of persons served, restricting the definition of who is "poor" enough to qualify for Medicaid, limiting the range and depth of coverage, and limiting the level of reimbursement paid to providers. For example, in 1985 Medicaid financial eligibility levels for a family of three with no other income ranged from $118 per month in Alabama to $719 per month in Alaska.

Medicaid is the largest and most complex of all need-based federal grant-in-aid programs. Basically, however, it is an entitlement program that generally "piggybacks" onto two cash-assistance programs for the poor, including Aid to Families with Dependent Children (AFDC)[2] and the Supplemental Security Income (SSI)[3] programs. The SSI program is a federally financed welfare program providing cash grants to aged, blind, and certain disabled persons, and its categorical and financial eligibility requirements are set by federal law. AFDC, on the other hand, is a federal grant-in-aid program that provides states with near total flexibility to establish financial eligibility criteria. In 1985 a single, noninstitutionalized SSI recipient received a living allowance of $336 per month in addition to Medicaid coverage.

That same year, however, the average AFDC benefit for a family of three was approximately $340 per month, or a pro-rated amount of approximately $113 per month for each family member. As Table 1 records, the 1985 monthly AFDC cash payment levels for a family of three were extraordinarily low.

The AFDC program represents the major test by which children's financial eligibility for Medicaid is determined. Over 95 percent of the more than 10 million children who received Medicaid in fiscal year 1984 were eligible as "dependent children." These children were covered by Medicaid either because they received AFDC or because they lived in families with countable incomes at or below AFDC payment levels (Health Care Financing Administration 1984a). Eighty-four percent of all children classified as "dependent" also received an AFDC cash grant. Another portion lived in families whose total incomes were at or below AFDC eligibility levels. About one million children were enrolled in Medicaid because, after incurred medical expenses were deducted, their families had countable incomes between 100 percent and 133 percent of their state's AFDC payment level (Health Care Financing Administration 1984a). Such recipients are known as the "medically needy" (Rosenbaum 1983b). Only about a quarter million children received Medicaid on the basis of SSI eligibility.

TABLE 1

Monthly Medicaid Eligibility Levels* for a Family of Three, as a Percentage of the Federal Poverty Level**

State	Medicaid eligibility level	As a percentage of the federal poverty level
Alabama	$118	16%
Alaska	719	97
Arkansas	192	26
California	555	75
Colorado	346	47
Connecticut	487	66
Delaware	287	39
District of Columbia	327	44
Florida	240	33
Georgia	223	30
Hawaii	468	63
Idaho	304	41
Illinois	302	41
Indiana	256	35
Iowa	360	49
Kansas	365	49
Kentucky	197	27
Louisiana	190	26
Maine	370	50
Maryland	313	42
Massachusetts	396	54
Michigan	372	50
Minnesota	524	71
Mississippi	120	16
Missouri	273	37
Montana	332	45

TABLE 1 (continued)

State	Medicaid eligibility level	As a percentage of the federal poverty level
Nebraska	350	47
Nevada	285	39
New Hampshire	378	51
New Jersey	404	55
New Mexico	258	35
New York	474	64
North Carolina	246	33
North Dakota	371	50
Ohio	290	38
Oklahoma	282	38
Oregon	386	52
Pennsylvania	348	47
Rhode Island	409	55
South Carolina	187	25
South Dakota	329	45
Tennessee	153	21
Texas	184	25
Utah	376	51
Vermont	531	72
Virginia	269	36
Washington	462	63
West Virginia	206	28
Wisconsin	533	72
Wyoming	360	49

Source: Social Security Administration, October, 1985: Data based on typical state maximum AFDC payments.
*Reflects categorically needy eligibility only for 1985 for families with no other income. Medically needy eligibility levels may be slightly higher in those states in which the actual AFDC payment amount is lower than AFDC payment standard.
**For 1985, annual federal poverty guidelines set poverty income levels for a family of 3 at $8,850 ($737.50 per month).

Thus, insofar as financial eligibility is concerned, AFDC is the determinant of children's eligibility for Medicaid. Federal law mandates coverage for all poor children under age five whose families are categorically ineligible for AFDC. Federal law also provides state Medicaid programs the option of covering any child under age 21 whose family does not meet AFDC categorical eligibility standards. Thirty states have exercised this option (Table 2). But even for children who are categorically ineligible for AFDC cash assistance, the AFDC program nonetheless provides the financial test by which their eligibility is measured.

Obviously, a program that incorporates financial eligibility criteria as restrictive as those found in the states' AFDC programs will result in the denial of aid to millions of extremely poor children. For example, were an AFDC recipient with two children to find full-time, minimum wage employment, her gross salary of about $575 per month, which equals two-thirds of the federal poverty level for a family of three, would give her a monthly income level greater than the 1985 AFDC payment level for a family of three in every state but Alaska (Table 1). Even her take-home pay, which would be somewhat lower (the federal tax system unfortunately taxes poor as well as nonpoor workers), would still exceed nearly all states' monthly AFDC payment levels. Her gross salary would also have exceeded the so-called "standard of need" in 30 states (Children's Defense Fund 1986b). The "standard of need" is the threshold point for determining AFDC and Medicaid eligibility for applicants with outside income.

De minimus AFDC financial eligibility standards thus result in a built-in bias against Medicaid coverage of poor workers and their families. Prior to 1981, only 12 percent states' AFDC caseloads included persons with earned income, and "excess" earnings, meager as they might be, have traditionally been one of the primary reasons why a family loses its AFDC coverage (Congressional Research Service 1985).

The traditional bias in public assistance programs against poor working families is particularly disturbing since two-thirds of all poor children in 1984 lived in families in which at least one member was in the labor force (Children's Defense Fund 1986a) and since firms that primarily employ minimum wage earners are likely to offer no health insurance as a fringe benefit (Monheit et al. 1984). Not surprisingly, it has been estimated that three-quarters of uninsured Americans are either in the labor force (and disproportionately working at lower-wage jobs) or are dependents for persons in the labor force

TABLE 2
Medicaid Coverage of Children under 18 and Medically Needy Children and Pregnant Women

State	State covers all poor children under 18 in 2-parent working families	State covers medically needy children and pregnant women
Alabama	No	No
Alaska	Yes	No
Arkansas	Yes	Yes
California	Yes	Yes
Colorado	No	No
Connecticut	Yes	Yes
Delaware	*	No
District of Columbia	Yes	Yes
Florida	Yes	**
Georgia	Yes	Yes
Hawaii	No	Yes
Idaho	No	No
Illinois	Yes	Yes
Indiana	No	No
Iowa	Yes	Yes
Kansas	Yes	Yes
Kentucky	No	Yes
Louisiana	No	Yes
Maine	Yes	Yes
Maryland	Yes	Yes
Massachusetts	Yes	Yes
Michigan	Yes	Yes
Minnesota	Yes	Yes
Mississippi	Yes	No
Missouri	Yes	No
Montana	No	Yes
Nebraska	Yes	Yes
Nevada	No	No
New Hampshire	No	Yes
New Jersey	Yes	Yes
New Mexico	No	No
New York	Yes	Yes
North Carolina	Yes	Yes

State	State covers all poor children under 18 in 2-parent working families	State covers medically needy children and pregnant women
North Dakota	No	Yes
Ohio	Yes	No
Oklahoma	Yes	Yes
Oregon	No	Yes
Pennsylvania	Yes	Yes
Rhode Island	No	Yes
South Carolina	Yes	Yes
South Dakota	No	No
Tennessee	Yes	Yes
Texas	Yes	Yes
Utah	Yes	Yes
Vermont	Yes	Yes
Virginia	No	Yes
Washington	***	Yes
West Virginia	No	Yes
Wisconsin	Yes	Yes
Wyoming	No	No

Source: State Medicaid plans and Children's Defense Fund survey, 1985.
*State provides Medicaid, under special waiver, to all children who receive state-funded general assistance, GA levels are lower than AFDC levels.
**Effective July 1986 (pending legislative approval).
***Has a state-funded medical assistance program for all low-income persons receiving general assistance, and who do not qualify for Medicaid. Children under 21 are covered under either this program or under Medicaid.

(Monheit et al. 1984). In 1980 poor children were over 3 times more likely than nonpoor children to be completely uninsured and only 33 percent of poor children had any private insurance coverage that year (Butler et al. 1985).

Since 1980 the limitations on children's Medicaid eligibility have been intensified by a series of congressional actions undertaken as part of the Reagan administration's fiscal year 1982 budget proposals. These proposals, which established new, mandatory federal limits on AFDC coverage for families with outside income were specifically designed to remove the working poor from the program. These limitations, which automatically apply to Medicaid, include the following:

- Prior to 1981 a working AFDC recipient had all necessary work-related expenses deducted form his earnings in calculating his or her eligibility for benefits. Since enactment of the Omnibus Budget Reconciliation Act of 1981 (OBRA),[4] states can now deduct only $75 of an individual's work-related costs each month, regardless of a worker's actual expenses.
- Prior to 1981 a worker could deduce all child care costs in applying for AFDC. OBRA limited the child care deduction to $160 per month, even for full-time workers.
- Prior to 1981 a set portion of a worker's wages were discounted, for as long as he or she worked, in computing his or her entitlement to AFDC benefits. After OBRA that portion of earned income could be disregarded only for a limited period of time.
- Prior to 1981 workers could apply for and receive AFDC and Medicaid no matter how high their gross earnings, so long as their countable earnings fell below payment eligibility levels. After OBRA a worker with gross earnings in excess of 150 percent of a state's "standard of need" could not even be considered for benefits, no matter how much his or her earnings might be reduced by work-related expenses.
- OBRA tightened the federal AFDC asset test from $2,000 to $1,000, thereby eliminating from coverage persons with more than $1,000 in personal resources.

In 1984, Congress softened some of these 1981 penalties.[5] First, the 150 percent "cap" on the "standard of need" was raised to 185 percent. Second, the period of time during which an AFDC-eligible worker could be credited with "disregards" earnings was slightly lengthened. Third, states were required to extend Medicaid for nine months for workers who lost coverage simply because certain AFDC disregards earnings expired (states were also given the option to extend this coverage for an additional six months).

However, these medications by no means restored AFDC's (and thus, Medicaid's) federal eligibility standards to modest, pre-1981 levels. As a result, millions of poor workers who previously might have been assisted by the AFDC and Medicaid programs now fail to quality for benefits.

The cumulative effects of the AFDC program's long-term financial stagnation and the federally imposed antiwork restrictions enacted in 1981 have been to limit severely the amount of time that a child's family can be expected to qualify for Medicaid (assuming that they can any longer qualify at all). Indeed, so severely have welfare stagnation and federal restrictions cut into children's Medicaid eligiblity that had state Medicaid programs in 1983 performed at their 1976 eligibility levels, two million additional children would have qualified for coverage that year (Children's Defense Fund 1985a). Moreover, in great measure because of fluctuating income, about one-third of all AFDC recipients lose eligibility within one year, and 50 percent lose eligibility within two years (McManus 1986).

Poor families with fluctuating earnings are extremely likely to be swept off the program for one or more reasons. A specialized study of the effects of the 1981 AFDC reductions found that, in five major cities surveyed, 66 to 86 percent of working AFDC recipients were affected by the reductions, compared to only 4 to 15 percent of those without earnings (U.S. General Accounting Office 1985). Among the employed, between 36 and 60 percent lost benefits outright. A year later half of these families had no health insurance. These five cities experienced approximately a two-thirds decline in the already low percentage of AFDC recipient families who had any earned income.

There can be no doubt as to Medicaid's impact on low-income children's access to and utilization of health care. One out of every three low-income children under the age of 6 with full-year Medicaid coverage, compared to one out of five uninsured low-income children, received any preventive health services in 1980. Furthermore, adjusted for health status, low-income uninsured children were significantly less likely to see a physician for any reason that year than Medicaid-covered children (Rosenbach 1985).

Thus, the most important public health financing program for poor children offers them increasingly attenuated coverage for services. Children in poor families, particularly families that work, may be eligible for Medicaid for a few months, if at all, only to lose coverage because of a slight increase in the otherwise-uninsured family head's earnings.

Thirty-five states do provide Medicaid to medically needy children whose family incomes slightly exceed AFDC eligibility levels but are insufficient to meet the cost of necessary medical care (Table 2). But these programs are of extremely limited usefulness. Like the basic Medicaid program, states' "medically needy" programs are tied to the AFDC payment level. Children living in minimum wage families would have to incur significant medical costs before their eligibility could begin—costs that in many instances far exceed the cost of a child's routine preventive and episodic health care needs.

The Early Periodic Screening Diagnosis and Treatment Program (EPSDT)

> We are a young nation. . . . Much of the courage and vitality that bless this land are the gift of young citizens. . . . What [young people] are able to offer the world as citizens depends on what their Nation offered them as youngsters (U.S. Congress 1967).

With these words, President Johnson transmitted to Congress the Social Security Amendments of 1967, containing certain "Recommendations for the Welfare of Children." These recommendations included a series of amendments to Medicaid and Crippled Children's programs[6] that were intended "to discover, as early as possible, the ills that handicap our children" and to provide "continuing followup and treatment so that handicaps do not go neglected." By the end of that year, after remarkably brief consideration, Congress had amended both statutes to include a new required service for all individuals under the age of 21 and eligible for Medicaid. This benefit was known as Early and Periodic Screening Diagnosis and Treatment (EPSDT).[7]

Thus, one of the most sweeping health guarantees for disadvantaged American children ever enacted by Congress was launched: a program that would locate children suffering from health problems and ensure that they received the continuous and comprehensive medical care they needed. Congress envisioned that working together, crippled children's agencies and other public agencies would identify children in need of care and would extend to them a program of preventive and remedial health benefits. The Medicaid program would finance the cost of the medical and remedial care provided by these agencies to Medicaid-eligible children.[8] Ultimately, Medicaid agencies would also themselves become responsible for case-finding and supportive activities in addition to financing medical care.[9]

As a required benefit for Medicaid beneficiaries under age 21, EPSDT finances a broad range of primary and preventive health services for children. The purposes of EPSDT are to provide a comprehensive and periodic assessment of a child's overall health, developmental, and nutritional status, to treat conditions and illnesses disclosed during the assessment process, and to provide vision, dental, and hearing care. Services contained in the EPSDT benefit package include: a detailed and comprehensive health examination that consists of a health and developmental history, an unclothed physical examination, appropriate vision and hearing testing, appropriate laboratory tests, and a direct referral to a dentist for children over the age of three; immunizations; vision, hearing, and dental care; the diagnostic and medical treatment for conditions disclosed during the screening process, to the extent that such treatment services are otherwise included in a state's general Medicaid plan.[10] Moreover, at their discretion, states may furnish special diagnostic and treatment services to children participating in the EPSDT program that are not otherwise made available to Medicaid-eligible persons.[11]

EPSDT assessment services must be furnished at periodic intervals specified in the state Medicaid plan (known as a periodicity schedule) that meet reasonable standards of medical care[12] (Table 3). Thus, for example, a reasonable EPSDT dental examination schedule would at a minimum call for annual exams and treatment.[13] Furthermore, each screening exam must meet reasonable content standards.[14] For example, all laboratory tests and developmental assessments must be age-appropriate.

In addition to furnishing this package of basic medical ser-

vices, state Medicaid agencies must also take affirmative action
to ensure that EPSDT-eligible children know about, and are
able to utilize, the benefits to which they are entitled. These
affirmative action requirements include "effective" programs
for informing families about EPSDT that combine oral and
written informing procedures,[15] provision of necessary scheduling and transportation assistance for both screening and treatment agencies;[16] arranging for free or reduced-cost care for
health services a child needs that are not covered by Medicaid;[17]
and the development of interagency agreements with agencies
funded under the Title V Maternal and Child Health Block
Grant and other agencies and institutions to ensure adequate
screening, diagnostic, and treatment providers.[18]

The EPSDT program's successes and failures have been extensively reviewed during the two decades since its enactment.
The program has assisted millions of children who otherwise
might never have received comprehensive basic preventive health
care. Children have received immunizations, eye exams, hearing

TABLE 3
State Periodicity Schedules

State	Infancy	Early Childhood	Late Childhood	Adolescence	Total
A.A.P.[1]	6	6	4	4	20
Alabama	1	4	1	2	8
Alaska	5	3	3	2	13
Arkansas	2	2	3	2	9
California	6	5	2	2	15
Colorado	6	7	2	3	18
Connecticut	5	3	3	2	13
Delaware	3	4	1	3	11
District of Columbia	5	3	2	2	12
Florida	5	6	3	2	16
Georgia	4	3	3	3	13
Hawaii	*	*	*	*	*
Idaho	1	1	1	1	4
Illinois	5	4	2	2	13
Indiana	5	6	7	5	23
Iowa	4	5	2	2	13

State	Infancy	Early Childhood	Late Childhood	Adolescence	Total
A.A.P.[1]	6	6	4	4	20
Kansas	3	5	2	3	13
Kentucky	5	5	4	3	17
Louisiana	2	3	2	3	10
Maine	6	5	3	3	17
Maryland	4	3	3	2	12
Massachusetts	*	*	*	*	*
Michigan	2	2	4	4	12
Minnesota	3	4	2	3	12
Mississippi	4	4	3	on request	12
Missouri	6	6	3	3	18
Montana	*	*	*	*	*
Nebraska	2	4	4	4	14
Nevada	*	*	*	*	*
New Hampshire	5	5	2	2	14
New Jersey	5	3	3	2	13
New Mexico	6	6	3	2	17
New York	6	6	4	4	20
North Carolina	6	5	2	3	16
North Dakota	1	4	7	8	20
Ohio	6	4	7	8	25
Oklahoma	1	1	2	1	5
Oregon	4	2	3	3	12
Pennsylvania	5	5	7	8	25
Rhode Island	4	5	4	3	16
South Carolina	4	4	3	3	14
South Dakota	6	3	2	2	13
Tennessee	6	4	2	3	15
Texas	4	4	1	2	11
Utah	3	5	2	2	12
Vermont	*	*	*	*	*
Virginia	5	4	3	2	14
Washington	6	4	7	8	25
West Virginia	5	6	7	3	21
Wisconsin	3	3	3	3	12
Wyoming	2	2	0	1	5

Source: Children's Defense Fund Survey, 1985.
[1]American Academy of Pediatrics, Guidelines for Supervision.
*Information not available.

tests, and dental care; and countless previously undiagnosed conditions have been disclosed and treated. EPSDT has contributed to a significant improvement in the health status of low-income children served by the program, and specialized studies have demonstrated its effectiveness and cost-effectiveness (Keller 1983; Irwin and Conroy-Hughes 1982).

At the same time, however, the program has faced serious problems. These problems have been extensively investigated by researchers (Foltz 1975; Children's Defense Fund 1977). No fewer than four separate sets of congressional hearings concerning the adequacy of the program have been held. No fewer than four major sets of federal rules have been issued.[19] Repeated litigation efforts have sought to enforce the entitlement and affirmative action aspects of the statute.[20] Numerous states have designed and redesigned their programs, as new generations of policy makers and agency heads have "discovered" EPSDT and seized upon it as an attractive programmatic initiative.

A number of researchers have pointed to various factors that impeded effective program implementation, including: the ambiguous nature of federal EPSDT directives and the ensuing confusion they have generated; the poor design of EPSDT programs at the state and local level that has resulted in ineffective implementation; and a general lack of political commitment on the part of many state officials to the program's aims (Foltz 1975; Children's Defense Fund 1977).

While these are all certainly important considerations in assessing the success of EPSDT, perhaps the single most important factor is the fact that, since EPSDT is a Medicaid benefit, its effectiveness rests upon children being eligible for Medicaid or an equivalent financing source (such as the Crippled Children's program) that incorporates all of the EPSDT standards and protocols. If there is no funding, then regardless of how committed or creative a program administrator is or how clear the federal directives, there will be no way to purchase the preventive, primary, and follow-up screening, diagnostic, and treatment services children need. Ultimately, Medicaid's failure to insure more than one-third of poor children for even a full year (Butler et al. 1985) is the greatest single impediment to achieving EPSDT's goals.

EPSDT has always been dependent upon the success of Medicaid. But the magnitude of the Medicaid program's shortcomings in 1986 undoubtedly was never envisioned by the drafters of the 1967 child health amendments. Indeed, the complete text of the 1967 Social Security Amendments (of which EPSDT was only a small part) and their legislative history suggest assumption on the part of Congress and the president that AFDC (and therefore, Medicaid) eligibility standards would remain relatively reasonable.

For example, the 1967 Social Security Amendments placed a ceiling on eligibility levels for state medically needy programs equal to 133 percent of the AFDC payment standard.[21] In 1967 state AFDC payment levels were approximately the same as those used under programs for the aged, blind, and disabled. Thus, the medically needy elderly would be left no worse off, and potentially slightly better off, than those elderly persons who received both cash and medical assistance.

Currently, however, most state AFDC payment levels are dramatically below the payment level under SSI (which was enacted in 1972 to replace prior, less generous state grant-in-aid programs for the aged, blind, and disabled). This discrepancy between AFDC and SSI has led to the anomalous situation in which medically needy eligibility levels for the elderly are significantly below those standards used to qualify the elderly for SSI. Elderly persons who receive welfare are often financially better off than medically needy elderly persons who do not receive cash assistance but who do need medical assistance to meet the high cost of health care. It is highly doubtful that the Congress would ever have used state AFDC payment standards to determine financial eligibility for the medically needy aged, had it anticipated how far behind cash assistance programs for the aged state AFDC benefits would ultimately fall.

State Response to EPSDT

Given poor children's tenuous insured status under the Medicaid program, the obvious question which arises is how can a state structure an effective EPSDT program that provides children with continuous access to the range of benefits EPSDT pays for if Medicaid itself is such an inadequate source of financing. Addressing children's volatile health financing dilemma is essential to EPSDT's success, not only because their uninsuredness frequently prevents them from securing EPSDT and other services, but also because low-income children who are not insured are less likely to receive preventive benefits at all (Rosenbach 1985). Medicaid has been shown to result in a greater use of preventive services and generally greater access to medical care (Rosenbach 1985).

Thus, for states to achieve EPSDT's objectives, as well as the broader goals of child health care, they must first stabilize poor children's health care financing arrangements. Low-income families who have health care coverage for their children on a continuous basis may prove to be more effective health care purchasers, and appropriate health outcomes for these children can be better assured.

During the summer of 1985, the Children's Defense Fund conducted a 50-state survey of EPSDT programs on a range of issues. A survey instrument was prepared to achieve the objectives of the study, which were to determine:

- the extent to which states are in compliance with basic program requirements;
- what program changes, if any, had been put into place as a result of changes in the federal regulations;
- if states have developed innovative programs, particularly in the areas of outreach, provider participation, and case management; and
- how effectively states were integrating various health care programs for low-income children.

The questionnaire was pretested and then administered by telephone. In all, more than 50 specific program-related questions were asked of each state, and an attempt was made in each case to speak with the EPSDT program coordinator. Follow-up materials, including a sample of participation data, provider protocols and agreements, periodicity schedules, and outreach materials were requested by mail and received from most states. Additional information was obtained from the EPSDT Program Report, for fiscal year 1984 prepared by the

Health Care Financing Administration, U. S. Department of Health and Human Services.

Several findings from this survey bear specifically on the issue of how adequately states have overcome Medicaid's financing dilemma for children and how adequately state supplemental financing mechanisms are integrated with the EPSDT program. Specifically, we sought information regarding the following: first, how many states have developed sources of funding to supplement Medicaid when a child in need of EPSDT screening, diagnostic, and treatment services is ineligible, or no longer eligible, for Medicaid coverage; and second, whether or not the EPSDT screening, diagnostic, and treatment protocols are incorporated into supplemental funding sources.

Supplemental EPSDT Funding for Children Who Are Ineligible for Medicaid

Our study revealed that no state has a uniform, statewide supplemental funding program to finance the range of EPSDT screening, diagnostic, and treatment services for low-income children who are ineligible for Medicaid. Nearly all states use some portion of the funds they receive from the federal government under the Title V Maternal and Child Health Block Grant Act to underwrite health screening activities for children through local health departments, although it is not uncommon for such screening programs to be limited to very young children. Moreover, there is no guarantee that even early childhood screening services are uniformly available throughout the state.

Supplemental state funding for treatment services for Medicaid-ineligible children (vision, dental, and hearing care and treatment for conditions disclosed through the assessment process) is almost nonexistent. Treatment services for certain problems may be available through Title V–funded Children and Youth (C&Y) projects (special comprehensive health clinics serving children and funded under the Maternal and Child Health Block Grant), but in no state are C&Y projects available statewide.

Other sources of funding for medical treatment for children who are Medicaid-ineligible include state Crippled Children's (CC) programs, also funded through the Maternal and Child

Health Block Grant. In 1983, however, state CC programs served only 620,000 children nationwide for selected medical problems, usually chronic and organic in nature (Association of State and Territorial Health Officials Foundation 1985). Crippled Children's programs are not commonly a source of funding for children's routine medical care needs, such as vision, hearing, and dental care. Furthermore, many state programs categorically exclude certain conditions, such as mental health problems, as treatable conditions.

Other residual sources of comprehensive health care for low-income children include Community and Migrant Health Centers.[22] These centers provide a range of primary health services in the areas in which they are located. Nearly 40 percent of all center users are children, an indication of their poverty and uninsuredness (National Association of Community Health Centers 1986). However, in 1985 the centers served only 5 million people, while 200 million more were unserved (National Association of Community Health Centers 1986).

In short, states do not have comprehensive supplemental health care financing arrangements for Medicaid-ineligible low-income children which can be used to advance EPSDT's goals. At any given time, one-third of America's 12.9 million poor children are completely ineligible for EPSDT benefits, while another third will have Medicaid coverage for less than one year (Butler et al. 1985). Implementing a program whose main thrust is providing access to long-term preventive services in such a context is virtually impossible.

EPSDT's incompatibility with Medicaid takes on ironic overtones, given policy makers' expectations for the program. In 1984 the U. S. Department of Health and Human Services issues EPSDT regulations that encouraged states to develop EPSDT programs that utilized the services of providers who could provide "continuing care"—that is, both preventive services and medical treatment for periodic, episodic, or chronic health care needs—to Medicaid-eligible children. The goal embodied in this rule of incorporating EPSDT services with comprehensive health care arrangements for children is certainly a laudable one. However, it is doubtful that "continuing care" arrangements of reasonable duration can be successfully developed if there is no way to finance a child's care over long periods of time.

Given the problems inherent in implementing "continuing care" programs for such poorly financed children, we were interested in discovering what actions the states had, in fact, taken to develop arrangements. Our findings indicate that while some states were pursuing continuing-care arrangements, none had tied such programs to supplemental funding sources. Instead, the states appeared to be entering into "continuing care" agreements as part of an overall effort to enroll Medicaid recipients in specialized primary care case-management arrangements, authorized under the Medicaid Act in 1981.

The primary purpose of these arrangements is to reduce state Medicaid expenditures, not to provide supplemental financing for poor families. Of 49 states responding to this survey question, 19 reported developing formal continuing-care initiatives. However, none of these initiatives reported the inclusion of supplemental funding mechanisms that could be triggered to retain a child's enrollment in the continuing-care program if his or her Medicaid eligibility ceased. Some states are recruiting into their continuing-care programs publicly funded providers with a legal obligation to serve the poor (such as Community Health Centers, Children & Youth projects, or public hospital outpatient clinics). In this way, children who lose Medicaid might continue to remain with the provider on a subsidized basis. However, in most states, enrollment in private physician arrangements is emphasized. These providers, of course, have no legal obligation to serve uninsured low-income children.

At least one state has now recognized that in the absence of a comprehensive supplemental financing program for poor children ineligible for Medicaid, it must more aggressively enroll public and quasi-public providers serving the poor into its EPSDT program. After an intensive review of its EPSDT program, a special task force in Massachusetts concluded that the Medicaid agency was doing an inadequate job of integrating its services with existing public health efforts, including Community Health Centers, school health programs, family planning clinics, and clinics providing general maternal and child health services, including supplemental food programs for women, infants, and children. Indeed, direct recruitment efforts by the Medicaid agency had been almost entirely limited to individual practitioners in private practice, rather than comprehensive, local agencies that could serve as a continuing-care provider's entity for uninsured poor children. The report recommended that integrated arrangements be developed with public health providers already furnishing health services to poor children in order to expand EPSDT's delivery system and to reach low-income children in their predominant health care entry points (Massachusetts Department of Public Welfare 1985).

TABLE 4
States Reporting Continuing-Care Arrangements

State	Status	State	Status
Alabama	No	Missouri	No
Alaska	No	Montana	No
Arizona	—	Nebraska	No
Arkansas	No	Nevada	Yes
California	Yes	New Hampshire	Yes
Colorado	Yes	New Jersey	Yes
Connecticut	Yes	New Mexico	No
Delaware	No	New York	Yes
District of Columbia	No	North Carolina	No
Florida	Yes	North Dakota	No
Georgia	No	Ohio	Yes
Hawaii	—	Oklahoma	No
Idaho	No	Oregon	Yes
Illinois	Yes	Pennsylvania	Yes
Indiana	No	Rhode Island	Yes
Iowa	No	South Carolina	*
Kansas	No	South Dakota	No
Kentucky	*	Tennessee	Yes
Louisiana	No	Texas	No
Maine	Yes	Utah	No
Maryland	No	Vermont	No
Massachusetts	Yes	Virginia	No
Michigan	Yes	Washington	Yes
Minnesota	Yes	West Virginia	No
Mississippi	No	Wisconsin	Yes
		Wyoming	No

Source: Children's Defense Fund survey, 1985.
*Under development or under consideration.

Application of EPSDT Standards to All Supplemental Funding Programs

No state provides supplemental funding for all EPSDT services. However, all states do underwrite at least some screening, diagnostic, or treatment services to Medicaid-ineligible children, either through their Maternal and Child Health Block Grant programs or other state-funded efforts. We, therefore, sought to determine how many states apply EPSDT assessment standards and protocols to all public programs.

Use of common standards would better assure the provision of health exams that include all of the elements outlined in the EPSDT rules. Common standards would also ensure that children participating in any publicly funded program are recalled for periodic exams in a consistent fashion and that common immunization schedules are used. Moreover, states would be better assured that children receiving any publicly subsidized health services throughout a year are receiving the medical care and services that Medicaid agencies are legally obligated to provide. Finally, providers delivering pediatric services in several different public programs would be guided by a single, standard set of protocols.

Our survey revealed, however, that rather than using EPSDT standards to unify and guide the range of publicly funded pediatric programs, state Medicaid agencies in fact have seriously diluted the EPSDT program by permitting pediatric providers to claim Medicaid reimbursement for child health exams that may fall short of the content and frequency requirements of the EPSDT program. Moreover, only a few states apply the EPSDT protocols to all publicly paid programs, such as Title V–funded well-child examination services furnished by local health departments.

We have termed these informal Medicaid provider–reimbursement arrangements that bypass the rigorous EPSDT requirements "shadow programs." In general, Medicaid agencies believe that children treated under these "shadow programs" are receiving care equivalent to that required under EPSDT and can, therefore, be considered to be enrolled in "continuing care" arrangements. However, adherence to EPSDT protocols is not a prerequisite to reimbursement of these "equivalent" providers. Thus, the states, in fact, have no way of ensuring that complete assessment and referral services have been furnished.

Without adherence to the articulated standards and detailed protocols embodied in EPSDT, the states have no means of verifying that "shadow" care provided to children is, in fact, equivalent to that furnished under EPSDT. Among the 44 states responding to our question regarding whether EPSDT standards apply to all primary pediatric care reimbursed by Medicaid, most explicitly permit "shadow" billing arrangements. Furthermore, in most states, these "shadow" billing arrangements are available only to private physicians. Evidently, rather than negotiating with private physicians to implement the full EPSDT screening package (the federal regulations for which are based on the American Academy of Pediatrics *Guidelines for Health Supervision*) states have instead permitted physicians to bill for routine pediatric health services outside the EPSDT program. In return, Medicaid agencies frequently pay somewhat less for a routine "shadow" health exam than they pay for the full EPSDT complement of services.

We suspect that "shadow" billing is tolerated if not explicitly permitted in almost every state, since it may not be uncommon for a physician to perform a "well-child" exam on a child who is being seen for diagnosis-related reasons. Thus, even states that do not expressly and separately reimburse providers for routine health "shadow" services may, in fact, allow such reimbursement if it is part of an otherwise diagnosis-related visit.

Several adverse effects flow from "shadow" programs. First, health exams may not meet the EPSDT program's quality and content protocols. For example, many state EPSDT screening protocols, in implementing the federal rules' requirement of an age-appropriate hearing exam, recommended the use of an audiometer in conducting a hearing exam for children over age three. Yet, many physicians do not utilize audiometers in their practices. As a result, children being treated by "shadow" providers may not receive a complete hearing exam.

An even more serious example involves conditions particularly threatening to poor children, such as lead poisoning. In *A Guide to Administration, Diagnosis and Treatment,* EPSDT, the

TABLE 5
States Reporting Shadow Programs

State	Status	State	Status
Alabama	Yes[1]	Missouri	Yes
Alaska	No	Montana	Yes
Arizona	—	Nebraska	Yes[3]
Arkansas	Yes	Nevada	No
California	—	New Hampshire	Yes
Colorado	No	New Jersey	Yes
Connecticut	Yes	New Mexico	No
Delaware	Yes	New York	Yes
District of Columbia	Yes	North Carolina	No
Florida	Yes	North Dakota	Yes
Georgia	No	Ohio	Yes
Hawaii	—	Oklahoma	Yes[4]
Idaho	Yes[2]	Oregon	Yes
Illinois	Yes	Pennsylvania	Yes[4]
Indiana	Yes	Rhode Island	Yes
Iowa	Yes	South Carolina	No
Kansas	Yes	South Dakota	Yes
Kentucky	No	Tennessee	No
Louisiana	Yes	Texas	No
Maine	Yes	Utah	No[5]
Maryland	Yes	Vermont	—
Massachusetts	Yes[6]	Virginia	No
Michigan	Yes	Washington	No
Minnesota	Yes	West Virginia	—
Mississippi	No	Wisconsin	Yes
		Wyoming	Yes

Source: Children's Defense Fund survey, 1985.
[1]one postpartum visit.
[2]birth to one year.
[3]birth to age three.
[4]one visit per year.
[5]if medically necessary or subject to review.
[6]limited to certain providers.
"Yes" indicates that state reports a shadow program without limitations on periodicity.
"No" indicates that state does not allow provider to bill for a well-child visit or examination outside of the EPSDT program.

U. S. Department of Health, Education, and Welfare, in cooperation with the American Academy of Pediatrics, specifically noted that:

> In the United States, 2.5 million children 1 through 5 years of age are at risk of undue lead absorption. Approximately 600,000 will be affected by the disease, generally as a result of living in old, deteriorated housing containing lead-based paint. Prevalence is lower in suburban areas and may be extremely low in areas with houses built after the 1950s and with little exposure to industrial sources of lead. Classical symptomatic lead poisoning is generally not seen. Approximately 6,000 will develop neurologic damage including slow learning, hyperactivity, and behavioral disorders even though the child is asymptomatic (HSM110-73-524).

Federal EPSDT assessment guidelines specifically call for lead poisoning testing as part of the basic exam. Yet, many physicians do not incorporate lead testing as part of their routine office practices. As a result, many children being seen by "shadow" providers may not be tested for lead poisoning.

A particularly serious problem has resulted in New York City, where plaintiffs, suing the city over its failure to identify and treat infants and children suffering from lead poisoning discovered that of all Medicaid-enrolled children in the city, only 5 percent could be certified as having received a full complement of EPSDT services, including lead poisoning exams.[23] With respect to the other 95 percent of Medicaid-eligible children, the city defendant noted that nearly all were under the care of an "equivalent" provider and were, therefore, not in need of EPSDT screens. However, according to affidavits of medical experts submitted in the case, it is not common practice outside of the EPSDT program for a physician in New York City to screen a child for lead poisoning. Therefore, because the state has failed to require adherence to the EPSDT protocol by all providers furnishing preventive Medicaid services to children, children potentially suffering from the effects of lead poisoning may be going unidentified and untreated.

Second, the use of "shadow" programs means that states cannot assure that all children are up-to-date with respect to health exams and immunizations in accordance with state periodicity schedules. Federal EPSDT regulations require that all states establish schedules that identify the ages at which children should be screened and the screening and treatment services (such as developmental assessments, dental care referrals, and immunizations) that are to be provided at each periodic interval (Table 3). However, "shadow" providers, who are not bound by state periodicity schedules, may follow individual schedules that call for screening at greater or closer intervals than those called for in the official state periodicity schedule. This practice may, in turn, lead to overutilization or underutilization of needed services.

A third implication of permitting "shadow" billing is the potential for poor quality care. For example, health experts emphasize that pediatric practitioners should not attempt to measure a child's overall health and development when the child is being seen for an acute or episodic illness, since a child's responsiveness and capabilities may be depressed as a result of illness. Moreover, experts also underscore the point that immunizations should not be provided when a child is ill. Since these practices constitute poor medical care, a reasonable EPSDT program by law would not permit reimbursement for an EPSDT exam conducted on a sick child. Yet, these practices might occur under "shadow" programs, which, by definition, fail to regulate provider practices.

A final problem created by the existence of a "shadow" program is its spillover effect on other agencies. A health department may have no real incentive to conform its provider standards for non-Medicaid pediatric programs to those used by the Medicaid agency, if the Medicaid agency itself does not requite adherence to rigorous protocols by all pediatric providers furnishing primary care and participating in Medicaid.

The problems created by the widespread use of "shadow" programs are complicated by the fact that not all states have developed detailed standards of practice even for providers willing to participate in the formal EPSDT program. In keeping with the tendency toward "shadow" billing, those that do maintain formal EPSDT protocols will frequently apply them only to selected groups of providers.

TABLE 6
EPSDT Provider Protocols

State	Written protocol*	Required applications
Alabama	manual	not all use
Alaska	manual	all use
Arizona	—	—
Arkansas	manual	all use
		not all components required
California	manual	all use
		not all components required
Colorado	—	—
Connecticut	yes	all use
Delaware	yes	all use
District of Columbia	yes	all use
Florida	no	—
Georgia	yes	all use
Hawaii	—	—
Idaho	yes	all use
Illinois	yes	all use
Indiana	yes	all use
Iowa	manual	only public providers use
Kansas	form	all use
Kentucky	yes	all use
Louisiana	yes	all use
Maine	no	rely on physician
Maryland	yes	all use
Massachusetts	yes	—
Michigan	yes	all use
Minnesota	yes	all use
Mississippi	form	all use
Missouri	form	all use
Montana	yes	all use
Nebraska	form	all use
Nevada	yes	all use
New Hampshire	revising	all use
New Jersey	yes	all use
New Mexico	yes	all use
New York	yes	all use
North Carolina	—	—
North Dakota	manual	all use

State	Written protocol*	Required applications
Ohio	yes	all use
Oklahoma	no	—
Oregon	yes	all use
Pennsylvania	manual	all use
Rhode Island	yes	all use
South Carolina	partial	—
South Dakota	yes	all use
Tennessee	partial	all use
Texas	partial	all use
Utah	yes	all use
Vermont	—	—
Virginia	no	—
Washington	—	—
West Virginia	yes	all use
Wisconsin	no	—
Wyoming	form	all use

*Where states provided an actual sample of the protocol, its status is described as form or manual or partial. In other cases, "yes" means a state reported having a protocol but did not send an example, and "no" means a state reported having no protocol.

Of the 45 states responding to our questions on provider standards, only 40 had developed provider standards that are to be used by all providers certified as formal EPSDT practitioners. Six states reported using no provider protocols at all.

Furthermore, of the 40 states using EPSDT provider protocols, 2 exempted private EPSDT providers from having to follow the protocols, even though health departments were required to follow written standards. Finally, the level of quality and detail in protocols varied greatly. For some states an extensive manual has been prepared; in others the standards may not include the full screening package. At least 5 of the 40 states are using only a claims form as a protocol, leaving the provider the discretion to interpret the requirements for which no details were provided. For example, officials in Maine report that they rely on physicians' judgments about the most appropriate manner in which to provide an EPSDT screen. Similarly, although the Texas agency requires all providers to use written protocols for the medical portion of the screen, it has developed no protocol for the dental exam.

In Wyoming and several other states, the claims form is the only written EPSDT guideline supplied to providers. The form is a single column listing beside which a provider might check off items such as "family health history/parents" or "physical examination/hearing." Such a form, while useful for determining the completeness of a provider's screen, does not tell the provider that an EPSDT hearing screen is to be conducted to certain specifications, such as with an audiometer.

Conclusion

Achieving the goals of high-quality health care for low-income children requires both adequate financing and adherence to sound standards of practice. The Medicaid program with its broad range of preventive, diagnosis and treatment-related services, and its open-ended financing mechanism, represents a powerful tool to reduce significantly uninsuredness and improve access among children. However, Medicaid suffers from serious limitations, some federally imposed and some created by the states. Years of stagnation in AFDC, whose eligibility methodology is used to determine nearly all children's eligibility for Medicaid, have seriously limited the program's reach. These limitations have been exacerbated since 1981 by federal restrictions designed to remove from Medicaid working-poor families who are least likely to be privately insured.

In recent years state and federal government response to Medicaid and children has been mixed. On the one hand, since 1980 about a dozen states have expanded categorical coverage of children under Medicaid to include all children under age 18 in families satisfying AFDC income and resources criteria. Another six have added coverage for "medically needy" children. Similarly, in 1984, Congress mandated Medicaid coverage of all children under age five whose families meet state AFDC financial eligibility standards; additionally, Congress softened somewhat the antiwork amendments incorporated into AFDC and

Medicaid in 1981. All of these actions are particularly notable in an era of great fiscal constraint.

On the other hand, the financial criteria used to determine children's Medicaid eligibility remain extraordinarily depressed, and punitive measures against the working poor have permanently disinsured millions of families from Medicaid. These highly restrictive eligibility conditions seriously undercut Medicaid's utility as a direct and stable insurer of poor children, thereby rendering such crucial programs as EPSDT far less useful than they might otherwise be. EPSDT's utility is further undercut by apparent state dilution of this all-important benefit.

We believe that two things must happen. First, the states must develop better public financing mechanisms for poor children. There are several ways this might be done. First and most obviously, the states might improve their Medicaid coverage significantly. Twenty states still do not extend benefits to all children under age 18 living in families with incomes below AFDC eligibility levels (Table 2). All should do so. The Health Care Financing Administration has recently estimated that such a program might add 4 percent to a state's annual Medicaid outlays (Health Care Financing Administration 1984b).

Fifteen states also currently fail to cover medically needy children (Table 2). In 1981 Congress amended Medicaid to permit states to establish limited medically needy programs only for pregnant women and children under 18, without having to cover other categories of medically needy individuals, as required under prior law.[24] Medically needy coverage of pregnant women and children only has been estimated to add no more than 4 percent to a state's annual Medicaid outlays (Wulsin 1984).

Most important, however, states should raise their AFDC payment levels. An AFDC increase would automatically increase Medicaid penetration rates. AFDC payment increases are vital not only because they improve children's access to Medicaid but also because of the strong link between children's overall standard of living and child health outcomes (Starfield 1982). In an era when the rate of progress in reducing infant mortality is declining and, even more important, the nation is experiencing an actual nationwide rise in postneonatal mortality, standard of living issues become particularly pressing (Children's Defense Fund 1986b).

We recognize, however, that AFDC increases are not easy to accomplish. The nation's conservative retrenchment and the widespread misconception that welfare benefits led to the explosion during the 1970s of out-of-wedlock births to teenage women (even though, in fact, the value of welfare declined dramatically as the out-of-wedlock birthrate grew) mean that the stigma of welfare is as strong today as it was 20 years ago.

Moreover, since by law Medicaid must be provided to anybody who receives AFDC, an AFDC increase means increased Medicaid coverage for adults as well as children and, therefore, a potential sizeable increase in Medicaid expenditures. Additionally, in states whose Medicaid plans include coverage of the medically needy, increased AFDC payments automatically push up medically needy eligibility standards, since AFDC serves as the basis for the states' medically needy eligibility levels. Many of these persons, including young adults, the elderly, and the disabled, have relatively high per capita costs (Health Care Financing Administration 1984b).

Thus, increasing Medicaid coverage by increasing AFDC may prove to be a politically and financially unpopular avenue for change. While state lawmakers might be persuaded to enact modest AFDC improvements, they may resist sizeable across-the-board AFDC increases, especially in those states with medically needy programs.

Given the political and financial difficulties in substantially increasing coverage of children under Medicaid by improving the program's eligibility criteria, we believe that states should explore several other approaches. First, states might supplement Medicaid with a state-financed public medical assistance entitlement or quasi-entitlement program for children whose family income falls between state AFDC payment levels and some outer limit (for example, 125 percent of the federal poverty level.) Children failing to qualify for or maintain Medicaid eligibility could be shifted onto coverage under this supplemental public-insurance program. Moreover, such a program could develop a more reasonable asset test than the one employed under the AFDC program (although welfare officials estimate that less than 5 percent of AFDC applicants are denied eligibility on the basis of excess resources).

A supplemental public-benefit health program for children makes both health and economic sense. Children who are stably insured could be enrolled over long periods of time with cost-effective providers, such as community health centers, HMOs, cost-efficient private group practices, or comprehensive public clinics. There is evidence that long-term enrollment in a stable preventive and primary health care system may actually reduce overall Medicaid costs (Keller 1983). Massachusetts has already established a supplemental public-benefit program for pregnant women with family incomes between that state's Medicaid eligibility level and 185 percent of the federal poverty level. This type of program could be extended to poor and near-poor children. Additionally, the governors of Arizona and New Jersey have included such plans for children in their fiscal year 1987 budget proposals, and Maryland lawmakers are considering a similar type of plan for pregnant teenagers.

Alternatively, states might consider making more aggressive use of their Medicaid flexibility more generously to finance public and quasi-public health care providers (such as community health centers) that are legally obligated to serve low-income children. Currently, many such clinical providers are poorly paid. Indeed, a number of state Medicaid programs fail to reimburse free-standing clinics for preventive, diagnostic, and treatment services rendered to Medicaid children unless the provider is a physician. These restrictive practices effectively give Medicaid agencies a "free ride" on the backs of health department clinics, community health centers, and other publicly obligated providers desperately in need of revenues to help offset their large caseloads of uninsured poor patients.

Instead of financially starving these providers, Medicaid agencies should include in their state plans coverage for all clinic services, not just those furnished by selected clinical staff. Reimbursement should be set on the basis of clinics' reasonable charges for the comprehensive health care they provide. This higher level of Medicaid reimbursement could provide clinics with greater revenues, thereby enhancing their operations.

Third, states might provide direct grants to providers giving ambulatory services to large numbers of low-income children. Massachusetts, Connecticut, Texas, Florida, South Carolina, Ohio, Rhode Island, and New York all currently provide direct grants to one or more types of comprehensive clinics serving the poor. Were such supplementation combined with enhanced

Medicaid reimbursement, a more comprehensive public health system for low-income children might be developed.

In the long run, states might consider establishing a program to provide publicly subsidized insurance coverage for poor and near-poor working families. A number of states, including New York, South Carolina, Florida, and West Virginia, have established revenue policy mechanisms for underwriting specific types of medical care, such as hospital services for poor and uninsured persons. Revenues for these pools are collected from a variety of sources, including taxes on hospitals, insurers, other types of taxes, and state and local contributions.

These pools might ultimately be used to underwrite a public insurance plan under which poor and near-poor families could buy coverage on an income-adjusted, sliding premium basis. Were such pooled money used simply to purchase private insurance for these families, problems might develop, since many private plans have poor coverage of preventive health benefits, utilize high coinsurance and deductibles, involve costly premiums, and provide coverage on an indemnity basis (which presents an impossible situation for low-income families, who cannot lay out cash first and collect from their insurer later). Publicly controlled plans would be less expensive to states and would permit states to control plan features. Massachusetts is currently considering such a plan.

We also strongly urge that *all* public child health financing mechanisms, whether Medicaid or supplemental public programs, utilize EPSDT protocols. While remedying the basic financing dilemma is crucial, equally as important is the quality and content of the care that is purchased with public funds. EPSDT is an enduring articulation of sound medical practice, and its provisions should be adhered to, not undercut.

We hope that some day all child health financing mechanisms, whether public or private, will incorporate a complete EPSDT-level schedule of preventive and primary health benefits. Congress is now, in fact, considering legislation, known as the Child Health Incentive Reform Plan (CHIRP) which would require all employer-purchased health insurance plans to include coverage for certain preventive pediatric services such as health examinations and immunizations, in order to qualify for federal tax treatment. There is precedent for legislation imposing conditions on the deductibility of employer-financed coverage. Recently enacted federal legislation requires employers to extend coverage at group rates to families of deceased or divorced workers as a condition of tax deductibility. Furthermore, many states now mandate minimum benefits for insurance plans.

We are hopeful about the potential for reform. Policy makers are increasingly recognizing the need to come to grips with the health care financing gap that confronts low-income children. Indeed, the National Governors Association has recently recommended a major expansion of federal Medicaid eligibility requirements for low-income women and children, with financing to be shared by the federal government and the states. This organization's commitment to maternal and child health, in an era of major fiscal retrenchment at all levels of government, is remarkable.

Without doubt, reshaping the health care financing and service delivery system for low-income children is one of the most sophisticated tasks facing state and federal policy makers. But we believe that the task of reconciling child health goals with program realities is one that can be successfully undertaken with patience, inventiveness, and relatively modest outlays.

NOTES

1. 42 U.S.C. sect. 1396d(b). By law, the federal medical assistance percentage rates range from 50 percent to 83 percent of funds expended by states.
2. 42 U.S.C. sect. 601, et. seq. (1985).
3. 42 U.S.C. sect. 1601, et. seq. (1985).
4. P.L. 97–35 (1981).
5. Sect. 2624 of the Deficit Reduction Act of 1984 (P.L. 96–369).
6. The Crippled Children's Program was originally codified as a separate authority within the Social Security Act. In 1967, however, it was consolidated with the Maternal and Child Health Program as Title V of the Social Security Act, 42 U.S.C. sect. 701, et seq. In 1981 Title V was expanded to include a series of previously categorical maternal and child health services programs including the Title V Maternal and Child Health and Crippled Children's Programs, and renamed the Maternal and Child Health Block Grant (P.L. 97–35, 95 Stat. 357 [1981]. (See also Rosenbaum 1983a).

7. 42 U.S.C. sect. 1396d(a)(4)(B); 42 U.S.C. section 705(a)(1968).
8. S. Rep. 744 to accompany H.R. 12080, the Social Security Amendments of 1967.
9. The affirmative action requirement of the Medicaid EPSDT program was originally added to the Social Security Act in 1972 in response to growing congressional concern over states' failure to implement EPSDT. The original provision withheld 1 percent of federal AFDC payments from any state that failed to inform, screen, and treat eligible children, 42 U.S.C. sect. 602(g) (1972). In 1981 this so-called AFDC "penalty" provision was removed and the Medicaid statute was amended to incorporate these affirmative action provisions as a state plan requirement, sect. 2181 of P.L. 97–35, 95 Stat. 357 (1981), codified at 42 U.S.C. sect 1396(a)(44) (1982).
10. 42 C.F.R. sect. 441.56(b) and (c) (1986).
11. 42 C.F.R. sect. 441.57 (1985). The originally proposed EPSDT regulations would have required states to provide all medically necessary diagnostic and treatment services for conditions disclosed during the screening process, even if such services were not included in the state's basic medical plan. After intense opposition by states to this rule, however, the Nixon administration chose to limit the EPSDT enriched services package to vision, dental, and hearing treatment only, despite the fact that the statute itself contains no such limitation.
12. 42 C.F.R. sect. 441.58 (1985).
13. *Mitchell v. Johnston* 701 F2d 337 (5th Cir. 1983) holding that the Texas EPSDT dental program, which used a dental examination schedule that called for routine dental exams only once every three years was unreasonable, not in accordance with accepted professional standards of practice and therefore in violation of federal Medicaid and EPSDT regulations.
14. 42 C.F.R. sect. 441.58 (1985).
15. 42 C.F.R. sect. 441.56(a) (1985).
16. 42 C.F.R. sect. 441.62 (1985).
17. 42 C.F.R. sect. 441.85 (1985).
18. 42 C.F.R. sect. 441.85 (1985).
19. 35 *Fed. Reg.* 18878 (December 11, 1970); 40 *Fed. Reg.* 3678 (August 20, 1975); 44 *Fed. Reg.* 29420 (May 18, 1974); and 49 *Fed. Reg.* 43654f (October 31, 1984).
20. See e.g., *Mitchell v. Johnston,* 701 F2d 337 (5th Cir. 1983); *Bond v. Stanton* 655 F2d 766 (7th Cir. 1981); *Bond v. Stanton*

630 F2d 1231 (7th Cir. 1980); *Brooks v. Smith* 356 A.2d 723 (Me. 1976); *Dominguez v. Milliken*, no. 9-198-72 (D. Mich. 1973) [reprinted at] C.C.H. Medicare/Medicaid Guide + 26,632; *Harris v. Candom*, no. 74–79 (D. Vt. 1978) [reprinted at] C.C.H. Medicare/Medicaid Guide 29, 099; *Philaae'phia Welfare Rights Org. v. Schapp* 602 F2d 1114 (3rd Cir., 1979); cert. den. 444 U.S. 1026 (1980).
21. Sect. 238 of P.L. 90–248.
22. Sects. 330 of 329 of the Public Health Service Act, respectively.
23. *New York City Coalition to End Lead Poisoning et al. v. Koch* (no. 42780 185, S.D.N.Y., 1985).
24. Sect. 2171 of P.L. 97–35, replacing 42 U.S.C. sect. 1396a (a) 10) (C) (1980).

American Academy of Pediatrics. 1981. *Guidelines for Health Supervision*. Evanston, Ill.

Association of State and Territorial Health Officials Foundation, 1985. *Public Health Agencies 1983: Services for Mothers and Children*. Vol. 3. Kensington, Md.

Budetti P., J. Butler, and P. McManus. 1982. Federal Health Program Reforms: Implications for Child Health Care. *Milbank Memorial Fund Quarterly/Health and Society* 60:155–81.

Butler, J., W. Winter, J. Singer, and M. Wegner. 1985. Medical Care Use and Expenditures Among U.S. Children and Youth: Analysis of a National Probability Sample. *Pediatrics* 76:495–503.

Children's Defense Fund. 1977. *EPSDT: Does It Spell Health Care for Poor Children?* Washington.

———. 1985a. *A Children's Defense Budget: An Analysis of the President's FY 1986 Budget and Children*. Washington.

———. 1985b. *Black and White Children in America: Key Facts*. Washington.

———. 1986a. *A Children's Defense Budget: An Analysis of the President's 1987 Federal Budget and Children*. Washington.

———. 1986b. *Maternal and Child Health Data Book: The Health of America's Children*. Washington.

Congressional Research Service. 1985. *Children in Poverty*. Document no. 46–869 0. Washington.

Davis, K., and C. Schoen. 1978. *Health and the War on Poverty: A Ten-Year Appraisal*. Washington: Brookings Institution.

Egbuonu, L., and B. Starfield. 1982. Child Health and Social Status. *Pediatrics* 69:550–57.

Foltz, A. 1975. The Development of Ambiguous Federal Policy: Early and Periodic Screening Diagnosis and Treatment (EPSDT). *Milbank Memorial Fund Quarterly/Health and Society* 4:35–64.

Health Care Financing Administration. 1984a. *Fiscal year 1984 Medicaid Recipient and Expenditure Data.* Baltimore.

————. 1984b. *Short Term Evaluation of Medicaid: Selected Issues.* U.S. Department of Health and Human Services, contract no. HHS-100-82-0038. Baltimore.

Irwin, P., and R. Conroy-Hughes. 1982. EPSDT Impact on Health Status: Estimates Based on Secondary Analysis of Administratively Generated Data. *Medical Care* 20:216–34.

Keller, W. 1983. Study of Selected Outcomes of the EPSDT Program in Michigan. *Public Health Reports* 28:110–18.

Kleinman, J. 1981. Use of Ambulatory Health Care by the Poor: Another Look at Equity. *Medical Care* 19:1011–19.

McManus, P. 1986. Medicaid Services and Delivery Settings for Maternal and Child Health. Washington: National Governors Association. (Unpublished.)

Massachusetts Department of Public Welfare. 1985. *Increasing Enrollment in Project Good Health: A Report to the Commissioner.* Office of Research, Planning, and Evaluation. Boston.

Monheit, A., M. Hogan, M Berk, and P. Farley. 1984. *The Employed Uninsured and the Role of Public Policy.* Washington: National Center for Health Services Research.

National Association of Community Health Centers. 1986. *Community and Migrant Health Centers: Two Decades of Achievement.* Washington.

President's Commission for the Study of Ethical Problems in Medicine and Biomedical and Behavioral Research. 1983. *Securing Access to Health Care: A Report on the Ethical Implications of Differences in the Availability of Health Services.* Vol. 1. Pub. no. 0-401-553 QL3. Washington.

Rosenbach, M. 1985. Insurance Coverage and Ambulatory Medical Care of Low-income Children: United States, 1980. *National Medical Care Utilization and Expenditure Survey*, series C., Analytical Report no. 1. Washington: National Center for Health Statistics.

Rosenbaum, S. 1983a. The Maternal and Child Health Block Grant Act 1981: Teaching an Old Program New Tricks. *Clearinghouse Review* 17:400–14.

————. 1983b. The Prevention of Infant Mortality: The Unfulfilled Promise of Federal Health Programs for the Poor. *Clearinghouse Review* 17:701–35.

Starfield, B. 1982. Family Income, Ill Health, and Medical Care of U.S. Children. *Journal of Public Health Policy* 3:244–59.

Swartz, K. 1985. Changes in the Uninsured Population Over Time: Implications for Public Policy. Paper presented at the annual meeting of the American Public Health Association, Washington, November 19.

U.S. Congress. 1967. *Message from the President of the United States*, 90th Cong. 1st sess., doc. no. 54. Washington.

U.S. General Accounting Office. 1985. *An Evaluation of the 1981 AFDC Changes: Final Report.* Pub. no. (GAO)PEMD-85-4. Washington.

Wulsin, L. 1984. Adopting a Medically Needy Program. *Clearinghouse Review* 18:841–55.

Acknowledgment: The authors are indebted to Sharon Weir, M.P.H., who, while an intern at the Children's Defense Fund, helped design and conducted the 50-state EPSDT survey reviewed in this article.

SECTION VI

MEDICINE AND THE QUALITY OF DYING

A. Euthanasia

B. Human Organ Procurement

A. Euthanasia

The Principle of Euthanasia

Antony Flew

M Y particular concern here is to deploy a general moral case
for the establishment of a legal right to voluntary euthanasia. The first point to emphasize is that the argument is about
voluntary euthanasia. [I do not advocate] the euthanasia of
either the incurably sick or the miserably senile except in so far
as this is the strong, constant, and unequivocally expressed wish
of the afflicted candidates themselves. Anyone, therefore, who
dismisses what is in fact being contended on the gratuitously
irrelevant grounds that he could not tolerate compulsory euthanasia, may very reasonably be construed as thereby tacitly
admitting inability to meet and to overcome the case actually
presented. . . . So what can be said in favour of the principle
[of the legalization of voluntary euthanasia]? There are two
main, and to my mind decisive, moral reasons. But before
deploying these it is worth pausing for a moment to indicate
why the onus of proof does not properly rest upon us. It may
seem as if it does, because we are proposing a change in the
present order of things; and it is up to the man who wants a
change to produce the reasons for making whatever change he
is proposing. This most rational principle of conservatism is in
general sound. But here it comes into conflict with the overriding and fundamental liberal principle. It is up to any person and
any institution wanting to prevent anyone from doing anything
he wishes to do, or to compel anyone to do anything he does

From *Voluntary Euthanasia: Experts Debate the Right to Die*. A. B. Downing and
Barbara Smoker, c. 1986. Reprinted with the Permission of Peter Owen.

not wish to do, to provide positive good reason to justify interference. The question should therefore be: *not* 'Why should people be given this new legal right?'; *but* 'Why should people in this matter be restrained by law from doing what they want?'

Yet even if this liberal perspective is accepted, as it too often is not, and even if we are able to dispose of any reasons offered in defence of the present legal prohibitions, still the question would arise, whether the present state of the law represents a merely tiresome departure from sound liberal principles of legislation, or whether it constitutes a really substantial evil. It is here that we have to offer our two main positive arguments.

(1) First, there are, and for the foreseeable future will be, people afflicted with incurable and painful diseases who urgently and fixedly want to die quickly. The first argument is that a law which tries to prevent such sufferers from achieving this quick death, and usually thereby forces other people who care for them to watch their pointless pain helplessly, is a very cruel law. It is because of this legal cruelty that advocates of euthanasia sometimes speak of euthanasia as 'mercy-killing'. In such cases the sufferer may be reduced to an obscene parody of a human being, a lump of suffering flesh eased only by intervals of drugged stupor. This, as things now stand, must persist until at last every device of medical skill fails to prolong the horror.

(2) Second, a law which insists that there must be no end to this process—terminated only by the overdue relief of 'death by natural causes'—is a very degrading law. In the present context the full force of this second reason may not be appreciated immediately, if at all. We are so used to meeting appeals to 'the absolute value of human personality', offered as the would-be knock-down objection to any proposal to legalize voluntary euthanasia, that it has become hard to realize that, in so far as we can attach some tolerably precise meaning to the key phrase, this consideration would seem to bear in the direction precisely opposite to that in which it is usually mistaken to point. For the agonies of prolonged terminal illness can be so terrible and so demoralizing that the person is blotted out in ungovernable nerve reactions. In such cases as this, to meet the patient's longing for death is a means of showing for human personality that respect which cannot tolerate any ghastly travesty of it. So our second main positive argument, attacking the present state of the law as degrading, derives from a respect for

the wishes of the individual person, a concern for human dignity, an unwillingness to let the animal pain disintegrate the man.

Our first main positive argument opposes the present state of the law, and the public opinion which tolerates it, as cruel. Often and appositely this argument is supported by contrasting the tenderness which rightly insists that on occasion dogs and horses must be put out of their misery, with the stubborn refusal in any circumstances to permit one person to assist another in cutting short his suffering. The cry is raised, 'But people are not animals!' Indeed they are not. Yet this is precisely not a ground for treating people worse than brute animals. Animals are like people, in that they too can suffer. It is for this reason that both can have a claim on our pity and our money.[1]

But people are also more than brute animals. They can talk and think and wish and plan. It is this that makes it possible to insist, as we do, that there must be no euthanasia unless it is the firm considered wish of the person concerned. People also can, and should, have dignity as human beings. That is precisely why we are urging that they should be helped and not hindered when they wish to avoid or cut short the often degrading miseries of incurable disease or, I would myself add, of advanced senile decay. . . .

It is time now to begin to face, and to try to dispose of, objections. This is the most important phase in the whole exercise. For to anyone with any width of experience and any capacity for compassion the positive reasons must be both perfectly obvious and strongly felt. The crucial issue is whether or not there are decisive, overriding objections to these most pressing reasons of the heart.

(1) Many of the objections commonly advanced, which are often mistaken to be fundamental, are really objections only to a possible specific manner of implementing the principle of voluntary euthanasia. Thus it is suggested that if the law permitted doctors on occasion to provide their patients with means of death, or where necessary to do the actual killing, and they did so, then the doctors who did either of these would be violating the Hippocratic Oath, and the prestige of and public confidence in the medical profession would be undermined.

As to the Hippocratic Oath, this makes two demands which in the special circumstances we have in mind may become mutually contradictory. They then cannot both be met at the same time. The relevant section reads: 'I will use treatments to help the sick according to my ability and judgment, but never with a view to injury and wrong-doing. I will not give anyone a lethal dose if asked to do so, nor will I suggest such a course.'[2] The fundamental undertaking 'to help the sick according to my ability and judgment' may flatly conflict with the further promise not to 'give anyone a lethal dose if asked to do so'. To observe the basic undertaking a doctor may have to break the further promise. The moral would, therefore, appear to be: not that the Hippocratic Oath categorically and unambiguously demands that doctors must have no dealings with voluntary euthanasia; but rather that the possible incompatibility in such cases of the different directives generated by two of its logically independent clauses constitutes a reason for revising that Oath.

As to the supposed threat to the prestige of and to our confidence in the medical profession, I am myself inclined to think that the fears expressed are—in more than one dimension—disproportionate to the realities. But whatever the truth about this the whole objection would bear only against proposals which permitted or required doctors to do, or directly to assist in, the actual killing. This is not something which is essential to the whole idea of voluntary euthanasia, and the British Euthanasia Society's present draft bill* is so formulated as altogether to avoid this objection. It is precisely such inessential objections as this which I have undertaken to eschew in this essay, in order to consider simply the general principle.

(2) The first two objections which do really bear on this form a pair. One consists in the contention that there is no need to be concerned about the issue, since in fact there are not any, or not many, patients who when it comes to the point want to die quickly. The other bases the same complacent conclusion on the claim that in fact, in the appropriate cases, doctors already

---

*Editors' Note: *Such a bill was presented in the House of Lords by Lord Raglan in 1969. It would have legalized voluntary, active euthanasia. The bill was defeated.*

mercifully take the law into their own hands. These two comfortable doctrines are, like many other similarly reassuring bromides, both entirely wrong and rather shabby.

(a) To the first the full reply would probably have to be made by a doctor, for a medical layman can scarcely be in a position to make an estimate of the number of patients who would apply and could qualify for euthanasia. But it is quite sufficient for our immediate purposes to say two things. First, there can be few who have reached middle life, and who have not chosen to shield their sensibilities with some impenetrable carapace of dogma, who cannot recall at least one case of an eager candidate for euthanasia from their own experience—even from their own peacetime experience only. If this statement is correct, as my own inquiries suggest that it is, then the total number of such eager candidates must be substantial. Second, though the need for enabling legalization becomes progressively more urgent the greater the numbers of people personally concerned, I wish for myself to insist that it still matters very much indeed if but one person who would have decided for a quick death is forced to undergo a protracted one.

(b) To the second objection, which admits that there are many cases where euthanasia is indicated, but is content to leave it to the doctors to defy the law, the answer is equally simple. First, it is manifestly not true that all doctors are willing on the appropriate occasions either to provide the means of death or to do the killing. Many, as they are Roman Catholics, are on religious grounds absolutely opposed to doing so. Many others are similarly opposed for other reasons, or by force of training and habit. And there is no reason to believe that among the rest the proportion of potential martyrs is greater than it is in any other secular occupational group. Second, it is entirely wrong to expect the members of one profession as a regular matter of course to jeopardize their whole careers by breaking the criminal law in order to save the rest of us the labour and embarrassment of changing that law.

Here I repeat two points made to me more than once by doctor friends. First, if a doctor were convinced he ought to provide euthanasia in spite of the law, it would often be far harder for him to do so undetected than many laymen think, especially in our hospitals. Second, the present attitude of the medical establishment is such that if a doctor did take the chance, was caught and brought to trial, and even if the jury, as they well might, refused to convict, still he must expect to face complete professional disaster.

(3) The next two objections, which in effect bear on the principle, again form a pair. The first pair had in common the claim that the facts were such that the question of legislative action need not arise. The second pair are alike in that whereas both might appear to be making contentions of fact, in reality we may have in each a piece of exhortation or of metaphysics masquerading as an empirical proposition.

(a) Of this second relevant pair the first suggests that there is no such thing as an incurable disease. This implausible thesis becomes more intelligible, though no more true, when we recall how medical ideologues sometimes make proclamations: 'Modern medicine cannot recognize any such thing as a disease which is incurable'; and the like. Such pronouncements may sound like reports on the present state of the art. It is from this resemblance that they derive their peculiar idiomatic point. But the advance of medicine has not reached a stage where all diseases are curable. And no one seriously thinks that it has. At most this continuing advance has suggested that we need never despair of finding cures *some day*. But this is not at all the same thing as saying, what is simply not true, that *even now* there is no condition which is at any stage incurable. This medical ideologue's slogan has to be construed as a piece of exhortation disguised for greater effect as a paradoxical statement of purported fact. It may as such be instructively compared with certain favourite educationalists' paradoxes: 'We do not teach subjects, we teach children!'; or 'There are no bad children, only bad teachers!'

(b) The second objection of this pair is that no one can ever be certain that the condition of any particular patient is indeed hopeless. This is more tricky. For an objection of this form might be given two radically different sorts of content. Yet it would be easy and is common to slide from one interpretation to the other, and back again, entirely unwittingly.

Simply and straightforwardly, such an objection might be

made by someone whose point was that judgments of incurability are, as a matter of purely contingent fact, so unreliable that no one has any business to be certain, or to claim to know, that anyone is suffering from an incurable affliction. This contention would relevantly be backed by appealing to the alleged fact that judgments that 'this case is hopeless, *period*' are far more frequently proven to have been mistaken than judgments that, for instance, 'this patient will recover fully, *provided that* he undergoes the appropriate operation'. This naïve objector's point could be made out, or decisively refuted, only by reference to quantitative studies of the actual relative reliabilities and unreliabilities of different sorts of medical judgments. So unless and until such quantitative empirical studies are actually made, and unless and until their results are shown to bear upon the question of euthanasia in the way suggested, there is no grounded and categorical objection here to be met.

But besides this first and straightforwardly empirical interpretation there is a second interpretation of another quite different sort. Suppose someone points to an instance, as they certainly could and well might, where some patient whom all the doctors had pronounced to be beyond hope nevertheless recovers, either as the result of the application of new treatment derived from some swift and unforeseen advance in medical science, or just through nature taking its unexpected course. This happy but chastening outcome would certainly demonstrate that the doctors concerned had on this occasion been mistaken; and hence that, though they had sincerely claimed to know the patient's condition to have been incurable, they had not really known this. The temptation is to mistake it that such errors show that no one ever really knows. . . .

First, in so far as the objection is purely metaphysical, to the idea that *real* knowledge is possible, it applies absolutely generally; or not at all. It is arbitrary and irrational to restrict it to the examination of the principle of voluntary euthanasia. If doctors never really know, we presumably have no business to rely much upon any of their judgments. And if, for the same metaphysical reasons, there is no knowledge to be had anywhere, then we are all of us in the same case about everything. This may be as it may be, but it is nothing in particular to the practical business in hand.

Second, when the objection takes the form of a pretended

refusal to take any decision in matters of life and death on the basis of a judgment which theoretically might turn out to have been mistaken, it is equally unrealistic and arbitrary. It is one thing to claim that judgments of incurability are peculiarly fallible: if that suggestion were to be proved to be correct. It is quite another to claim that it is improper to take vital decisions on the basis of sorts of judgment which either are in principle fallible, or even prove occasionally in fact to have been wrong. It is an inescapable feature of the human condition that no one is infallible about anything, and there is no sphere of life in which mistakes do not occur. Nevertheless we cannot as agents avoid, even in matters of life and death and more than life and death, making decisions to act or to abstain. It is only necessary and it is only possible to insist on ordinarily strict standards of warranted assertability, and on ordinarily exacting rather than obsessional criteria of what is beyond reasonable doubt.

Of course this means that mistakes will sometimes be made. This is in practice a corollary of the uncontested fact that infallibility is not an option. To try to ignore our fallibility is unrealistic, while to insist on remembering it only in the context of the question of voluntary euthanasia is arbitrary. Nor is it either realistic or honourable to attempt to offload the inescapable burdens of practical responsibility, by first claiming that we never really *know*, and then pretending that a decision not to act is somehow a decision which relieves us of all proper responsibility for the outcome.

(4) The two pairs of relevant objections so far considered have both been attempts in different ways to show that the issue does not, or at any rate need not, arise as a practical question. The next concedes that the question does arise and is important, but attempts to dispose of it with the argument that what we propose amounts to the legalization, in certain circumstances, of murder, or suicide, or both; and that this cannot be right because murder and suicide are both gravely wrong always. Now even if we were to concede all the rest it would still not follow, because something is gravely wrong in morals, that there ought to be a law against it; and that we are wrong to try to change the law as it now subsists. We have already urged that the onus of proof must always rest on the defenders of any restriction.

(a) In fact the rest will not do. In the first place, if the law were to be changed as we want, the present legal definition of 'murder' would at the same time have to be so changed that it no longer covered the provision of euthanasia for a patient who had established that it was his legal right. 'Does this mean,' someone may indignantly protest, 'that right and wrong are created by Acts of Parliament?' Emphatically, yes: and equally emphatically, no. Yes indeed, if what is intended is *legal* right and *legal* offence. What is meant by the qualification 'legal' if it is not that these rights are the rights established and sanctioned by the law? Certainly not, if what is intended is *moral* right and *moral* wrong. Some moral rights happen to be at the same time legal rights, and some moral wrongs similarly also constitute offences against the law. But, notoriously, legislatures may persist in denying moral rights; while, as I insisted earlier, not every moral wrong either is or ought to be forbidden and penalized by law.

Well then, if the legal definition of 'murder' can be changed by Act of Parliament, would euthanasia nevertheless be murder, morally speaking? This amounts to asking whether administering euthanasia legally to someone who is incurably ill, and who has continually wanted it, is in all relevant respects similar to, so to speak, a standard case of murder; and whether therefore it is to be regarded morally as murder. Once the structure of the question is in this way clearly displayed, it becomes obvious that the cases are different in at least three important respects. First, whereas the murder victim is (typically) killed against his will, a patient would be given or assisted in obtaining euthanasia only if he steadily and strongly desired to die. Second, whereas the murderer kills his victim, treating him usually as a mere object for disposal, in euthanasia the object of the exercise would be to save someone, at his own request, from needless suffering, to prevent the degradation of a human person. Third, whereas the murderer by his action defies the law, the man performing euthanasia would be acting according to law, helping another man to secure what the law allowed him.

It may sound as if that third clause goes back on the earlier repudiation of the idea that moral right and wrong are created by Act of Parliament. That is not so. For we are not saying that this action would now be justifiable, or at least not murder morally, simply because it was now permitted by the law; but rather that the change in the law would remove one of possible reasons for moral objection. The point is this: that although the fact that something is enjoined, permitted, or forbidden by law does not necessarily make it right, justifiable, or wrong morally, nevertheless the fact that something is enjoined or forbidden by a law laid down by established authority does constitute one moral reason for obedience. So a doctor who is convinced that the objects of the Euthanasia Society are absolutely right should at lease hesitate to take the law into his own hands, not only for prudential but also for moral reasons. For to defy the law is, as it were, to cast your vote against constitutional procedures and the rule of law, and these are the foundations and framework of any tolerable civilized society. (Consider here the injunction posted by some enlightened municipal authorities upon their public litter bins: 'Cast your vote here for a tidy New York!'—or whatever it may be.)

Returning to the main point, the three differences which we have just noticed are surely sufficient to require us to refuse to assimilate legalized voluntary euthanasia to the immoral category of murder. But to insist on making a distinction between legalized voluntary euthanasia and murder is not the same thing as, nor does it by itself warrant, a refusal to accept that both are equally immoral. What an appreciation of these three differences, but crucially of the first, should do is to suggest that we ought to think of such euthanasia as a special case not of murder but of suicide. Let us therefore examine the second member of our third pair of relevant objections.

(b) This objection was that to legalize voluntary euthanasia would be to legalize, in certain conditions, the act of assisting suicide. The question therefore arises: 'Is suicide always morally wrong?'

The purely secular considerations usually advanced and accepted are not very impressive. First, it is still sometimes urged that suicide is unnatural, in conflict with instinct, a breach of the putative law of self-preservation. All arguments of this sort, which attempt directly to deduce conclusions about what *ought* to be from premises stating, or mis-stating, only what *is* are—surely—unsound: they involve what philosophers label, appropriately, the 'Naturalistic Fallacy'. There is also a peculiar viciousness about appealing to what is supposed to be a descriptive law of nature to provide some justification for the prescription to obey that supposed law. For if the law really obtained as a description of what always and unavoidably happens, then there would be no point in prescribing that it should; whereas if the descriptive law does not in fact hold, then the basis of the supposed justification does not exist.[3] Furthermore, even if an argument of this first sort could show that suicide is always immoral, it could scarcely provide a reason for insisting that it ought also to be illegal.

Second, it is urged that the suicide by his act deprives other people of the services which he might have rendered them had he lived longer. This can be a strong argument, especially where the suicide has clear, positive family or public obligations. It is also an argument which, even in a liberal perspective, can provide a basis for legislation. But it is irrelevant to the circumstances which advocates of the legalization of voluntary euthanasia have in mind. In such circumstances as these, there is no longer any chance of being any use to anyone, and if there is any family or social obligation it must be all the other way—to end your life when it has become a hopeless burden both to yourself and to others.

Third, it is still sometimes maintained that suicide is in effect murder—'self-murder'. To this, offered in a purely secular context, the appropriate and apparently decisive reply would seem to be that by parity of reasoning marriage is really adultery—'own-wife-adultery'. For, surely, the gravamen of both distinctions lies in the differences which such paradoxical assimilations override. It is precisely because suicide is the destruction of oneself (by one's own choice), while murder is the destruction of somebody else (against his wishes), that the former can be, and is, distinguished from the latter.

Yet there is a counter to this own-wife-adultery-move. It begins by insisting, rightly, that sexual relations—which are what is common to both marriage and adultery—are not in themselves wrong: the crucial question is, 'Who with?' It then proceeds to claim that what is common to both murder and suicide is the killing of a human being; and here the questions of 'Which one?' or 'By whom?' are not, morally, similarly decisive. Finally appeal may be made, if the spokesman is a little old-fashioned, to the Sixth Commandment, or if he is in the contemporary swim, to the Principle of the Absolute Sanctity of Human Life.

The fundamental difficulty which confronts anyone making this counter move is that of finding a formulation for his chosen principle about the wrongness of all killing, which is both sufficiently general not to appear merely question-begging in its application to the cases in dispute, and which yet carries no consequences that the spokesman himself is not prepared to accept. Thus, suppose he tries to read the Sixth Commandment as constituting a veto on any killing of human beings. Let us waive here the immediate scholarly objections: that such a reading involves accepting the mistranslation 'Thou shalt not kill' rather than the more faithful 'Thou shalt do no murder'; and that neither the children of Israel nor even their religious leaders construed this as a law forbidding all war and all capital punishment.[4] The question remains whether our spokesman himself is really prepared to say that all killing, without any exception, is morally wrong.

It is a question which has to be pressed, and which can only be answered by each man for himself. Since I cannot give your answer, I can only say that I know few if any people who would sincerely say 'Yes'. But as soon as any exceptions or qualifications are admitted, it becomes excessively difficult to find any presentable principle upon which these can be admitted while still excluding suicide and assistance to suicide in a case of euthanasia. This is not just because, generally, once any exceptions or qualifications have been admitted to any rule it becomes hard or impossible not to allow others. It is because, particularly, the case of excluding suicide and assisting suicide from the scope of any embargo on killing people is so strong that only some absolutely universal rule admitting no exceptions of any sort whatever could have the force convincingly to override it.

Much the same applies to the appeal to the Principle of the Absolute Sanctity of Human Life. Such appeals were continually made by conservatives—many of them politically not Conservative but Socialist—in opposition to the recent efforts to liberalize the British abortion laws. Such conservatives should be, and repeatedly were, asked whether they are also opponents of all capital punishment and whether they think that it is always wrong to kill in a 'just war'. (In fact none of those in

Parliament could honestly have answered 'Yes' to both questions.) In the case of abortion their position could still be saved by inserting the qualification 'innocent', a qualification traditionally made by cautious moralists who intend to rest on this sort of principle. But any such qualification, however necessary, must make it almost impossible to employ the principle thus duly qualified to proscribe all suicide. It would be extraordinarily awkward and far-fetched to condemn suicide or assisting suicide as 'taking an innocent life'.

Earlier . . . I described the three arguments I have been examining as secular. This was perhaps misleading. For all three are regularly used by religious people: indeed versions of all three are to be found in St. Thomas Aquinas's *Summa Theologica*, the third being there explicitly linked with St. Augustine's laboured interpretation of the Sixth Commandment to cover suicide.[5] And perhaps the incongruity of trying to make the amended Principle of the Absolute Sanctity of Innocent Human Life yield a ban on suicide is partly to be understood as a result of attempting to derive from secularized premises conclusions which really depend upon a religious foundation. But the next two arguments are frankly and distinctively religious.

The first insists that human beings are God's property: 'It is our duty to take care of God's property entrusted to our charge—our souls and bodies. They belong not to us but to God';[6] 'Whoever takes his own life sins against God, even as he who kills another's slave sins against that slave's master';[7] and 'Suicide is the destruction of the temple of God and a violation of the property rights of Jesus Christ.'[8]

About this I restrict myself to three comments here. First, as it stands, unsupplemented by appeal to some other principle or principles, it must apply, if it applies at all, equally to *all* artificial and intentional shortening *or* lengthening of any human life, one's own *or* that of anyone else. Alone and unsupplemented it would commit one to complete quietism in all matters of life and death; for all interference would be interference with someone else's property. Otherwise one must find further particular moral revelations by which to justify capital punishment, war, medicine, and many other such at first flush impious practices. Second, it seems to presuppose that a correct model of the relation between man and God is that of slave and slave-master, and that respect for God's property ought to be the fundamental principle of morals. It is perhaps significant that it is to this image that St. Thomas and the pagan Plato, in attacking suicide, both appeal. This attempt to derive not only theological but all obligations from the putative theological fact of Creation is a commonplace of at least one tradition of moral theology. In this derivation the implicit moral premise is usually that unconditional obedience to a Creator, often considered as a very special sort of owner, is the primary elemental obligation.[9] Once this is made explicit it does not appear to be self-evidently true; nor is it easy to see how a creature in absolute ontological dependence could be the genuinely responsible subject of obligations to his infinite Creator.[10] Third, this objection calls to mind one of the sounder sayings of the sinister Tiberius: 'If the gods are insulted let them see to it themselves.' This remark is obviously relevant only to the question of legalization, not to that of the morality or the prudence of the action itself.

The second distinctively religious argument springs from the conviction that God does indeed see to it Himself, with a penalty of infinite severity. If you help someone to secure euthanasia, 'You are sending him from the temporary and comparatively light suffering of this world to the eternal suffering of hell.' Now if this appalling suggestion could be shown to be true it would provide the most powerful moral reason against helping euthanasia in any way, and for using any legislative means which might save people from suffering a penalty so inconceivably cruel. It would also be the strongest possible prudential reason against 'suiciding oneself'.[11] (Though surely anyone who knowingly incurred such a penalty would by that very action prove himself to be genuinely of unsound mind; and hence not *justly* punishable at all. Not that a Being contemplating such unspeakable horrors could be expected to be concerned with justice!).

About this second, peculiarly religious, argument there is, it would seem, little to be done except: either simply to concede that for anyone holding this belief it indeed is reasonable to oppose euthanasia, and to leave it at that; or, still surely conceding this, to attempt to mount a general offensive against the whole system of which it forms a part.

(5) The final objection is one raised, with appropriate modifications, by the opponents of every reform everywhere. It is that

even granting that the principle of the reform is excellent it would, if adopted, lead inevitably to something worse; and so we had much better not make any change at all. Thus G.K. Chesterton pronounced that the proponents of euthanasia now seek only the death of those who are a nuisance to themselves, but soon it will be broadened to include those who are a nuisance to others.[12] Such cosy arguments depend on two assumptions: that the supposedly inevitable consequences are indeed evil and substantially worse than the evils the reform would remove; and that the supposedly inevitable consequences really are inevitable consequences.

In the present case we certainly can grant the first assumption, if the consequence supposed is taken to be large-scale legalized homicide in the Nazi manner. But whatever reason is there for saying that this would, much less inevitably must, follow? For there are the best of reasons for insisting that there is a world of difference between legalized voluntary euthanasia and such legalized mass-murder. Only if public opinion comes to appreciate their force will there be any chance of getting the reform we want. Then we should have no difficulty, in alliance doubtless with all our present opponents, in blocking any move to legalize murder which might conceivably arise from a misunderstanding of the case for voluntary euthanasia. Furthermore, it is to the point to remind such objectors that the Nazi atrocities they probably have in mind were in fact not the result of any such reform, but were the work of people who consciously repudiated the whole approach to ethics represented in the argument of the present essay. For this approach is at once human and humanitarian. It is concerned above all with the reduction of suffering; but concerned at the same time with other values too, such as human dignity and respect for the wishes of the individual person. And always it is insistent that morality should not be 'left in the dominion of vague feeling or inexplicable internal conviction, but should be . . . made a matter of reason and calculation'.[13]

NOTES

1. Thus Jeremy Bentham, urging that the legislator must not neglect animal sufferings, insists that the 'question is not "Can they *reason*?" nor "Can they *talk*?" but "Can they

suffer?" ' (*Principles of Morals and Legislation,* Chap. XVII, *n.*)

2. The Greek text is most easily found in *Hippocrates and the Fragments of Heracleitus*, ed. W.H.S. Jones and E.T. Withington for the Loeb series (Harvard Univ. Pr. and Heinemann), Vol. 1, p. 298. The translation in the present essay is mine.

3. I have argued this kind of point more fully in *Evolutionary Ethics* (London: Macmillan, 1967). See Chap. IV, 'From *Is* to *Ought*'.

4. See, f.i., Joseph Fletcher, *Morals and Medicine* (1954; Gollancz, 1955), pp. 195–6. I recommend this excellent treatment by a liberal Protestant of a range of questions in moral theology too often left too far from liberal Roman Catholics.

5. Part II: Q. 64, A5. The Augustine reference is to *The City of God*, I, 20. It is worth comparing, for ancient Judaic attitudes, E. Westermarck's *Origin and Development of the Moral Ideas,* Vol. I, pp. 246–7.

6. See the Rev. G.J. MacGillivray, 'Suicide and Euthanasia', p. 10; a widely distributed Catholic Truth Society pamphlet.

7. Aquinas, loc. cit.

8. Koch-Preuss, *Handbook of Moral Theology*, Vol. II, p. 76. This quotation has been taken from Fletcher, op. cit., p. 192.

9. Cf., for convenience, MacGillivray, loc. cit.; and for a Protestant analogue the Bishop of Exeter quoted by P. Nowell-Smith in *Ethics* (Penguin, 1954), pp.37–8 *n.*

10. I have developed this contention in *God and Philosophy* (Hutchinson, 1966), §§2.34ff.

11. This rather affected-sounding gallicism is adopted deliberately: if you believe, as I do, that suicide is not always and as such wrong, it is inappropriate to speak of 'committing suicide'; just as correspondingly if you believe, as I do not, that (private) profit is wrong, it becomes apt to talk of those who 'commit a profit'.

12. I take this quotation, too, from Fletcher, op. cit., p. 201: it originally appeared in *The Digest* (Dec. 23, 1937). Another, much more recent specimen of this sort of obscurantist flim-flam may be found in Lord Longford's speech to the House of Lords against Mr. David Steel's Abortion Bill as originally passed by the Commons. Lord Longford (formerly Pakenham) urged that if that bill were passed, we might see the day when senile members of their lordships' House were put down willy-nilly.

13. J.S. Mill's essay on Bentham quoted in F.R. Leavis, *Mill on Bentham and Coleridge* (Chatto & Windus, 1950), p. 92.

Euthanasia and the Law

Richard L. Trammell

One advocate of the legalization of positive euthanasia has said that it "matters very much indeed if but one person who would have decided for a quick death is forced to undergo a protracted one."[1] It matters also, of course, if but one person who would have decided to live longer is pressured into accepting a quick death. A prudent utilitarian will weigh carefully the overall impact of any bill legalizing euthanasia.

For some people any appeal to utility in considering the desirability of legalizing euthanasia will seem cruel and inappropriate. Some advocates of euthanasia, Marvin Kohl complains, ". . . have written as if the question of fiscal utility were of prime importance. They argue that there is a need to save the young from the great cost of caring for those who are irremediably ill and to save the general public from staggering and unnecessary medical expense, adding that euthanasia legislation 'might save the country a few billion dollars a year.' "[2] But there is a type of appeal to utility which is important in evaluating any proposal to legalize euthanasia, and which is consistent with Kohl's claim that euthanasia should be legalized (if at all) only for the benefit of the recipients. The type of appeal I have in mind is not purely utilitarian because it excludes certain kinds of utility from consideration, such as inconveniences to the healthy. On the other hand, considerations of utility go beyond the person actually being euthanatized. The utility to be

From *Journal of Social Philosophy*, vol. 9, Jan. 1978. Reprinted by permission of the author and the *Journal of Social Philosophy*.

taken into account is the utility of the class of people who are eligible for euthanasia.

In the discussion which follows, only voluntary positive euthanasia will be considered. Negative euthanasia will not be considered, in part because some kind of negative euthanasia is inevitable. To insist that every patient's life be extended to the last possible moment, with ever quickening series of operations and restrictions to mechanical devices, in direct contradiction to the patient's desires, is a policy with few defenders. Furthermore, it should not be forgotten that the doctor's self-interest (monetarily) lies in continuing medical treatment. Thus it is not only a matter of the patient's liberty but the need to protect *his* self-interest, which demands that the patient have the right to refuse treatment. Consideration will be given to voluntary euthanasia, in part because this is the type of positive euthanasia which is currently being most actively promoted by the proponents of the legalization of positive euthanasia.

It would seem that any proposed law legalizing positive euthanasia would be undesirable for the class of people who are eligible for euthanasia if the following condition is met:

> Given the law, it is more probable that euthanasia will result in negative utility to any person to whom it is administered than it is that it will result in positive utility.

This condition might still not be sufficient to achieve the result claimed above if negative utilities on the average were very small for those cases when euthanasia is erroneously applied whereas positive utilities on the average were very high for those cases euthanasia is correctly applied. It might be argued that if the legalization were restricted to diagnosed terminal cases where the people involved voluntarily request it, positive utility if life continues could not be very high. Yet by the same reasoning, if the case is really "terminal" and death imminent, and if humane and efficient use of pain-relieving measures are employed, then negative utility will not be extremely high either if the person is allowed to die by natural means rather than being deliberately and directly put to death. Cases of prolonged and unavoidable pain are paralleled by cases of mistaken diagnosis, temporary depression, etc. The net result seems to be that when mistakes do occur, the loss of utility on the average will be just as much per person, and perhaps even more, as the gain of utility when euthanasia is rightly applied. For example, a 50-year-old victim of a handicapping stroke might in a period of depression request euthanasia and yet if allowed time to adjust to his new limitations discover that he has many years of meaningful life ahead.

At first it might seem unlikely that the condition given above would be met by a law which stipulates that euthanasia must be voluntary and performed only if the doctor agrees with the patient's assessment of his future (i.e., the case is "terminal," the patient is not suffering from temporary depression, he has not been unduly pressured by members of family or otherwise, etc.). Under such a legalization, meeting the above condition (assuming that the degree of negative utility for mistaken applications would be the same on the average as the degree of positive utility for correct application) would require that both the patients and those administering euthanasia be wrong more often that at least one of them is right concerning what is beneficent treatment for the patients involved.

Yet any bill legalizing euthanasia would inevitably create certain pressures for it to be used. Suppose a doctor has the attitude of Marya Mannes. Mannes states in her book *Last Rights* that she believes that she would want her life ended if she were deprived of "independent mobility," or if she had to use for more than two weeks "mechanical equipment for breathing, heart action, feeding, dialysis or brain function without a prognosis of full recovery of my vital organs," or if a stroke impaired her ability to speak, or if her vision became too impaired to read. Although she disclaims her position being a "model" or "example," she does hope that it will give "direction and courage" to other people.[3]

Proponents of legalization of voluntary positive euthanasia will assert that what Marya Mannes would want under such conditions is her own business; and that if any of these conditions were realized and she did indeed want her death, then the probability of positive euthanasia being the most beneficent action would be very high. Yet we must not overlook a very important difference between the position of Marya Mannes and the position of the average person if a bill legalizing active voluntary euthanasia were passed. Mannes's choice of euthanasia for herself under the conditions mentioned above, takes place in a society in which such a choice, if acted upon by others, would be illegal, and in which the majority of social, medical, moral and religious pressures are against such a decision. Thus when Mannes announces her decision we can feel relatively confident that this represents a decision which has not been unduly influenced by external pressures. The decision is truly voluntary. But in a society in which active euthanasia for such cases were legalized, and socially, medically and religiously accepted, the pressures would be reversed. If father or mother faces a serious and costly illness, few children now expect father or mother to drink the hemlock in order that the family fortune will be preserved for the children. But how will things be if active euthanasia is legalized?

If positive euthanasia becomes legally and morally accepted, it is inevitable that strong pressures will be put on many patients who, in Yale Kamisar's words, "do not really want to die, but who feel they should not live on, because to do so when there looms the legal alternative of euthanasia is to do a selfish or a cowardly act." Mannes will be looking over their shoulders, giving them "direction and courage." Serious internal discords and pressures will develop in many families concerning whether or not to encourage the patient to live or to be put to death. As Kamisar asks, "Are these the kind of pressures we want to inflict on any person, let alone a very sick person? Are these the kind of pressures we want to impose on any family, let alone an emotionally shattered family? And if so, why are they not also proper considerations for the crippled, the paralyzed, the quadruple amputee, the iron-lung occupant and their families?"[4]

The impact of euthanasia legislation must be weighed not only on those who actually choose it but also on the whole class of people who would be eligible to choose it. In addition to the person who is pressured into doing what is not really in his best interest, weight must also be given to the person who chooses *not* to undergo active euthanasia but whose life is made less happy because euthanasia is legal. There are various reasons why the old or sick who do not choose positive euthanasia might live less happy lives than they would have lived if such a possibility had not been a legal option for them. Perhaps their unhappiness will stem from guilt, or from resentment of friends or family, or from neglect by other people generated by the attitude that if a person could choose euthanasia and does not, then things must not really be so bad for that person. Even today, when those confined to bed or home have little or no choice but to accept their restricted conditions, most of us find it very easy to neglect doing simple things which could make their lives more meaningful and happy.

Contrast these two cases. Mrs. X has a stroke which leaves her speech somewhat impaired and one side paralyzed. Still she can talk and walk, but not nearly as well as before. In society A there is no legal means for Mrs. X to choose positive euthanasia, and neither Mrs. X nor her family will consider this possibility. Because their hopes and expectations are focused on her continued life, even in restricted conditions, it will in fact be beneficent to Mrs. X that she continue to live. In society B, there is the legal means for Mrs. X to choose euthanasia. Both Mrs. X and her family know this and seriously consider the possibility. Because her continued life will place certain restrictions on her family, Mrs. X will feel guilty if she chooses to live, and the family will feel resentment if she chooses to live, all knowing that she could choose otherwise. This combined guilt and resentment, with negative impact on many aspects of Mrs. X's situation, might actually result in the fact that it would not be beneficent to Mrs. X that she continue to live.

Now let us return to the condition which we asserted, if met, would provide a utilitarian justification of a prohibition of positive euthanasia, confining our consideration to the class or people eligible to choose such euthanasia. This condition needs to be reformulated. To the extent that a law legalizing euthanasia would create conditions which would change a person's life from "worth living" to "not worth living," even a correct decision under that law that a person's life is "not worth living" is not justification for the law, since that person's life would have been worth living were it not for the law. We can reformulate the condition as follows:

> Given the law, it is more probable that positive euthanasia will not be to the benefit of any person to whom it is administered *or would not have been to the benefit of the person if that law had not been enacted*, than it is that positive euthanasia will be to the benefit of that

> person *and would have been to the benefit of that person even if that law had not been enacted.*[5]

Obviously this revised condition will be more easily met than the initial condition. Furthermore, the more accepted the practice of positive euthanasia becomes, the more likely it is that people will be euthanatized who, if the law did not permit positive euthanasia, would have had worthwhile lives ahead. In addition, the revised formulation still does not take into account people whose lives are made less happy by the law even though they do not choose euthanasia. It would seem that the vast majority of people who go through an agonizing process of deciding whether or not to be euthanatized, and choose not to, would have been happier if this agonizing choice had not been put before them.

It is worth noting that not all legalizations of exceptional kinds of killing help create conditions which lead to the killing needing to be done. In this respect, as in others, the effect of legalization of the right to kill in self-defense is quite different from the effect of legalization of positive euthanasia. If people intent on violence knew that their victims could not retaliate against them without incurring legal penalties, the likelihood of situations arising in which self-defense is needed would certainly increase. Thus the law permitting self-defense makes it less likely that the situation will arise in which people need to use self-defense. However, precisely the reverse would be true of a law legalizing positive euthanasia. As far as I know, no advocate of euthanasia has ever maintained that legalization of euthanasia will make it less likely that situations will arise in which euthanasia is needed, Rather it seems clear that the opposite would be true, for reasons such as those indicated above.

It might be thought that the same kind of argument can be used against the legalization of abortion, since there will be many people who would have been careful enough not to get pregnant if they had known there were no legal right to abortion, but who will get pregnant knowing that the legal right to abortion is guaranteed. It is true that the legalization of abortion helps create conditions which lead to the need for abortion to be done. However, there is a disanalogy between abortion and euthanasia in regard to the existence of the subject if the law is not passed.[6] In the case of abortion, the fetus which would not have been conceived and aborted if the law legalizing abortion did not exist, would not, by hypothesis, even have been conceived if the law legalizing abortion did not exist. But a person who needs to be euthanatized only because the law legalizing euthanasia has created a climate in which his life is not worth living, by hypothesis will not need to be euthanatized if the law does not exist. But still the person will exist.

The above discussion, based solely on utility of those who would be eligible to choose positive euthanasia, has not considered the very deep and persistent intuition that it is more wrong to kill unjustly than to fail to kill justly, i.e., that it is more wrong to kill someone whose life is worth living, than to fail to kill someone whose life is not worth living. Even without considering this and other intuitions about killing, it seems doubtful that any of the prevalent proposals for legalized positive and voluntary euthanasia would result in overall positive utility for the class of people eligible to choose. The pressures such legalization would create are both many and subtle, and would become greater and greater the more "socially accepted" the practice of euthanasia became.

NOTES

1. Antony Flew, "The Principle of Euthanasia," in *Euthanasia and the Right to Death: the Case for Voluntary Euthanasia,* edited by A.B. Downing (Peter Owen: London, 1969), p. 36.
2. Marvin Kohl, *The Morality of Killing* (Humanities Press: Atlantic Highlands, New Jersey, 1974), p. 99.
3. Marya Mannes, *Last Rights* (Morrow, Williams & Co., Inc: New York, 1974), pp. 133–135.
4. Yale Kamisar, "Euthanasia Legislation: Some Non-Religious Objections," in *Euthanasia and the Right to Death*, op. cit., pp. 96–97.
5. If *A* represents the society without legalization of euthanasia and *B* the society with legalization of euthanasia, then the logic of the revised principle can be stated as follows: in order for a specific case of euthanasia to be morally justified, it must be in the best interest of the person euthanatized in *both A* and *B*; if it is not in the person's best interest in *either* A *or* B, then euthanasia is *not* justified. The require-

ment to justify legalization (both A and B) is more stringent than the requirement to justify non-legalization. (either A or B).

6. Abortion obviously is a very complex moral issue. In pointing out the partial disanalogy with euthanasia, I am considering only one minor factor in this complexity.

Do Not Go Slowly
into That Dark Night:
Mercy Killing in Holland

Gregory E. Pence, Ph.D.

THE Dutch are known for practicality, fierce independence, moral integrity, free-thought, and defense of civil liberties. Under Nazi occupation, Dutch physicians successfully resisted Hitler's programs.[1] Holland is nominally Catholic but 27 percent of Dutch citizens claim no religious affiliation, and Dutch Catholicism is very democratic and aggressively anti-Vatican. Moreover, the Dutch seem to distrust elaborate technology and wish to die at home more than Americans, 80 percent of whom die in hospitals.[2]

Seventy-five percent of Dutch citizens now endorse mercy killing by physicians after requests by terminal patients.[3] These attitudes have changed Dutch medical practices. It is estimated that Dutch physicians have now killed between 5,000 and 8,000 terminal patients. This new development in the history of medicine needs to be carefully studied.

The Dutch national movement for decriminalization began in 1971 when a female physician accepted her mother's repeated requests for death. Geertruida Postma's mother had had a cerebral hemorrage that left her partially paralyzed, deaf, and mute. After the stroke, Postma's mother lived in a nursing home, where she was tied to a chair for support. Dr. Postma said, "When I watched my mother, a human wreck, hanging in that chair, I couldn't stand it anymore."[4] So she injected her mother with morphine and killed her. Postma then told the

From *American Journal of Medicine*, 1988; 84; 139–41. Reprinted by permission of the *American Journal of Medicine* and the author.

director of the nursing home, who called police. Postma was found guilty of murder, but was given only a symbolic sentence. Postma's lawyer argued that "rational suicide" assisted by a physician should be a legal defense. The judge rejected this defense but nevertheless specified some guidelines. The 1973 case of physician Piet Schoonheim also concerned mercy killing, but of patients who were not immediately terminal.[5] Schoonheim was eventually cleared.

Two Dutch euthanasia societies grew after such cases. One group sought legislative reform, like the American Society for the Right to Die, and the other helped terminal patients to die, like the American Hemlock Society.

In 1973, the Dutch Medical Association softened its condemnation of mercy killing by physicians. While stating that euthanasia by request should still be a crime, it urged that courts should decide whether physicians could be justified in particular cases. Public support for euthanasia dramatically increased over the next decade, and in 1984 the Dutch Medical Association advocated new guidelines stating that: (1) only a physician may implement requests for euthanasia, (2) requests must be made by competent patients, (3) patients' decisions must be free of doubt, well documented, and repeated, (4) the physician must consult another independent physician, and (5) a determination must be made that no one pressured patients into their decisions. Two other guidelines were more vague: (6) the patient must be in unbearable pain and suffering without prospect of change, and (7) no measures can be available that could improve the patient's condition or render his or her suffering bearable.

Dutch medicine had long before rejected the American view that actively killing a terminal patient differs ethically from withdrawing care. In the past decade, Americans have increasingly accepted withdrawing heroic treatment, standard treatment, and most recently, food and water. Groups such as the Hemlock Society now campaign in California for a bill to let the terminally ill request a voluntary physician's assistance in dying.

In 1985, the *Final Report of the Netherlands State Commission on Euthanasia* appeared with 13 of 15 Commissioners recommending a new exception to the criminal code covering homicide.[6] Mercy killing by physicians was proposed as a legal excuse to homicide, like self-defense or insanity. The remaining two Commissioners disagreed because of beliefs about the sanctity of life and slippery slopes. The final report created emotional debate in Holland. Politically, a majority of the Dutch parliament accepted the recommendations, but the Christian Democratic party strongly opposed them.

Between the spring and summer of 1986, opposition formed to a bill in Parliament accepting the report's recommendations for decriminalization. Opposition was led by anti-abortion groups and Catholic bishops, who called the bill "a descent into barbarity." Evangelical religious groups produced a television show featuring old pictures of victims in concentration camps and emphasizing the "slippery-slope" under Nazi medicine from initial killing of mental defectives to the "final solution" for "lebensunwertes Leben" (life unworthy of life). They said physicians would push the outer edges of legal euthanasia, generalizing to different but similar cases. They claimed that euthanasia by patient request was "murder" and people are the creatures of God who do not have the right to end their own lives.[7]

Champions of the bill retorted that the Nazis practiced murder, which had nothing to do with their cause. They said that using sophisticated medical technology is a physician's right but it imposes an obligation to end life when no purpose is served, that physicians too often merely prolong dying, that the slippery slope metaphor wrongly implies that society cannot make small changes without creating moral nihilism, that physicians are not eager to kill patients, that personal physicians can be trusted, and that if decriminalized euthanasia created bad results, it could be re-criminalized.

In the spring of 1987, while the euthanasia bill was being debated in Holland, ABC's *Nightline* staged a live debate between Dutch physician Peter Admiraal, Betty Rollin, author of *Last Wish*, and Father Robert Barry, a religion professor.[8] Admiraal, an anesthesiologist and oncologist who practices in a large Catholic hospital, speaks for Dutch physicians favoring mercy killing. As of the spring 1987 and since 1972, he has performed mercy killing on more than 100 patients. Father Barry criticized Admiraal's work, claiming that if patients were really in "unbearable pain and suffering," they couldn't make rational decisions to die. Father Barry accused Ms. Rollin (in the death of her mother described in *Last Wish*) of a "failure to care" in allowing her mother to die quickly. Father Barry also accused Rollin's physician of not knowing how to treat cancer pain, and predicted that if euthanasia were decriminalized, the "immature and the desperate" would increasingly choose suicide.

Admiraal agreed that pain in cancer patients could be stopped and was not the real issue. Instead, Admiraal said (in another interview):

> But there is severe dehydration, uncontrolled itching and fatigue. These patients are completely exhausted. Some of them can't turn around in their beds. They become incontinent. All these factors make a kind of suffering from which they only want to escape.
>
> And of course you are suffering because you have a mind. You are thinking about what is happening to you. You have fears and anxiety and sorrow. In the end, it gives a complete loss of human dignity. You cannot stop that feeling with medical treatment.[9]

Some Dutch physicians disagreed, such as Dr. Karel Gunning who claims to know "quite a number of cases" where "we thought patients would die in 34 hours" but were mistaken and they "lived 30 more years." He said on *Nightline* that a medical prognosis of a terminal condition is only "a guess" about the time of death.

Two more recent developments grew out of the first cases and make some people uneasy. First, the Dutch Medical Association allows terminal children to die even if their parents oppose it. The argument is that dying children do not understand why they have to live to suffer and that prolonging life is too often merely for the parents. Second, Dutch physicians and judges have now accepted other cases for mercy killing covering paraplegia, multiple sclerosis, and gross physical deterioration at advanced age. Some see these developments as a slippery slope, others as logical consistency. In all these cases, patients themselves must repeatedly request a physician's assistance to end their lives.

Contrary to many reports in the media, Holland has not legalized mercy killing. To understand what has happened, some features of Holland's judicial system different from those of America need to be mentioned. In Holland, trials are decided by judges without juries; judges are professional and unelected, ruling for life and often making decisions unpopular with vocal minorities. The discretionary power of Dutch district attorneys to not prosecute surpasses that of American prosecutors. What has happenend is that Holland has a de facto agreement among its powerful judges and public prosecutors not to prosecute physicians who perform (officially illegal) mercy killing done according to precise guidelines.

Performing euthanasia appears to have been accepted as an occasional duty by Dutch physicians. One study discovered that most physicians have two patients every three years who request mercy killing, one of which is performed.[10] Another found that nearly 80 percent of general practitioners in Holland had "experience with" mercy killing.[11] The preferred method appears to be injection of morphine followed after deep unconsciousness with curare.

Famous American decisions about euthanasia differ from these changes in Holland in two ways. First, they concern withdrawing treatment—respirators in Quinlan, chemotherapy in Saikewicz, and food/water in Conroy—not terminating life as such, and second, they concern incompetent patients whose wishes could only be inferred. The American cases should be called "euthanasia by inference of a patient's wishes," not voluntary euthanasia among competent adults. In America, the case distantly similar to the Dutch cases concerns Elizabeth Bouvia who had no terminal disease and who wanted to starve to death painlessly with medical assistance. In New Jersey this year, Beverly Requena sued to be allowed to remain to die at a nursing home run by St. Clare/Riverside Hospital, which agreed to allow her to be transferred to remove feeding and hydration tubes but which would not allow it in their residence.[12] But none of these cases involved active killing, and how Americans feel about such actions is uncertain.

Physicians in Holland dislike the current situation because they are told, "You will probably not go to jail for something which is officially a crime but which you have an obligation to occasionally perform." They would rather have a new statute telling them exactly when they can mercy kill and not be prosecuted. As things stand, misinterpretations are possible. One Dutch physician who failed to document a patient's request for euthanasia received a one-year prison sentence, and three nurses who secretly killed comatose patients received longer sentences.[13,14,15]

Moreover, the Dutch program seems to be personally difficult for Dutch physicians. It is rare for them to encounter the idealized terminal patient who is intelligent, in untreatable pain, and with supportive relatives. Instead, they find ordinary people, usually quite alone or with one relative who visits on weekends, who are not in acute pain or at death's door, but who are otherwise very badly off, e.g., after losing 70 pounds to esophageal cancer. Helping these patients die is not easy. In contrast to a slippery slope of mass-killings, few Dutch physicians seem eager to kill.

What will happen in the future is difficult to predict. A statute won't solve all problems because it can't be drafted both broadly enough to cover all patients and precisely enough to close loopholes ("terminal condition," "unbearable suffering"). In any case, the Dutch experience may show whether mercy killing leads to Auschwitz, civilized death, or somewhere in between.

NOTES

1. Alexander L: Medical science under dictatorship. N Engl J Med 1949; 241: 39–47.
2. President's Commission for the Study of Ethical Problems in Medicine and Biomedical and Behavioral Research: Deciding to forego life-sustaining treatment. Washington, DC: Superintendent of Documents, 1983; 17–18. See also Bowling A: Should more people die at home? J Med Ethics 1983; 9: 158–161.
3. De Ligny R: Voluntary euthanasia grows at fast pace in Netherlands. Associated Press story. April 4, 1987.
4. Humphrey D, Wickett A: The right to die: understanding euthanasia. In: Euthanasia in the Netherlands. New York: Harper & Row, 1986; 170–180.
5. Parachini A: A Dutch doctor carries out a death wish. Los Angeles Times. July 5, 1987, 6, p. 1.
6. Final report of the Netherlands State Commission on Euthanasia: an English summary. Bioethics 1987; 1: 2: 163–174.
7. Clines FX: Dutch are quietly taking the lead in euthanasia. New York Times. October 31, 1986, A4.
8. Nightline, February, 1987.
9. Parachini A: The Netherlands debates the legal limits of euthanasia. Los Angeles Times. July 5, 1987, 6, p.9.

10. Gevers JKM: Legal developments concerning active euthanasia on request in the Netherlands. Bioethics 1987; 1: 2: 156–162.
11. Euthanasie in de huisartspraktijk. Medisch Contact, 1986; 41:691; cited in Gevers, JKM, op cit.
12. Society for the Right to Die Newsletter, Fall, 1986, p.4.
13. Dawson J: Easeful death. Br Heart J 1986; 293: 1187–1188.
14. Cody E: Dutch weigh legalizing euthanasia. Washington Post. March 16, 1987, A12.
15. Sagel J: Voluntary euthanasia (letter). Lancet 1986; ll: 691.

B. Human Organ Procurement

Protecting Autonomy in Organ Procurement Procedures: Some Overlooked Issues

David A. Peters

VERSIONS of the 1968 Model Uniform Anatomical Gift Act[1] (UAGA) are now law in all 50 states and the District of Columbia. Most state UAGAs follow the Model Act in giving paramount authority to individuals to decide whether their medically acceptable bodies or parts shall be made available after death for research, education, therapy, or transplantation. These statutes declare that if an individual has validly signed a donation instrument, or given prior notice of objection to serving as a posthumous donor, the person's positive or negative declarations concerning personal donation cannot be vetoed by his or her family.

Despite the first authority given by the UAGA to individuals to control the use of their own bodies or parts after death for various medical purposes, organ retrieval in the United States is carried out in a manner that fails to give due recognition and protection to this paramount right of individuals. This is illustrated in two ways. First, procurement staff routinely ask families of brain-dead potential donors for permission to remove organs from these individuals, whether they have signed donor cards or not. In most cases, families of registered donors (i.e., those who have signed donation documents) are not even in-

The Milbank Quarterly, Vol. 64, No. 2, 1986. Reprinted by Permission of The Milbank Quarterly, Milbank Memorial Fund.

formed of the legal rights of these donors and the corresponding rights of donees that are controlling in the situation. Second, while the UAGA declares that organs shall not be taken from the bodies of those who before death have given "actual notice of contrary indication" concerning donation, current procurement policy provides no effective means for objectors to register dissent so as adequately to protect themselves against unwanted removal of their body parts after death.

In the first section of this article, I show that pre-UAGA American case law has been indecisive on the question of whose wishes take precedence when there is a conflict between the premortem declarations of a decedent concerning the posthumous disposition of his or her body and the wishes of that individual's family. In the following section, I demonstrate that the UAGA settles this issue with respect to organ donation by giving paramount authority to individuals to control postmortem organ removal and transfer from their own bodies. I argue that this legal right of individuals plausibly rests on the deeper theoretical claim that a person's body is his or her property in a significant sense. This warrants the further assertion that the person has first right to control its disposition before and after death. This places a weighty burden on procurement personnel to justify continuing current retrieval policy that regularly ignores this right under the UAGA.

I then examine a number of plausible explanations and justifications of current rights-ignoring retrieval policy and attempt to isolate the strongest set of considerations that could support it. I conclude that these considerations are not weighty enough to justify continuing present policy that blindly disregards the rights of declared donors and donees.

In the final section of the article, I offer two policy proposals. One is designed to effect a more appropriate balance between three principal competing values at stake when a deceased potential donor has authorized posthumous donation: (1) the rights of the donor and donee generated by this formal authorization, (2) the needs of the declared donor's grieving family to pay proper respect to the body of their loved one, and (3) the general interest of society and the medical profession in maximizing the number of lives saved through organ transfer. The other proposal is aimed at pro-

viding better protection than is available under current procurement policy to those who do not wish to serve as posthumous
donors.

Family versus Decedent's Wishes Concerning the Disposition of the Body in Anglo-American Common Law

A principal aim of the 1968 Model Uniform Anatomical Gift
Act (UAGA) was to increase the availability of cadaveric organs and tissues for transfer to end-stage organ disease (ESOD)
victims facing imminent death absent these replacement body
parts. In developing this model legislation, drafters were faced
with the task of balancing this interest in saving lives against a
variety of competing interests, including respecting the wishes
of individuals concerning the postmortem disposition of their
own bodies, the state interest in conducting autopsies in cases
of suspect deaths (coroner's inquiries), the interests of families
in possessing the bodies of dead relatives for the purpose of
burial, etc. The particular balance among these interests achieved
by the UAGA may be fairly said to represent a consensus
concerning the relative weight of these interests that had emerged
in American case law by 1968. Some of this pre-UAGA legal
history needs to be understood to appreciate fully the seriousness and complexity of the issue that is the principal focus of
this inquiry, namely, current procurement policy's routine failure to acknowledge the paramount authority vested in individuals by the UAGA to control the disposition of their own bodies
and body parts after death. I have rehearsed elsewhere (Peters
1985) details of the history of the treatment of cadavers in
English and American law. I will simply summarize here some
of the main principles and interpretive trends that have emerged
since the seventeenth century in adjudicating conflicts between
a decedent's premortem declarations concerning the disposition
of his or her corpse and claims of the decedent's family.

Rules Governing the Treatment of Cadavers in English Common Law

The eminent jurists Coke (1552–1634) and Blackstone (1723–1780) are usually credited with establishing in English common law the rule that dead bodies are not a type of commercial property.[2,3] That is, a cadaver is not the kind of thing with respect to which anyone could have property rights—rights which permit the "owner" to dispose of a body, abandon it, maintain exclusive possession of it, etc. The genesis of this rule appears to be partly explained by the fact that in seventeenth-century England matters pertaining to burial and sepulture were under the jurisdiction of ecclesiastical courts established during the reign of William the Conqueror (1028–1087). These courts comprised a separate judicial system from the temporal courts which held exclusive power of review over property disputes. Coke's reasoning seems to have been that since the treatment of corpses was not by convention within the cognizance of civil courts, corpses could not be commercial property.

In an early English grave-robbing case, the court ruled that theft of or tampering with a corpse is not a crime. On the other hand, the court declared that stealing or disturbing burial accouterments like tombstones or grave-clothes is a crime. These items are bonafide property. They belong to those who laid the decedent to rest.[4] In a later case, a "Resurrectionist" who disinterred and removed a body for the purposes of dissection was convicted on the charge of offending public decency rather than for property theft.[5] While the court makes no reference to the "no property" rule concerning dead bodies, a later court inferred from the absence of a larceny charge in the case that the original court tacitly accepted this rule.[6]

A further implication of the rule that corpses are not property in a commercial sense was enunciated by a nineteenth-century English court which ruled that a person has no legal right to direct by will the disposition of his or her body after death. The court declared that the executor of a person's estate was legally empowered to possess the decedent's body for the purpose of burial.[7]

Rules Governing the Treatment of Cadavers in American Common Law

No ecclesiastical court system like that in England was ever established in this country. Matters pertaining to the disposition of the dead always came under the jurisdiction of American civil courts. These courts took over, with some modifications, the basic tradition of English common law.

One prominent and far-reaching American modification of British legal tradition occurred in a landmark mid-nineteenth-century case where the court expressly rejected the English principle that the executor of a decedent's will has primary authority to possess the body for interment. The court ruled that this authority is vested in the decedent's *family*.[8]

American common law reflects its English heritage insofar as the right of family members to possess a relative's corpse for burial is not considered to be a property right in a commercial sense.[9] Rather, the right is described as a "quasi-property" interest in the body,[10,11] a right conferred on the family pursuant to the exercise of its *duty* to provide the deceased with a decent burial.[10,12] This family duty is, in turn, generated by the *decedent's right* to a decent burial.[11] Courts have frequently spoken of the family's right to possess the body of a dead relative as grounded on natural affection and moral obligations, on the "sensibilities of the living."[11]

One of the most vexatious problems in American law pertaining to the treatment of cadavers has been the problem of deciding whose interests take precedence when there is a conflict between the premortem directives of a decedent concerning the posthumous disposition of his or her body (e.g., concerning the manner or place of burial) and the wishes of the surviving family. Courts have regularly and vigorously asserted that first authority concerning the disposition of a dead body rests with the person whose body it is. The antemortem wishes of an individual concerning the treatment of his or her corpse should be respected if at all possible.[9,12] However, in many cases in which a decedent's declarations concerning the posthumous disposition of his or her body have been challenged by surviving kin, courts have found some reason, however feeble, to side with the family's petition.[13] The testamentary directives of decedents concerning the manner or place of their burial have been upheld against family objections in cases where state statute expressly grants individuals the right to control by will the posthumous disposition of their bodies.[14] The safest generalization that can be made concerning the authority granted by American common law to the stated premortem wishes of individuals concerning the disposition of their bodies after death is this: Case law rhetorically affirms the paramount authority of individuals to control the treatment of their dead bodies (within the standards of public decency), but in absence of statutory authority, individuals cannot be confident that their expressed desires concerning the treatment of their corpses will prevail over the contrary views of relatives if the controversy is brought before a court of equity.

The provisions of the Model UAGA are founded on the frequently enunciated but also frequently excepted principle in American case law that a person has paramount authority concerning the disposition of his or her body after death. This author is unaware of any case that has been litigated since the adoption by states of the UAGA in which a decedent's positive or negative declarations concerning posthumous donation have been opposed by the decedent's family.

In the next section I will show that the text of the UAGA is unequivocal in giving individuals paramount authority to decide whether their organs shall be available for specified medical uses after death. The Act gives families no legal power to veto deceased relatives' decisions concerning this matter. Given the explicit provisions of the UAGA and the textual clarifications provided by drafters in the commentary portion of the Model Act, it is hard to imagine how a family's veto of a dead relative's written declarations concerning posthumous donation (whether positive or negative) could be granted legal validity without patent interpretive legerdemain. Nevertheless, the history of American case law on the disposition of cadavers hardly gives reason for optimism concerning the ultimate triumph of decedent's wishes over family objections under judicial review.

Provisions of the UAGA Concerning the Use of Bodies and Body Parts and Current Procurement Policy

Statutory Priority of Decedent's Antemortem Declarations over Family Wishes

The anatomical gift acts adopted by all 50 states and the District of Columbia by and large duplicate in wording and substance the provisions of the Model Uniform Anatomical Gift Act drafted in 1968 by representatives of the American Bar Association and the Commissioners on Uniform State Laws. The following interpretation of sections of the Model Act pertaining to the paramount authority of a decedent's premortem declarations concerning the use of his or her body or body parts after death applies then to most current state versions of the model legislation. I intend to show that the current practice in most United States hospitals of *asking permission* of next of kin to remove organs from a brain-dead individual when that individual has properly signed a donation document is contrary to both the spirit and the letter of the Model Act and all state versions of it that retain in unqualified form the specific provisions of the Model Act discussed below.

Section 2 of the Act identifies those persons who may execute an anatomical gift. Listed first (Section 2(a)) is "any individual of sound mind and 18 years of age." Such an individual "may give all or any part of his body for any purpose specified in Section 3, the gift to take effect upon death." Listed second, (Section 2(b)), and in descending order of priority, are various classes of individuals related to the decedent by legal and blood ties. Section 2(e) declares: "The rights of the donee created by the gift are paramount to the rights of others except as provided in Section 7(d)."

This provision states that once valid consent to provide a body or body parts is given by a donor, this consent confers on the donee, that is, the institution or individual authorized to receive the gift, the right to possess the gift for those uses specified by the donor. This right of the donee is "paramount to the rights of others" and is preempted only by the rights of coroners, medical examiners, and physicians to conduct autopsies under conditions described in the state's death laws, the substance of Section 7(d) of the Model Act. Of particular importance here is the commentary on Section 2(e) supplied by the drafters of the original act: "Subsection (e) recognizes and gives legal effect to the right of the individual to dispose of his own body without subsequent veto by others." There can hardly be a stronger assertion of the first priority granted to a person's own premortem declarations concerning the disposition of his or her body after death.

Section 3 specifies, among other things, persons who may become donees, i.e., accepted recipients of anatomical gifts. Subsection (c) of Section 4—"Manner of Executing Anatomical Gifts"—speaks to the usual circumstance of organ donation:

> The gift may be made to a specified donee or without specifying a donee. If the latter, the gift may be accepted by the attending physician as donee upon or following death. If the gift is made to a specified donee who is not available at the time and place of death, the attending physician, upon or following death, in the absence of any expressed indication that the donor desired otherwise, may accept the gift as donee. The physician who becomes a donee under this subsection shall not participate in the procedures for removing or transplanting a part.

In other words, if an individual has validly signed a donation document, and has not specified a particular organization or individual to be the recipient of his or her body or parts, the attending physician (a category expressly excluding any physician removing or implanting a body part from the deceased) is legally empowered to function as donee. The rights of a donee include the right to *accept* or *decline* the gift (see Section 2(c)). Taken together, these provisions yield the following conclusions.

First, once an individual has validly signed a donation document, that positive declaration of donative intent *cannot be overruled by the person's family*. Official consent to donation by the individual confers on the donee (whoever that might be) the right to take the person's body or parts for the purposes indicated by the donor. This right of the donee is preempted only by the rights of coroners, pathologists, and physicians to conduct an autopsy under certain statutorily defined conditions.

Second, the donee's right of access to the body or parts of a decedent who has, prior to death, authorized the bequest, may be *waived by the donee*. If, for example, the tissues or organs of the decedent are not medically acceptable for transplant because of infection, injury, malignancy, etc., the donee is prohibited from accepting them (see, e.g., Section 2(d)). If the donee is aware that the family of a consenting donor disapproves of organ or tissue removal from their brain-dead loved one, presumably the donee is permitted to waive his or her right of access to the authorized donor's body or parts in deference to the opposed wishes of the family. (Whether the donee has a moral obligation to defend and uphold the legal-moral rights of a registered donor against a dissenting family is another matter.) But it is important to understand what actually takes place in such a circumstance. The appropriate description of what happens is that the donee waives legal right of access to the authorized donor's body or parts for those purposes specified by the donor. The family is not nullifying the donation by exercising some supposed right it has to override the premortem declarations of the deceased. The family has no such right under the provisions of most state UAGAs.

Current Procurement Policy's Failure to Acknowledge the Paramount Legal Rights of Declared Donors

Despite the paramount authority given by the UAGA to an individual's decision to be a posthumous donor (which confers on the donee a corresponding right of access to the individual's organs after death), current procurement procedure routinely overlooks the interlinked rights of declared donors and donees. Procurement personnel approach surviving families of declared donors in the same way they approach families of potential donors who have not signed donor cards; they ask families for permission to excise organs from their deceased loved ones. Relatives of declared donors are seldom even *informed* about the legal rights of these kin (and of the donees) that are applicable in the situation. Families are given the impression that they have final legal authority to control the removal and transfer of body parts from dead relatives, even when the latter have expressly authorized this in writing before death. By not apprising families of registered donors of these rights, and by regularly asking such families for permission to remove organs from such individuals, hospital staff lead these families to believe that signed donor cards function simply as nonbinding expressions of what their loved ones "would have wanted," i.e., as mere "advisorial" documents, which families should consider as they decide whether to grant the request for organ removal from their deceased relatives. Under present policy, then, the interlinked rights of declared donors and donees are ignored completely.

How serious is this problem? Of those interviewed in a recent survey, only 14 percent carried signed donor cards. Six percent of the respondents had never heard about organ transplantation, and of the 94 percent who had, only 19 percent carried completed donor cards (Manninen and Evans 1985). One might conclude from this data that the problem of recognizing and protecting the rights of registered donors is not an issue of particular importance.

Three replies can be made to this assessment. First, the number of declared donors may increase in the future, even if they never comprise a majority of the population. "Blitz" recruitment campaigns such as were conducted in April 1985 by the American Council on Transplantation and the National Kidney Foundation during Organ Donor Awareness Week met with some success in enlisting additional registered donors, though the overall yield was probably small (Medical World News 1985). Other recruitment efforts have had impressive results, however. Sixty percent of the licensed drivers in Colorado are designated donors according to a recent report (Overcast et al.1984). In Washington, D.C., the number of people signing donor cards in conjunction with driver's license application or renewal has risen from 25 a month in 1982 to 600 a month in 1985 (Levine 1985).

A second and more telling reply to the claim that the rights-protection issue we are considering is insignificant is this: The gravity of rights violations is not appropriately measured by reference to the incidence of occurrence of these violations. In the next section, I argue that the legal rights of declared donors and objectors under the UAGA plausibly rests on the premise that a person's body is his or her property in a significant sense. This premise licenses the further claim that a person is properly vested with paramount authority to control the disposition of his or her body or parts before and after death. If this argument holds, then procurement personnel bear a burden to show why current retrieval policy, which routinely ignores these rights, should continue. The fact that this disregard of rights occurs in only a few cases is irrelevant to assessing its significance. The practice still demands moral-legal justification in those cases where it occurs, small in number as they may be.

Third, the rights-recognition and protection issue we are focusing upon is likely to become more confused as more states enact what is called "required request" legislation (Caplan 1984; *American Medical News* 1985b). These laws mandate that all hospitals ask families of brain-dead potential donors about the possibility of organ removal from these individuals before disconnecting them from respirators and issuing death certificates. People are likely to assume that if families of *all* potential donors must be asked about donation from these ex-patients— irrespective of whether the latter have signed donor cards— then families must have final legal authority concerning the disposition of organs from these individuals. With the exception of Florida and New York, whose UAGAs permit families to override positive declarations of donative intent by dead relatives,[15] no state grants families of declared donors this authority. Required-request legislation will lend increased authority to the view that surviving families *do* have this legal power, and the rights-recognition issue here under examination will become increasingly difficult even to clarify. The issue should be addressed before it becomes too obscure to appreciate.

Declared Donors' Rights under the UAGA: "Deeper" Considerations

If the paramount legal rights of registered donors under the UAGA are to be provided with a deeper theoretical justification, such a justification cannot rest simply on the principle that the decision of a declared donor ought to be respected because it is an autonomous decision. My autonomous decision to give 10 percent of my neighbor's salary to charity carries no weight because his income is not mine to give. Something else must be added to an autonomous decision to donate anything before such a decision can command first authority: a legitimate "property" interest in the donated thing on the part of the decision maker. If someone can make a posthumous "gift" of his or her body or parts, these items are by implication personal property in some sense.

The body-as-personal-property claim is not without its problems, however. The following considerations seem to count against it:

1. If someone injures my body, ordinarily I do not say that the person has damaged a piece of my "property."
2. The strongest form of property interest is "ownership" which embraces a distinct set of rights. These rights include the right to possess the thing, the right to manage the thing, the right to receive income from it, the right to transfer the thing, the right to exclude others, etc. (Honoré 1961). But it is odd to speak about a person having this type of rights in his or her body or parts. Therefore, a person's body or parts cannot be coherently regarded as property.

These objections can be countered as follows:

Consider the first claim. Suppose my hand is severed in a machinery accident and is stolen before it is regrafted. Do I not have a possessory interest in this detached member justifying a claim of theft of personal property? To be sure, once the hand is reattached it would then be odd to speak of injury to it as property damage rather than assault. But as a detached part of my body it certainly seems natural and appropriate to speak of it as my "property."

In a 1974 British case,[16] the defendant, who gave a urine sample to police in compliance with the provisions of the Road Traffic Act, was convicted on the charge of theft of the urine from the police because he poured the sample into a sink, prohibiting analysis. A recent commentator argues:

> [If] a urine or blood sample can be stolen from the police when they have statutory possession, presuma-

bly it can be stolen from the provider of it himself (or anyone to whom he has transferred it) where no statute interferes. The person producing the substance has the *first right to it*, subject to statute (Matthews 1983 [emphasis added]).

Other variations on this example are conceivable. Suppose I have one of my kidneys removed for transfer to a blood relative, or to another histocompatible end-stage renal disease victim, and the kidney is stolen or damaged before implantation in the designated recipient. Isn't it coherent to speak of the excised organ as somebody's property (mine, or that of the hospital, transplant surgeon, or recipient to whom I have transferred it) such that one of these parties, as owner or trustee, can reasonably institute property theft or damage proceedings against the responsible party? Indeed, wouldn't a legal system be inadequate if it failed to permit such claims?

With respect to objection 2, it's far from clear that *all* the rights that ownership embraces become ungrammatical and hence nonsense when applied to the relationship of a person to his or her body or body parts. In many jurisdictions, individuals can legally sell certain body substances like plasma, semen, or hair, and also receive compensation for body services like surrogate mothering ("rent a womb"). The commercial sale of these substances/services implies an "income" interest in these items— one of the standard "incidents" of ownership. Most people, upon reflection, would probably consider a legal system inadequate if it prohibited the sale of these substances/services. (This contention has interesting implications for the question of the propriety of a commercial market in human organs and tissues [Peters 1984].) The legal doctrine of informed consent certainly suggests, and may be even said to imply that a person's body is personal property from which he or she can "exclude others," —yet another incident of ownership. These cases, combined with the earlier theft-of-body-substances examples, indicate that while *all* the incidents of ownership may not intelligibly apply to the relationship of a person to his or her body (what would the right to "manage" one's body consist in?), enough do apply to warrant the claim that a person's body or parts is (are) that person's property in an important sense. At the very least they support the claim that a person has a property right (interest) in his or her body or parts even if that right is a lesser right than that of full-fledged ownership. (The law, too, recognizes lesser property interests than ownership, e.g., an easement or a lease.)

Does or ought a person have property interests in his or her *dead* body such that he or she has or should have rights to control by premortem declarations what shall be done with it after death? Bellioti (1979) has convincingly shown that the claim that dead human beings cannot be rights bearers, simply because they're dead, cannot withstand philosophical scrutiny. The following example concerning the treatment of President Franklin D. Roosevelt's body shows the intuitive plausibility of the claim that a person should have first authority to control the posthumous disposition of his or her own corpse. In a four-page letter, Roosevelt gave specific instructions concerning the manner of his burial. He directed that "the casket be of absolute simplicity, dark wood, that the body not be embalmed or hermetically sealed, and that the grave not be lined with brick, cement, or stones" (Mitford 1963). Despite these instructions the body was embalmed, placed in a bronze casket, and interred in a cement vault. One is led to ask: Why does this treatment of Roosevelt's corpse seem illicit? We're strongly tempted to reply: Well, it was Roosevelt's body, so his word should have been respected. This general view is enunciated in the 1978 case, *Matter of the Estate of Moyer*,[17] where the court said:

> It is our view that the laws relating to wills and the descent of property were not intended to relate to the body of a deceased; and that it forms no part of the "property" of one's estate in the usual sense, as other chattels or property. Nevertheless, we agree with the petitioner's contention that a person has some interest in his body, and the organs thereof, of such a nature that he should be able to make a disposition thereof, which should be recognized and held to be binding after his death, so long as that is done within the limits of reason and decency as related to the accepted customs of mankind. However, because of the involvement of the public interest and rights and responsibilities of survivors, this is a property right of a special nature; and we do not desire to be under-

stood as saying that this right should be regarded as an absolute property right by which a person could give absurd or preposterous directions that would require extravagant waste of useful property or resources, or be offensive to the normal sensibilities of society in respect for the dead.

It is plausible to hold, then, that a person has a legitimate and primary proprietary interest in his or her living or dead body. This claim warrants the further assertion that a person has first right to control what happens to his or her body before and after death. A person's legal right under the UAGA posthumously to donate or retain personal body parts without veto by his or her family arguably rests on this plausible premise. This adds significant weight to the claim that present policy ought to be revised in favor of a policy in which families of registered donors are explicitly apprised of the rights of these donors in the standard interview situation and recognizable limits placed on the de facto authority now given to families to expedite or prevent donation from relatives who are declared donors.

Explanations and a Possible Justification of Current Rights-ignoring Procurement Policy

What explanations or justification might be given for present retrieval policy that routinely ignores the rights of declared donors and donees? Some individuals involved in organ procurement may simply be misinformed about what the UAGA says. They may think that the law requires that a person's family "validate" his or her premortem decision to donate before organ removal can take place. Others may be aware of what the law says concerning the rights of declared donors yet believe that if the law was tested, e.g., if a family challenged organ removal from a relative who was a declared donor absent their consent or over their dissent, that the courts would rule in favor of the family. (The foregoing history of Anglo-American case law concerning the disposition of cadavers lends some support to this view.) On the basis of this belief procurement staff may judge that it is pointless to tell an authorized donor's family about the legal rights of their deceased relative since these rights would never be granted priority anyway under judicial review.

I suspect, however, that few procurement personnel are even aware of the fact that the current procedure of regularly asking families of all potential donors—declared and undeclared—for permission to remove organs from these expatients is contrary to both the spirit and the letter of the UAGA. The nonacknowledgment of the rights of registered donors and donees under present procurement practice, therefore, stems from ignorance and may be pardoned. Nonetheless, I think it will be instructive to consider one initially plausible argument for continuing the present rights-disregarding retrieval policy, despite what the law says. The argument consists of three premises:

1. The practice of regularly seeking consent from families of all potential donors—whether the latter have signed donor cards or not—and letting a family's decision (whether positive or negative) control the disposition of body parts, will not subject procurement personnel to legal challenge. (Call this the " 'no liability' claim.")
2. Revising present policy so that families of declared donors are routinely informed about the rights of these individuals will not yield more organs than are retrieved under present policy. Such a revision would have no practical value; hence, it would be useless. (Call this the " 'useless revision' claim.")
3. Revising present policy so that families of declared donors are routinely informed about the rights of these individuals may jeopardize the long-term goal of the organ procurement movement, namely, securing the maximum amount of organs for transfer to ESOD victims who will die without them. (Call this the " 'risky revision' claim.")

Let us examine each of these assertions.

The "No Liability" Claim This claim seems to embrace two subclaims: (a) The provisions of the UAGA do not provide grounds for challenging current procurement practice; and (b) even if the UAGA provides grounds for challenging present retrieval practice, it is unlikely that anyone will bring suit against procurement personnel on these grounds.

The following counterargument might be made against sub-claim (a): If an individual has validly signed a donation document, and, if his or her organs are medically acceptable for transfer to one or more needy ESOD victims after death, then the most readily available person authorized to function as donee (usually the attending physician) is under an affirmative legal obligation to initiate the necessary procedures to get the decedent's organs into the "distribution system." (Minimally, this would require notifying the nearest organ procurement agency of the donor's availability.) The drafters of the Model UAGA never intended to permit a donee to decline an anatomical gift for just any reason. The UAGA expressly says that an anatomical gift from a registered donor must be declined if it is medically unacceptable for use for those purposes specified by the donor. And it is equally certain that the drafters of the Model Act never intended family objection to stand as an acceptable reason for a donee's refusing a gift from a declared donor. The following statement from the commentary on Section 2(e) of the Model Act makes this abundantly clear: "[This] subsection . . . recognizes and gives legal effect to the right of the individual to dispose of his own body without subsequent veto by others."

If there are other legitimate reasons for a donee refusing a gift from a declared donor (besides medical unacceptability of the donor's body or parts), these are for a court of law to determine. The attending physician must, therefore, make a good-faith effort to see to it that the body or parts of a declared donor get into the available organ pool. Under the provisions of the UAGA the role of the donee is analogous to that of an executor of a will and the class of waiting ESOD patients is analogous to a group of heirs to an estate. Whether a court would accept this line of reasoning is far from certain. Subclaim (a), therefore, is at least debatable.

How about subclaim (b)? Even if the foregoing interpretation of the UAGA is cogent, would anybody ever bring suit against organ procurement staff on these grounds? The possibility is remote but nonetheless conceivable. Suppose someone dying of an ESOD discovers that organs from a deceased histocompatible declared donor were not taken because the donee (the attending physician) failed to initiate retrieval procedures in deference to family objection to organ removal from their relative. This potential recipient, recognizing that under existing allocation rules he or she would not have been *guaranteed* to receive the needed organ from the deceased (histocompatible) donor, might nonetheless band together with a representative group of other potential recipients and bring a class action against the attending physician on the grounds cited above. While this is a conceivable scenario, it is an improbable one. It must be conceded, then, that subclaim (b) is plausible.

The "Useless Revision" Claim The full argument for this proposition might go like this: Under present procurement policy, whenever a family knows or is informed that a deceased relative has signed a donor card, the family almost always agrees to permit organ donation from their loved one. It is unlikely, then, that telling families of declared donors about the legal rights of these donors will increase the number of organs retrieved from such individuals by family consent. The procedure will be a useless exercise.

This argument simply misses the point. If a person is vested with paramount legal authority to give his or her organs away at death, and if he or she exercises this authority (a right) by signing a donor card, then the family and all other parties are under a corresponding legal obligation to refrain from actions that stop or impede the process of giving effect to the decedent's stated wishes. According to Feinberg's (1973) by now classic exposition of the nature and value of rights, a right is a valid claim under some system of rules, moral or legal, for actions of forbearance or positive assistance from others. The particular type of behavior that the right obliges others to provide is behavior that is owed to the rights-bearer as his or her "due" under the system of rules. The behavior can be legitimately demanded by the rights-bearer or a proxy, and coercing those who fail to comply is thought to be justified. Whether the interests of the individual within the scope of the right are to be served by others (by actions of forbearance or assistance) is not at all dependent on whether those who owe this behavior to the rights-bearer are positively disposed to serve these interests from motives of love, self-interest, a sense of noblesse oblige, etc.

Under the UAGA, the family has no legal right to control the disposition of organs from a dead relative who is a declared donor. On the contrary, they have a duty to "stand out of the way" so that the decedent's desire can be given effect by those authorized to perform the necessary removal and transfer procedures. Leading the family of a declared donor to believe that they have disposing authority over organ removal from the deceased by asking their permission to do this is pure deception; it misrepresents the legal topography of the situation. From this new perspective, seeking consent from the family of a declared donor is a "pointless procedure." But this just shows that the "useless revision" claim implicitly invokes the following procedural rule: Unless there is good reason to believe that giving recognition to the rights of declared donors will increase the organ "harvest," there is no point in revising current family interview procedures to include it. But then it's natural to ask: If acknowledging declared donors' rights will not jeopardize the goal of securing the greatest number of organs for the benefit of dying ESOD victims, why not go ahead and apprise families of these rights and avoid perpetuating the current rights-ignoring policy?

One answer to this query might be that a revised procurement policy that expressly acknowledges and protects the rights of declared donors would pose more risk to the long-term success of the organ procurement effort than present policy which keeps these rights "under wraps." This is the substance of the next proposition.

The "Risky Revision" Claim One tempting argument for this claim might be this: It is pointless to inform families of declared donors about the rights of these individuals unless one is prepared to follow through with appropriate rights-acknowledging/ protecting behavior, e.g., orally defending the donor's rights against a dissenting family, taking medically acceptable organs from the deceased over the family's objection and being prepared to defend this action in court if necessary, etc. But this type of follow-through behavior will surely alienate the families of declared donors. Procurement personnel will gain the reputation of being "organ vultures" who care little about the feelings and values of surviving families. The procurement movement will get a bad press which may result in fewer donations of organs by families in circumstances where they are legally permitted to decide whether organs will be taken from deceased relatives, in cases, namely, where the decedents have not signed donor cards and there is no known objection by the decedents to this procedure. Even if procurement personnel are acquitted of legal wrongdoing for taking organs from a declared donor without consulting the family or over their objection, they will have won a legal battle but probably at the cost of ultimately losing the procurement "war." Follow-through procedures are bound to be counterproductive. Therefore, families of declared donors should not be informed as a matter of policy of the legal rights of their deceased kin.

This argument assumes that appropriate rights-acknowledging/ protecting behavior is an all-or-nothing affair. It maintains that unless one is prepared to go to court to defend the rights of a declared donor and donee against an objecting family, there's no point in apprising families of these rights to begin with. But this is an extreme position.

Admittedly, an equally unacceptable option would be to provide mere "token recognition" of the rights of declared donors. This would involve simply telling the family about the applicable rights of the donor and donee in the situation and then proceeding to deal with the family as under present policy by asking their permission to remove organs from the decedent. This policy would communicate the following message to the family: These rights are operative in this circumstance but we (procurement personnel) don't take them seriously and we don't expect you to either. So we'll treat this case as if your loved one had not signed a donor card and defer to your judgment about the acceptability of taking his or her organs. This policy doesn't completely sell out the paramount authority of the decedent in the way current policy does. Some recognition is afforded the declared donor's rights. But the distinction between this policy and current policy is vanishingly small. It's an almost complete sellout.

Practical Proposals

A Revised
Rights-acknowledging/Protecting Policy

I suggest that the following revised policy be adopted in cases where potential donors have authorized posthumous organ removal from their own bodies.

The family of a medically acceptable declared donor should be informed that the hospital is about to take the necessary steps to give effect to the decedent-authorized donation. The family is not asked to consent to this activity since such a request is both unnecessary and inappropriate. The family is simply informed, as a matter of courtesy, about standard hospital procedure. This approach is reportedly used by transplant coordinators in California, Florida, Colorado, and Wyoming (Overcast et al. 1984). It would be proper and salutary for the procurement staff person to convey to the family that they have reason to be proud that their deceased relative was generous and practical-minded enough to make this bequest before he or she died. (Most people dread thinking about matters pertaining to their own death. Few even make out a will.) The interviewer will, of course, provide the family with answers to the kinds of questions most often asked by lay persons about organ removal: Will it disfigure the body and preclude open casket viewing? What is meant by "brain death"? Will organ removal jeopardize the possibility or quality of life in the hereafter? etc.

If, after such questions have been responded to by the interviewer, the family still objects to organ removal from the declared-donor relative, and it appears that more information will not persuade them to the contrary, then the interviewer will ask the family to sign a "written declaration of dissent" form. This document will be a formal request to the donee (usually the attending physician) to decline the decedent-approved gift. The form will state that family members understand that the decedent has authorized the gift, and it will require that the family state briefly the nature of their objection. I suggest that the interviewer leave the room to permit the family to complete this short document in private. This will give the family an opportunity to reflect about what they're doing without the coercive presence of a hospital functionary who is not a member of the "inner circle." It will be understood that the donee will perfunctorily sign the document and that will be the end of the matter. The form, completed by the donee and family members, will become part of the patient's hospital record. (This policy assumes the truth of the "no liability" claim above.)

There are a number of advantages to this policy. First, it gives stronger recognition to the rights of declared donors vis-à-vis their dissenting families than does the "token recognition" approach. It requires that the family assume a modest burden of proof by declaring in writing why the decedent-authorized bequest should not be honored. The consciences of family members serve as the final judge of whether their reasons are adequate. The exercise will make them aware of the seriousness of what they're doing and also leave no doubt that the decedent-authorized gift will be "aborted" not by a legal action performed by them, but by a legal action of the *donee*, namely, the donee's waiving right of access to the decedent's body or parts.

Second, I doubt whether such a policy will alienate the public from the organ procurement movement. The family gets their way (the donee's waiver is automatic) without having to bow and scrape in a face-to-face interchange with the donee and without having to go to court. But the family does have to assume some burden of proof in deference to the decedent's rights.

It might be objected that this policy still permits "selling out" a declared donor's rights in capitulation to his or her family's contrary wishes. In reply I ask: Are the predictable long-term consequences of adopting a policy of *never* "selling out" a declared donor's rights and going to court if necessary really worth it? Given the current state of public knowledge and opinion about organ donation, an unyielding rights-protection policy might endanger further the lives of those awaiting transplants because an alienated public will make fewer organs available for transfer to needy ESOD victims.

The compromise policy I recommend might still be opposed on other grounds, however. It might be urged that telling families about the rights of deceased relatives who have signed donor cards will simply add to the stress these families experience as a result of the sudden deaths of their loved ones. They already feel an overwhelming sense of powerlessness. God, fate, destiny, or chance has struck them a devastating blow. Now they have to be told that one more thing is out of their control: the disposition of body parts from their relatives. This information will hardly be therapeutic. It also risks giving the procurement staff person a bad image as the bearer of more bad tidings. This is surely not conducive to engendering and maintaining good relations between the organ procurement movement and the public.

This objection can be countered in a number of ways. First, when the family of an undeclared donor is asked about donation from a relative, that question also doubtless increases family stress. It confronts them with the fact that the end has indeed come. There is no ground for further hope. The message is hardly therapeutic. But honesty demands that it be spoken. Second, it probably adds to a family's stress to tell them that an autopsy must be performed on a relative because of insurance contract provisions or because there is reason to believe that the death may have been caused by criminal action. But despite the upset this information may cause the family, this information must be provided because legal rights of insurers and/or coroners are controlling in the circumstance. Similar reasons warrant telling the family of a declared donor about the latter's rights after he or she has died.

Another objection to adopting the policy I have recommended might be that the policy will deprive families of registered donors of an opportunity to be generous and to experience the therapeutic benefits associated with performing an act that benefits others. The argument here is that if the family of a declared donor is told that organ transfer procedures will be set in motion as a result of an action performed by the decedent (his or her signing a donor card), then the family is put in the position of being a mere spectator to a chain of events aimed at a lifesaving result. The family will be deprived of an opportunity of understanding that an action of theirs contributes to bringing some good out of their tragic loss—a perception which carries with it positive therapeutic effects.

This argument says, in effect, that we should continue to hide the rights of registered donors from their surviving families so that the latter will be provided with an opportunity to exercise charitable impulses with attendant emotional benefits. We should perpetuate a charade, in other words, for the sake of advancing the psychological welfare of such families.

I doubt, however, whether families of declared donors would themselves approve of this deception if they became aware of it. So, in addition to the fact that the policy sells out entirely the rights of registered donors, it would also likely be rejected by those whom the policy is designed to benefit, namely, the families of these potential donors. These two reasons count heavily against this argument for maintaining present policy rather than adopting a policy that expressly acknowledges these rights.

The revised family-interview "script" I have recommended is offered as a political compromise among the triad of conflicting interests at stake when families are approached about organ donation from registered donors: (1) saving the lives of the maximum number of ESOD victims, (2) acknowledging and protecting the rights of declared donors, and (3) respecting the needs of the grieving family. This resolution is hardly a "clean" one on a strict moral assessment—the moral-legal rights of registered donors should trump the needs and wishes of the grieving family—but it is probably the most socially acceptable balance among these interests we can hope for at present.

Formal Procedures Protecting Objectors

Up to now the discussion has focused on issues connected with protecting the rights of donors and donees in cases where decedent-donors have expressed a positive desire to donate their bodies or parts for medical uses after death. There is another aspect of organ retrieval procedure, however, which so far we have bracketed from consideration: providing adequate respect and protection to a person's premortem decision *not* to serve as a donor.

An individual opposed to being a donor will naturally refrain from signing a donation document. But an unsigned driver's license donor card is ambiguous. It fails to distinguish between various classes and subclasses of unsigned card carriers such as: (A) individuals who have never thought about donating their organs; (B) individuals who have considered (momentarily or reflectively) donating their own organs, including (1) individuals who in fact favor donating their organs but who (a) do not know that their license contains a donation form, or (b) haven't taken the time to sign the form; (2) undecided individuals who, because they haven't made up their minds, have refrained from signing their driver's license donor cards; and (3) individuals definitely opposed to donation who have resolutely refrained from signing the donor forms on their licenses.

The three basic subcategories under (B) (favor donation, undecided, oppose donation) are a standard minimum-classification scheme. If those in category (A) reflected about personal donation, the results of their deliberations would fall under one of these subcategories. In a recent survey, approximately 19 percent of those interviewed were definitely opposed to donating their own organs after death (Manninen and Evans 1985). (Some of the undecided doubtless expect that if they don't make a commitment one way or the other before death, their bodies will be given the standard form of interment, viz., intact burial underground.)

What protection does the UAGA afford dissenters? The relevant sections of the Model Act are the following:

> 2(b) Any of the following persons . . . *in the absence of actual notice of contrary indication by the decedent* . . . may give all or any part of the decedent's body . . . [emphasis added];
> 2(c) If the donee has *actual notice of contrary indications by the decedent* . . . the donee shall not accept the gift . . . [emphasis added].

If a person does not wish to be a posthumous donor the Act informally requires that he or she inform others about this decision before death. Refraining from signing a donor card is clearly insufficient because unsigned cards are ambiguous. An "actual notice of contrary indication" would have to be either a written declaration or an oral statement of dissent made to someone—a family member, a friend, a physician, attorney, minister, etc. But it is plausible to believe that, in real life, individuals who do not want to be posthumous donors may never inform anyone about their views. It is naive to think that many objectors will take the time to put their objection in writing, and many might not make an oral declaration of their opposition because the "right moment" never comes up. Other objectors may be too embarrassed to reveal their reasons for refusing to donate. For example, some individuals may not want to donate because they just don't like the idea of being cut up after death. But they may think that others will view this as a silly fear and a weak excuse for not making organs available when these body parts might save one or more ESOD victims from impending death. Thus, in order not to be put on the defensive, such objectors never give "actual notice" of their dissent.

If data from a number of recent surveys can be trusted, however, tacit objectors appear to be at some risk of actually having their organs removed after death against their true desires. A majority of people express a willingness to donate organs from deceased relatives (Manninen and Evans 1985; *American Medical News* 1985a). In actual practice, the majority of white families (60 to 80 percent) do consent to organ removal from deceased kin when asked (Prottas 1983). But less than a majority of individuals (42.1 percent in a recent study) (Manninen and Evans 1985) believe that their own families would give permission to remove organs if asked.

There is reason to believe, then, that the provisions of the UAGA offer insufficient protection to objectors. This situation could be remedied by two revisions in current policy:

1. Provide an "objection box" on driver's license donor cards which individuals can check if they do not want to be donors at death. A revised donor form might read as follows:
   "I hereby declare my desire to provide at death, if medically acceptable,
   _____ any needed organs or parts
   _____ only the following organs or parts
   _____
   for the purposes of transplantation, therapy, medical research, or education.
   _____ my body for anatomical study, if needed
   Limitations or special wishes, if any: _____
   _____ I oppose the use of my body or parts for any of the purposes enumerated above."
2. Place an affirmative obligation on all hospitals to conduct a reasonable search for evidence of a po-

tential donor's objection to donation before organ removal procedures are initiated. This would require looking for a donor card carried by the decedent, or, if such a document cannot be located or proves uninformative (it is blank), querying the family about the decedent's views on donation.

This entire process could be simplified if at the time of driver's license application or renewal an individual's positive or negative decision about donation was entered into a computer registry. After a potential donor is pronounced dead, authorized procurement staff could consult the registry to determine whether the individual is a declared donor or an objector. The computer registry device could be combined with the practice of requiring licensees to state explicitly whether they agree or object to serving as posthumous organ donors. Under this policy a license application would be considered incomplete without this information.

An objection to the procedure of mandatory choice might be that the threat of withholding driver's licenses from individuals until they have registered an official "yes" or no" decision about donation is an unjustifiable infringement of personal liberty; or, at any rate, it is too strong a penalty to impose for such an omission. Suppose a person doesn't want to make a decision? Wouldn't a policy that required such a decision be coercive? Isn't it like forcing a person to vote in a public election?

I do not believe that the analogy to voting is apt. The degree of imposition on an individual in the two situations is not comparable. Voting may require a substantial expenditure of time and effort that a person might not otherwise undertake. But those who apply for or renew driver's licenses usually have to appear at a department of motor vehicles office to take a vision test, pay fees, etc. Requiring a person to check one more box on an application or renewal form that must be completed anyway hardly seems an onerous burden. Indeed, my suspicion is that the general public would probably not object to such a requirement. After all, if a person isn't sure about whether he or she wants to serve as a posthumous donor, such a person can protect his or her interests simply by checking the objection box, that is, by saying "no." And many might do this.

But now we can see why it is likely that those who would most strenuously oppose a policy of mandated choice would be organ-procurement staff who might worry that a sizable number of undecided people would register negative decisions concerning donation. Assuming that the decisions of these nay-sayers would be honored (no family would or could be asked if they wished to override the decedent's refusal), the number of organs retrieved under such a policy might be less than under current policy. At present, if undecided individuals do not sign driver's license donor cards, and if they have not given "actual notice" of opposition to this procedure, then their families can make this decision for them after death. And, as we have seen, most (white) families do consent to organ donation from deceased relatives when asked. The speculative risks connected with a policy of mandated choice are ones that procurement personnel would probably prefer not to run. Procurement staff might also argue that the policy unfairly oversimplifies the actual spectrum of possible views people may have about personal donation. Some people may really be undecided about the issue. If from motives of self-protection these individuals register a "no" decision, or out of disingenuous altruism they indicate a "yes" decision, the policy has forced them to make an inauthentic declaration.

These are formidable objections to a policy of mandated choice. Only further debate will reveal whether they are decisive. The policy of adding an "objection box" to donor cards, however, quite independent of a system of mandated choice, I believe, stands on its own merits and deserves adoption.

Summary

Organ procurement personnel in the United States appear to be unaware that the standard practice of asking the surviving families of all classes of potential donors (declared and undeclared) for permission to remove organs and tissues from these individuals is inconsistent with the provisions of most state UAGAs. The majority of these Acts vest first authority concerning the donation of body parts in those individuals whose organs and tissues are needed and judged medically acceptable for removal and transfer. These laws do not give families the right to veto the positive written declarations of dead relatives who have authorized the posthumous taking of their own body parts. Hence, seeking family consent for the removal of body parts from registered donors is unnecessary and inappropriate according to the provisions of most state UAGAs.

The primary authority given to individuals under this legislation to control the taking of organs and tissues from their bodies after death arguably rests on the plausible premise that a person's body is his or her property in a significant sense. This gives individuals first authority to control the posthumous disposition of their body parts. Under current retrieval practice, however, families of deceased registered donors are seldom informed about the paramount rights of these individuals and are led to believe that they have final legal authority over the disposition of organs and tissues from these expatients. This is, in effect, an unwitting but nonetheless serious "sellout" of the moral-legal rights of these potential donors.

I have attempted to show the weakness of one plausible line of argument for the claim that current retrieval practice with its family priority orientation ought to be continued in unamended form, irrespective of what the law says. I suggested an alternative procedure for approaching the surviving families of registered donors which I believe offers a socially acceptable compromise among three values which enter into competition at the death of a declared donor: (1) saving the maximum number of lives of ESOD victims, (2) respecting and protecting the rights of declared donors, and (3) honoring the needs of the grieving family.

Finally, I called attention to the manner in which current procurement practice provides insufficient protection to those who do not wish to serve as donors after death. A practical solution to this problem, I urged, would be to include on standard donation documents (e.g., driver's license donor cards) a box that card carriers check to register officially their objection to serving as posthumous donors. A person's positive or negative decision concerning donation made in conjunction with driver's license renewal or application could also be recorded in a computer registry which procurement personnel can consult after the death of the individual.

The revised policy I recommended for approaching the families of registered donors, as well as the suggested addition of an "objection box" to standard donation forms, would, I believe, provide more adequate recognition of and protection to the paramount rights accorded individuals under state UAGAs to control the posthumous disposition of their own bodies or parts than is available under present retrieval policy.

NOTES

1. Model Uniform Anatomical Gift Act, *Uniform Laws Annotated,* master ed., vol. 8A., 1983. St. Paul: West.
2. 3 Coke *Institutes* 203.
3. 4 Blackstone *Commentaries* 236; 2 *Commentaries* 429.
4. *Rex v. Haynes,* 12 Coke Reprints 113, 77 E.R. 1389 (1614).
5. *Rex v. Lynn,* 2 TR 733, 100 E.R. 394 (1788).
6. *Rex v. Price* 12 Q.B.D. 247, 254–55.
7. *Williams v. Williams,* XX Chancery 659 (1882).
8. *In re Widening of Beekman Street,* 4 Bradford 503 (N.Y. 1857).
9. *Larson v. Chase,* 47 Minn. 307, 50 N.W. 238 (1891).
10. *Koerber v. Patek,* 123 Wis. 453, 102 N.W. 40 (1905).
11. *Pierce v. Swan Point Cemetery,* 10 R.I. 227 (1872).
12. *Pettigrew v. Pettigrew,* 207 Pa. 313 (1904); *Wood v. Butterworth & Sons,* 65 Wash. 344, 18 P. 212 (1911); *Estate of Henderson* 13 Cal. App. 2d 449 (1936); *In re Johnson's Estate,* 169 Misc. 215, 7 N.Y.S. 2d 81 (1938).
13. *Enos v. Snyder,* 131 Cal. 68, 63 P. 170 (1900); *Fidelity Union Trust Company v. Heller,* 16 N.J. Sup. 285, 84 A.2d 485 (1951); *In re Estate of Angela C. Kaufman,* 158 N.Y.S. 2d 376 (surr.); *Holland V. Metalious* 105 N.H. 290, 198 A.2d 654 (1964).
14. *In re Eichner's Estate* 173 Misc. 644, 18 N.Y.S. 2d 573 (1940).
15. *Florida Statutes Annotated,* Sec. 732.911(3); New York. *McKinney's Public Health Law,* Sec. 4301.
16. *Rex v. Welsh,* R.T.R. 478 (1974).
17. *Matter of Estate of Moyer,* 577 P. 2d 108, Utah (1978).

American Medical News 1985a. Poll: Not Many Donate Organs. May 10, p. 64.
———. 1985b. New York Hospitals Required To Ask About Organ Donation. September 27, p.21.

Bellioti, R. 1979. Do Dead Human Beings Have Rights? *Personalist* 60 (April): 201–10.

Caplan, A. 1984. Ethical and Policy Issues in the Procurement of Cadaver Organs for Transplantation. *New England Journal of Medicine* 311 (15):981–83.

Feinberg, J. 1973. *Social Philosophy*. Englewood Cliffs, N.J.: Prentice-Hall.

Honoré, A.M. 1961. Ownership. In *Oxford Essays in Jurisprudence,* First series, ed. A.G. Guest, 107–47. London: Oxford University Press.

Levine, C. 1985. Why Blacks Need More Kidneys but Donate Fewer. *Hastings Center Report* 15 (4):3.

Manninen, D., and R. Evans. 1985. Public Attitudes and Behavior regarding Organ Donation. *Journal of the American Medical Association* 253 (21):3111–15.

Matthews, P. 1983. Whose Body? People As Property. *Current Legal Problems* 36:193–239.

Medical World News. 1985. Withholding Transplant Funding while Pushing for Organ Donations. 26:(10):23–24.

Mitford, J. 1963. *The American Way of Death*. New York: Simon and Schuster.

Overcast, T., R. Evans, L. Bowen, M. Hoe, and C. Livak. 1984. Problems in the Identification of Potential Donors. *Journal of the American Medical Association* 251 (12): 1559–62.

Peters, D., 1984. Marketing Organs for Transplantation. *Dialysis & Transplantation* 13(1):40, 42.

———. 1985. Competing Legal Interests in the Treatment of Dead Bodies. Stevens Point, Wis.: Institute for Health Policy & Law. (Unpublished.)

Prottas, J. 1983. Encouraging Altruism: Public Attitudes and the Marketing of Organ Donation. *Milbank Memorial Fund Quarterly/Health and Society* 61(2):278–306.

Acknowledgment: A brief passage in this article is reprinted from my article "Required Request: A Practical Proposal for Increasing the Supply of Cadaver Organs for Transplantation," *Wisconsin Medical Journal* 84: 10–13 (1985), and is used by permission of the State Medical Society of Wisconsin.

The Mistreatment of Dead Bodies

Joel Feinberg

IT is a very good thing that people have higher-level sensibilities, that some things are dear to them, even sacred to them, and that the symbols of these things too are taken with comparable seriousness and held to be beyond legitimate mockery. It gives one pause to think of what life would be like if no one ever held anything to be precious or dear or worthy of profound respect and veneration. If most people held nothing to be sacred, then I suspect that the rest of us would be less secure even from personal harm, and social stability would have a soggy and uncertain foundation. Granted that it is important that we respect certain symbols, it is even more important that we do not respect them too much. Otherwise we shall respect them at the expense of the very values they symbolize, and fall into the moral traps of sentimentality and squeamishness.

Few people subject dead human bodies to harsh treatment out of personal taste (cannibalism, necrophilia, misanthropy, personal rage). Moral disagreements in the real world arise when bodies are harshly treated out of at least a fancied necessity. The motive is invariably to help individual living human beings even at an acknowledged cost to a precious natural symbol of humanity. In their characteristic modern form, ethical controversies about the treatment of corpses began when scientists discovered how useful the careful study of human bodies could be. A Benthamite Member of Parliament in 1828

From *Hastings Center Report,* 1985, Vol. 15, no. 1. Reprinted by Permission of the Author and the Hastings Center.

introduced what became known as the Dead Body Bill to permit the use of corpses for scientific purposes when the death occurred in a poorhouse, hospital, or charitable institution maintained at public expense, and the body was not claimed within a specified time by next of kin. This bill was eventually passed but not before it was emphatically denounced by its opponents as unfair to poor people. So powerful was the dread of posthumous dissection it was predicted that the aged poor would be led by this bill to "avoid the hospitals and die unattended in the streets"![1]

Similar political battles, with similar results, occurred later in the nineteenth century over proposals to make autopsies mandatory when needed for crime detection or public health. These controversies died down until the recent spurt in medical technology but now they are coming back. One recent example was the controversy in 1978 between a California Congressman and the Department of Transportation. The government had contracted with several university laboratories to test designs for automobile air bags in actual crashes of cars at varying velocities. Dummies had proved unsatisfactory for measuring the degree of protection for living passengers, so some researchers had substituted, with the consent of next of kin, human cadavers. Congressman Moss addressed an angry letter to the Secretary of Transportation charging that "the use of human cadavers for vehicle safety research violates fundamental notions of morality and human dignity, and must therefore permanently be stopped."[2] And stopped it was, despite the Department's feeble protest that prohibition of the use of cadavers would "set back progress" on safety protection for "many years."[3]

Moral philosophers might well ponder the question why the use of cadavers for trauma research would seem to violate "morality" and "decency" more than their use in pathological examinations and autopsies. The answer probably has something to do with the perceived symbolism of these different uses. In the air bag experiments cadavers were violently smashed to bits, whereas dissections are done in laboratories by white-robed medical technicians in spotless antiseptic rooms, radiating the newly acquired symbolic respectability of professional medicine. One might protest that there is no "real difference" between these two uses of cadavers, only symbolic ones, but symbolism is the whole point of the discussion, the sole focus of concern and misgiving. The decision in the collision experiments to exclude cadavers did not involve the criminal law. But if the decision had been up to legislators considering whether to pass a criminal statute forbidding this kind of research on cadavers, the offense principle would not have warranted their interference with the experimenters' liberty. No workers were made to participate without their consent, and there is no record of subtle coercion employed against them. Next of kin, the group most vulnerable to deeply wounded feelings, were consulted, and all voluntarily agreed. The experiments were in a relevant sense done in private. That is, they were not held in a place open to widespread and random public observation like the city streets or a public park, though the superintending officials did not exclude members of the public from witnessing if they wished. Still, no effort was made to keep the fact of the experiments a secret, and the work was done on such a large scale that in effect the experiments were "open and notorious." Therefore, a great many people had bare knowledge of them to be offended by. Very likely then the experiments produced a large amount of profound offense among the members of this knowledgeable group. But that offense would register on each offended psyche in an impersonal way, not in the manner of an offensive nuisance merely which is a wholly personal grievance. The normal argument for legal protection from the profound kind of offense is based on the principle of legal moralism, not on the offense principle, and the liberal will not accept legal moralism. But the harm principle too can be invoked and that principle *is* endorsed by the liberal. The harm principle would underlie the argument, for example, of the person who speaks of the social utility of there being widespread respect for certain natural symbols. That real but diffuse value would be outweighed, however, in the present case (if the Department of Transportation was to be believed) by the clear and present prospect of saving lives and preventing injuries.

The most widespread and persistent current controversies over treatment of dead bodies are probably those concerning procedures for transplanting organs from the newly dead to ailing patients who desperately need them. We are familiar, from the ingenious work of recent philosophers,[4] with the hypothetical moral problems raised by the new possibility of taking organs for transplant from *living* persons, thus setting back their interests or taking their lives with or without their consent. But the problems to which I call attention here involve possible conflicts not between interest and interest, or life and life, but between interest or life on one side and symbolism and sentiment on the other.

Should a dying person or his next of kin have the legal right to deny another the use of his organs *after* he has died a natural death? Few writers, even among those of marked utilitarian bent, would make the salvaging of organs compulsory over the protests of dying patients or their next of kin. In many cases this would override deep religious convictions, and in this country, probably violate the freedom of religion guaranteed by the First Amendment. A more frequently joined issue is whether organs should be salvaged routinely unless the deceased had registered his objection while alive or his next of kin objects after his death. The routine method would produce more organs for transplant and experimentation, thus leading both directly and indirectly to saving more lives in the long run. On the other side, writers have objected that since a person's body is essential to his identity while alive, it becomes a "sacred possession" whose fate after his death he must actively control, and that these facts are properly recognized only by a system that renders a body's transfer to others into a freely given *gift*. Failing to make objection to the posthumous use of one's organs is not the same thing, the argument continues, as "real giving." "The routine taking of organs," Paul Ramsey protests, "would deprive individuals of the exercise of the virtue of generosity,"[5] On the one side of the scale is the saving of human lives; on the other is the right of a person—not simply to grant or withhold his consent to the uses of his body after his death (that right is protected under either scheme)—but his power by the use of a symbolic ritual to convert his consent into a genuine "gift." Even in this extreme confrontation of interest with symbol, Ramsey gives the symbol more weight. If the subject were not itself so grim I might be tempted to charge him with sentimentality.

Sentimental actions very often are excessive responses to mere symbols at great cost to genuine interests, one's own or others'. In the more egregious cases, the cherished symbol is an emblem of the very class of interests that are harmed, so that there is a kind of hypocritical inconsistency in the sentimental behavior. William James's famous example of the Russian lady who weeps over the fictitious characters of a play while her coachman is freezing to death on his seat outside the theatre is an instance of sentimentality of this kind. The error consists of attaching a value to a symbol, and then absorbing oneself in the sentiments evoked by the symbol at the expense of real interests, including the very interests the symbol represents. The process is not consciously fraudulent, for the devotion to sentiment may be sincere enough. Nor does it consist simply in a conflict between avowal and practice. Rather the faulty practice is partly *caused* by the nature of one's commitment to the ideal. Sentimental absorption in symbols distracts one from the interests that are symbolized.

Even honest and true, profoundly worthwhile sentiments then can fail as decisive reasons for legislative actions when the restrictions they support invade legitimate interests of others. If acting out of sentiment against interest is one of the things called "sentimentality" in the pejorative sense, then many of the appeals to sentiment in practical ethics are in fact appeals to sentimentality. A fetus is a natural symbol of a human being and as such should be respected, but to respect it by forbidding abortion to the twelve-year-old girl who becomes pregnant and contracts a life-threatening venereal disease because of a gang rape is to protect the symbol of humanity at the expense of the vital human interests of a real person. Similarly, a newly dead human body is a sacred symbol of a real person, but to respect the symbol by banning autopsies and research on cadavers is to deprive living human beings of the benefits of medical knowledge and condemn unknown thousands to illnesses and deaths that might have been prevented. That is a poor sort of "respect" to show a sacred symbol.

The balancing tests that mediate application of the offense principle dictate that appeals to interest, both of the "offensive actor" and those he might be helping, have greater weight and cogency than appeals to offended sentiment, and should take precedence when conflict between the two is unavoidable. The point applies more obviously when the sentiment itself is flawed in some way (contrived, artificial, false, or inhuman), but it applies in any case, no matter how noble or pure the sentiment. Justice Cardozo once wrote, in a civil case involving the reburial of a body, that "sentiments and usages devoutly held as sacred, may not be flouted for caprice."[6] I would agree but qualify the judgment in the obvious way: lifesaving, medical research, criminal detection, and the like are not capricious.

The most dramatic confrontation between interest and sentiment in connection with newly dead bodies probably lies in the future. It has been clearly anticipated in Willard Gaylin's remarkable article "Harvesting the Dead."[7] Gaylin has us imagine some consequences of the new medical technology combined with new definitions of death as irrevocable loss of brain function or loss of higher cortical function. Under these new definitions a body may be pronounced dead even though its heart continues to beat, its lungs breathe, and all other visceral functions are maintained. If there is total brain death then these physiological functions depend on the external support of respirators, but if only the cortex is dead, then the irrevocably comatose bodies might function on their own. As Gaylin puts it, "They would be warm, respiring, pulsating, evacuating, and excreting bodies requiring nursing, dietary, and general grooming attention, and could probably be maintained so for a period of years."[8]

Gaylin then has us imagine institutions of the future—he calls them "bioemporiums"—where brain-dead bodies, now euphemistically called "neomorts," are maintained and put to various important medical uses. The bioemporiums would resemble a cross between a pharmaceutical laboratory and a hospital ward. Perhaps there will be hospital beds lined up in neat rows, each with a freshly scrubbed neomort under the clean white sheets. The neomorts will have the same recognizably human faces they had before they died, the same features, even the same complexions. Each would be a perfect natural symbol not only of humanity in general but of the particular person who once animated the body and had his life in it. One might not even notice at first that the person was dead, his body lives on so efficiently.

But now along comes a team of medical students being taught the techniques of rectal or vaginal examination without fear of disturbing or embarrassing real patients with their amateur clumsiness. Later an experiment is scheduled to test the efficacy or toxicity of certain drugs in a perfectly reliable way—by judging their effects on real human bodies without endangering anyone's health or life. Elsewhere in the ward other neomorts are proving much better experimental subjects than live animals like dogs and mice would be, and they feel no pain, unlike living animals who would be tortured if treated the same way. Other neomorts serve as living organ banks or living storage receptacles for blood antigens and platelets that cannot survive freezing. From others are harvested at regular intervals blood, bone marrow, corneas, and cartilage, as needed for transfusion or transplant by patients in an adjacent hospital. Still others are used to manufacture hormones, antitoxins, and antibodies to be marketed commercially for the prevention or cure of other medical ailments.

Even if we use the whole brain death criterion, Gaylin estimates that our population could produce at least 70,000 suitable neomorts a year from cerebrovascular attacks, accidents, homicides, and suicides. Some of the uses of these bodies would be commercially profitable, thereby supporting the uses that were not, and the net benefit in the struggle against pain, sickness, and death would be incalculable. Yet when I asked my class of philosophy and third-year law students for a show of hands, at least half of them voted that the whole scheme, despite its benefits, was too repugnant to take seriously. Gaylin himself poses my question eloquently. After describing all the benefits of bioemporiums, he writes—

> And yet, after all the benefits are outlined, with life-saving potential clear, the humanitarian purposes obvious, the technology ready, the motives pure, the material costs justified—how are we to reconcile our emotions? Where in this debit-credit ledger of limbs and livers and kidneys and costs are we to weigh and enter the repugnance generated by the entire philanthropic endeavor?[9]

Repugnance alone will not outweigh the humanitarian benefits Gaylin describes. There is a possibility, however, that where the offense principle falters, other liberty-limiting principles, including the liberal harm principle, can pick up the justificatory loan on behalf of prohibition. That is the possibility to which we now turn.

Moral Sensibility, Sentimentality, and Squeamishness

Three types of argument designed to bolster or supplement the appeal to profound offense come to mind. The first tacitly appeals to the liberty-limiting principle we shall call "perfectionism" that criminal prohibitions can be supported by their expected effect in improving, elevating, or "perfecting" human character. The second applies the offense principle but in a sophisticated manner designed to take account of the subtle but serious offenses that come from inappropriate "institutional symbolism." The third is an appeal to the public harm that comes indirectly from the widespread weakening of respect for certain natural symbols. That argument, of course, contains an appeal to the harm principle. All three arguments are deployed in a very useful article by William May supporting the deliverances of offended sentiment against utilitarian calculations of public gain in order to oppose the routine salvaging of organs and the "harvesting of the dead."[10] May's arguments support moral conclusions about what ought and ought not to be done, not political-moral conclusions about what prohibitive legislation it would or would not be legitimate to enact (our present concern). Nevertheless, his arguments can be easily recast as political-moral ones simply by adding the appropriate liberty-limiting principle as a premise. (There is no reason to think that May would approve of this recasting of his arguments, and I attribute no views to him at all about the legitimacy of criminal legislation.) I shall now attempt to reconstruct, adapt to the legal-legislative context, and criticize three arguments derived from May.

1. *The argument that the offended sentiment is essential to our humanity.* May recalls the Grimm brothers' tale about the young man incapable of experiencing horror:

> He does not shrink back from the dead—neither a hanged man he encounters nor a corpse with which he attempts to play. From one point of view, his behavior

seems pleasantly childish, but from another angle, inhuman. His father is ashamed of him, and so the young man is sent away "to learn how to shudder." Not until he learns how to shudder will he be brought out of his nameless, undifferentiated state and become human.[11]

May plausibly suggests that this story testifies to "our deepgoing sense of the connection between human dignity and a capacity for horror."[12] The practice of routinely salvaging the re-usable organs of the newly dead, he contends, is to be rejected for its "refusal to acknowledge the fact of human horror." "There is a tinge of the inhuman," he writes, "in the humanitarianism of those who believe that the perception of social need easily overrides all other considerations and reduces the acts of implementation to the everyday, routine, and casual."[13] We can acknowledge the second-level horror, implied in May's remarks, that consists of the perception that the primary horror has been rubbed off a practice to which it naturally belongs, so that what was formerly a morally shocking occurrence now becomes routine and normal. Recall the daily television news during the Vietnam War when deliberate shootings, mangled babies, and regular "body counts" became mere routine occurrences portrayed in a humdrum fashion as if they were commonplace sporting events.

We can reconstruct May's argument so that it fits what can be called "one standard form of the argument from sentiment." The argument runs as follows:

1. Whatever leads to the weakening or vanishing of a natural, honest, human sentiment thereby degrades ("dehumanizes") human character and is in that way a bad thing.
2. There are natural, honest, human sentiments toward dead human bodies.
3. Routine salvaging of organs and harvesting of the brain-dead would lead to the weakening and eventual vanishing of these sentiments.
4. Therefore, these practices would degrade human character, and in that way be a bad thing.
   Now we can add—

5. It is always a good and relevant reason in support of a proposed criminal prohibition that it is necessary to improve (or prevent the degrading of) human character. (Legal Perfectionism)
6. Therefore there is good and relevant reason to prohibit routine salvaging of organs and harvesting of the brain-dead.

I have several comments about this argument. First, it is to be distinguished from the moral use of the offensive principle, with which it might otherwise be confused. The offense principle argument takes as its first premise the proposition that whatever causes most people, or normal people, deep revulsion is for that reason a bad thing. (It is unpleasant to experience revulsion, and wrong to cause others unpleasantness.) Professor May's argument, in contrast, is that whatever weakens the tendency of most people, or normal people, to experience revulsion in certain circumstances is a bad thing. He is less concerned to protect people from revulsion than to protect their "humanity" to which the capacity for spontaneous revulsion is essential.

Similarly, Professor May's argument should be contrasted with the "causal substitute" argument that assumes natural causal connections between watching and shrinking from, and between shrinking from and judgments of disapproval. The latter, if thought of as an argument, would be a kind of *argumentum ad hominem*. The person in whom the appropriate sort of repugnance is naturally induced needs no further argument; one can simply appeal to the disapproval he feels already. Obviously that tactic will not do for Professor May since the thought of routine salvaging and the like does not cause his opponents to shrink away and disapprove, and Professor May does not want to impugn *their* humanity (although he does discern a "tinge of the inhuman" in their proposals).

My first objection to the above argument is that it proceeds in a kind of vacuum, abstracted from the practical world to which it is directed. There is no qualifying clause in premise or conclusion to acknowledge even the bare relevance of benefits gained and harms prevented, as if "the promise of cures for leukemia and other diseases, the reduction of suffering, and the maintenance of life"[14] were of no account at all. Indeed, both May and Ramsey, whose earlier argument against routine salvaging rested on a subtle preference for symbolic gift-giving and guaranteed consciousness of generosity, approach these urgent questions more in the manner of literary critics debating the appropriateness of symbols than as moralists. One wants to remind them forcibly that while they distinguish among symbols and sentiments, there are people out there suffering and dying. William James's sentimental Russian countess too may have been experiencing genuine human feelings toward the characters on the stage, but the point of the story is not *that,* but the death of her coachman.

To be properly appreciated May's argument should be further recast. At most, the data from which he draws his premises show that *insofar* as a practice weakens natural human sentiment, it is a bad thing, so that *unless* there is some countervailing consideration on the other side, that practice is bad on balance and should not be implemented. Very well, one can accept that proposition, while pointing to the prevention of deaths and suffering as a countervailing reason to weigh against the preference for untarnished symbols.

Why do May and like-minded writers seem so dismissive of appeals to the reduction of suffering and the saving of lives? I suspect it is because they assimilate all such consequentialist considerations to the most vulnerable kind of utilitarianism, as if weighting life-saving over sentiment were a moral misjudgment of the same category as sacrificing an unwilling individual to use his organs to save the lives of others. It simply won't bear rational scrutiny to claim that there is a right not to be horrified, or not to have one's capacity to be horrified weakened, of the same order of priority as the right not to be killed and "disorganized."[15] May speaks dismissively of those who let mere "social needs" override all other considerations, as if a desperate patient's need for an organ transplant were a mere social need like a city's call for an additional public library or improved public transportation. In another place he uses in a similar way the phrase "the social order," adding the suggestion of disreputable ideology. There he writes of the routine salvaging scheme that "one's very vitals must be inventoried, extracted, and distributed by the state on behalf of the social order."[16] The moral conflict, as May sees it, is between honest human sentiment and an inferior kind of value, often called "merely utilitarian." What is overlooked is that the so-called "social utility" amassed on one side of the controversy is itself partly composed of individual *rights* to be rescued or cured. If, opposed to these, there are rights derived from sentiment, one would think that they are less weighty than the right to life and to the relief of suffering. Jesse Dukeminier makes the point well. He objects to labeling one of the conflicting interests "the need of society of organs." "Organs," he protests, "are not transplanted into society, organs are transplanted into people!"[17]

To give substance to this point, let us consider the following scenarios: Patient A dies in his hospital room, not having said anything, one way or the other, about the disposition of his cadaver. B, in the next room, needs his organ immediately to survive. A's next of kin refuses to grant permission for the transplantation of his kin's organ, so B dies. Were B's rights violated? Was an injustice done or was mere "social utility" withheld? Perhaps we would call this not merely an inutility but an injustice because B is a specific known person, a victim, and not a mere unknown possibility or abstraction. But consider a second scenario. Patient C dies in his hospital room not having said anything, one way or the other, about the disposition of his cadaver. D, at just that moment, is in an automobile crash. Five minutes later he arrives in an ambulance at the hospital in desperate need, as it turns out, of one of C's organs to survive. At the time of C's death no one knew anything about D who was a total stranger to all involved parties. At that moment C's next of kin gives his blanket refusal to let anyone use C's organs, so D, ten minutes later, dies. Were D's rights violated or mere social utility diminished? To argue for the latter, it would not be relevant to point out that no one knew who D was; no one knew his name; no one had any personal intention in respect to him. That would be to treat him as if he *had* no name, no identity, and no rights, as if his unknown and indeterminate status at the time of C's death deprived him of personhood, concerting him into a mere impersonal component of "social utility."

Even in its full recast form with its more tentative conclusion ("insofar as . . ."), May's first argument causes misgivings. I have no problem with premise 2, that there are natural human sentiments toward newly dead bodies that are in no way flawed when considered in their own right. But I have reservations about premises 1 and 3. Premise 1 needs qualifying. It states that whatever leads to the weakening or vanishing of such a sentiment is a bad thing. What is important, I think, is not only our capacity to have such sentiments but our ability to monitor and control them. To be sure persons sometimes need to "learn how to shudder," but it is even more commonly the case that people have to learn how *not* to shudder. Newly dead bodies cannot be made live again, nor can they be made to vanish forever in a puff of smoke. Some of us can shudder and avert our eyes, but others must dispose of them. Pathologists often must examine and test them, surgeons in autopsies skin them open like game, cutting, slicing, and mutilating them; undertakers embalm them; cremators burn them. These professionals cannot afford to shudder. If they cultivate rather than repress their natural feelings in order to "preserve their humanness," then their actions will suffer and useful work will not be done. There is an opposite danger, of course, that these persons' work will be done at the expense of their own humanity and the extinction of their capacity for essential feeling. What is needed is neither repression nor artificial cultivation, the one leading to inhumanity, the other to sentimentality. Instead what is called for is a careful rational superintendency of the sentiments, an "education and discipline of the feelings."[18]

I must take stronger exception to the partially empirical premise number 3, that routine salvaging of organs (and *a fortiori* "harvesting the dead") would lead to the general weakening or vanishing of essential human sentiments. These medically useful practices need not be done crudely, indiscreetly, or disrespectfully. They are the work of professionals and can be done with dignity. As for the professionals themselves, their work is no more dehumanizing than that of pathologists and embalmers today. Other professionals must steel their feelings to work on the bodies of *living* persons. I wonder if Professor May would characterize abdominal surgeons as "inhuman," as various writers in the 19th century did? Does their attitude of the everyday, routine, casual acceptance of blood, gore, and pain lead them inevitably to beat their wives, kick their dogs, and respond with dry-eyed indifference to the loss of their dear ones? That of course *would* render them inhuman.

This is the point where I should concede to Professor May that complete loss of the capacity for revulsion *is* dehumanizing. To be incapable of revulsion is as bad a thing as the paralysis of succumbing to it, and for the same kind of reason. The perfect virtue is to have the sensibility but have it under control, as an Aristotelian man of courage has natural fear in situations of danger (otherwise *he* would be "inhuman") but acts appropriately anyway.

   2. *The argument from institutional symbolism.* Hospitals traditionally have been places where the sick and wounded are healed and nursed. The modern hospital mixes the therapeutic function with a variety of ancillary ones, leading in the public mind to a conflict of images and an obscuring of symbolism. Hospitals now are training facilities, places of medical research and experiment, warehouses for the permanently incapacitated and terminally ill and so on. Now, Professor May warns us, "The development of a system of routine salvaging of organs would tend to fix on the hospital a second association with death . . . the hospital itself becomes the arch-symbol of a world that devours."[19] Perhaps it is fair to say that all institutions are in their distinctive ways symbols, and that the mixing of functions within the institution obscures the symbolism, but it is hard for me to see how this is necessarily a bad thing, much less an evil great enough to counter-balance such benefits as life-saving and relief of suffering. Schools are traditionally places of book learning. Now they host such diverse activities as driver training and football teams. Prisons are traditionally places of punishment and penitence; now they are also manufacturing units and occupational therapy centers. Churches, which are essentially places of worship, now host dances and bingo games. One might regret the addition of of new functions on the ground that they interfere with the older more important ones, but that is not the nub of Professor May's argument. He does not suggest that the healing function of the hospital will be hurt somehow by the introduction of routine organ salvaging. Rather his concern is focused sharply on the institutional symbolism itself. Like a skilled and subtle literary critic, he argues for the superiority of one kind of symbolism to another, just as if such benefits as life-saving were not involved at all.
   Of course May's fear for the hospital's benign image is not for a symbol valued as an end in itself. With the change he fears, hospitals will come to be regarded in new ways by the patients. The prospect of an eventual death in a hospital is bad

enough; now the patient has to think also of the hospital as a place where dead bodies are "devoured." It is just as if we landscaped hospital grounds with cemeteries and interspersed "crematorium wards" among the therapeutic ones. That would be rubbing it in, and as prospective hospital patients we might all register our protest. These examples show that May does have a point. But the disanalogies are striking. It is not necessary that burial and cremation be added to the functions of a hospital. There would be hardly any gain, and probably a net loss, in efficiency, and a very powerful change for the worse in ambience. Organ transplating, however, *requires* hospital facilities; its beneficiaries are sick people already hospitalized and its procedures are surgical, requiring apparatus peculiar to hospitals. The most we can say for the argument is that if the change in symbolism is for the worse, that is a reason against the new functions, so that if the change is capricious—not required for some tangible benefit—then it ought not be allowed. But greater life-saving effectiveness is not a capricious purpose.

Professor May's ultimate concern in this argument, however, may not be so much with symbolic ambience as with the morale of patients who are depressed by the bare knowledge that organ salvaging occurs routinely in their hospital, even though it will not occur in their case because they have registered their refusal to permit it. But it is difficult to understand how the thought of bodies having their organs removed before burial can be more depressing than the thought of them festering in the cold ground or going up in flames. Only the morale of a patient with a bizarre "sentimental belief," or an independently superstitious belief similar to one once analyzed by Adam Smith[20] would be hurt by such bare knowledge, and such beliefs are nearly extinct.

3. *The argument that the threatened sensibility has great social utility.* The argument I have in mind is the familiar "rule-utilitarian" one. It is only suggested in Professor May's article but it has been spelled out in detail by other writers discussing other topics in practical ethics, notably abortion and infanticide. The argument I have in mind differs from May's first argument from sentiment in that it appeals in its major premise not to the intrinsic value of a threatened sentiment, its status as the "best" or "most human" feeling, but to the high social

utility of this sentiment being widespread. Formulated in a way that brings out a structure parallel to May's first argument, it goes as follows:

1. Whatever leads to the weakening or vanishing of a socially beneficial (harm-preventing) human sentiment is socially harmful and in that way a bad thing.
2. There are sentiments toward dead bodies which, when applied to things other than dead bodies, promote actions that have highly beneficial consequences and whose absence would lead to harmful consequences.
3. Routine salvaging of organs and harvesting brain-dead bodies would lead to the weakening or vanishing of these sentiments.
4. Therefore, these practices would lead to widespread harm and in that way would be a bad thing. Now we can add—
5. It is always a good and relevant reason in support of a proposed criminal prohibition that it is necessary to prevent harm. (The Harm Principle)
6. Therefore, there is good and relevant reason to prohibit routine salvaging of organs and harvesting of the brain-dead.

Stanley Benn has a similar but more plausible argument about infanticide and abortion.[21] Benn concedes that fetuses and even newborn infants may not be actual persons with a right to life, but points out that their physical resemblance to the undoubted human persons in our everyday experience evokes from us a natural tenderness that is highly useful to the species. If we had a system of "infanticide on demand," that natural tenderness toward the infants we did preserve and raised to adulthood would be weakened, and the consequences both for them and the persons they later come in contact with would be highly destructive. As infants they would be emotionally stunted, and as adults they would be, in consequence, both unhappy and dangerous to others. The argument, in short, is an appeal to the social disadvantages of a practice that allegedly coarsens or brutalizes those who engage in it and even those who passively acquiesce to it. Benn cites the analogy to the similar argument often used against hunting animals for sport. Overcoming the sentiment of tenderness toward animals, according to this argument, may or may not be harmful on balance to the animals; but the sentiment's disappearance would be indirectly threatening to other human beings who have in the past been transferred beneficiaries of it. The advantage of this kind of argument is that it permits rational discussion among those who disagree, in which careful comparisons are made between the alleged disadvantages of a proposed new practice and the acknowledged benefits of its introduction.

The weakness of the argument consists in the difficulty of showing that the alleged coarsening effects really do transfer from primary to secondary objects. So far as I know, doctors who perform abortions do not tend to be cruel to their own children; the millions of people who kill animals for sport are not markedly more brutal even to their own pets than others are; and transplant surgeons are not notably inclined to emulate Jack the Ripper in their off hours. I think that the factual premise in arguments of this form usually underestimates human emotional flexibility. We can deliberately inhibit a sentiment toward one class of objects when we believe it might otherwise motivate inappropriate conduct, yet give it free rein toward another class of objects where there is no such danger.[22] That is precisely what it means to monitor the intensity of one's sentiments and render them more discriminating motives for conduct. Those who have not educated their sentiments in these respects tend to give in to them by acting in ways that are inadvisable on independent grounds, and then cite the "humanness," "honesty," or "naturalness" of the sentiment as a reason for their action. This pattern is one of the things meant by "sentimentality" in the pejorative sense. Fortunately, it does not seem to be as widespread as some have feared, and in any event, the way to counter it is to promote the education of the feelings, not to abandon the fruits of lifesaving technology.

In summary, I find no unmanageable conflict between effective humanitarianism and the maintenance, under flexible control, of the essential sentiments. I hope that conclusion is not too optimistic.

NOTES

1. M.J. Durey, "Bodysnatchers and Benthamites," *London Journal* 22 (1976) as quoted in Thomas C. Grey, ed., *The Legal Enforcement of Morality* (New York: Random House, (1983), p. 111.
2. N. Wade, "The Quick, the Dead, and the Cadaver Population," *Science*, March 31, 1978, p. 1420.
3. *Loc. cit.*
4. See *inter alia.* Philippa Foot, "The Problem of Abortion and the Doctrine of Double Effect," John Harris, "The Survival Lottery," Richard Trammel, "Saving Life and Taking Life," Nancy Davis, "The Priority of Avoiding Harm," and Bruce Russell, "On the Relative Strictness of Negative and Positive Duties," all in Bonnie Steinbock, ed. *Killing and Letting Die* (Englewood Cliffs, NJ: Prentice-Hall, 1980).
5. Paul Ramsey, *The Patient as a Person* (New Haven: Yale University Press, 1970), p. 210.
6. *Yome v. Gorman,* 242 N.Y. 395 (N.Y. Court of Appeals, 1926). For reference to this case and all the other materials mentioned in this section on dead body problems, I am indebted to Professor Thomas C. Grey and his excellent anthology, *The Legal Enforcement of Morality* (New York: Random House, 1983).
7. Willard Gaylin, "Harvesting the Dead," *Harper's Magazine,* Sept. 1974.
8. *Ibid.*, p. 26.
9. *Ibid.*, p. 30.
10. William May, "Attitudes Toward the Newly Dead." *The Hastings Center Studies* I (1972):3–13.
11. *Ibid.*, p.5.
12. *Loc. cit.*
13. *Loc. cit.*
14. Jesse Dukeminier, "Supplying Organs for Transplantation," *Michigan Law Review* 68 (1968):811.
15. This word for having one's organs taken for transplant without one's consent was introduced by John Harris in his "The Survival Lottery," *Philosophy* (1975).
16. May, *op. cit.*, p. 6.
17. Jesse Dukeminier, *op. cit.*
18. Michael Tanner, "Sentimentality," *Proceedings of the Aristotelian Society* 77 (1976-77):135.
19. May, *op. cit.*, p. 6.

20. When we sympathize with the dead (i.e., with corpses), Smith wrote, "the idea of that dreary and endless melancholy which the fancy naturally ascribes to their condition [or did in an earlier age] arises altogether from our lodging . . . our own living souls in their inanimated bodies, and thence conceiving what would be our emotions in this case." Adam Smith, *The Theory of Moral Sentiments*, 6th ed. (1970). Reprinted in Selby-Bigge, *British Moralists* (New York: Bobbs-Merrill, 1964), vol. I, pp. 262–263.

21. Stanley I. Benn, "Abortion, Infanticide, and Respect for Persons" in Joel Feinberg, ed., *The Problem of Abortion*, 2d ed. (Belmont CA: Wadsworth, 1983), pp. 135–144.

22. Where there is little perceived difference between the two classes, however, the strain on emotional flexibility may be intolerable. It is hard not to sympathize, for example, with the nurses mentioned by Jane English ("Abortion and the Concept of a Person" in J. Feinberg, ed., *The Problem of Abortion, op. cit.*) who were "expected to alternate between caring for six-week premature infants and disposing of viable 24-week aborted fetuses . . ." The danger here, however, is not that the nurses will be brutalized, but that they will be severely distressed or even psychologically damaged.

Do Dead Human Beings Have Rights?

Raymond A. Belliotti

A person who claims that dead humans have interests and rights places himself in the position of being considered either a sentimental crackpot, or a likely candidate for a mental sanity test, or perhaps even worse, a beguiling, philosophically seductive sophist. I shall risk being so labeled by making just such an assertion: human beings have interests that can be satisfied after they are dead and they have rights which can be violated or respected after they are dead. In arguing in defense of this claim I shall make no appeal to any form of a personal immortality thesis. That is, I shall not conjecture that we personally survive the cessation of earthly experience, or that there is a supernatural being who metes out punishment/reward in response to our earthly deeds.

I

A human being's interests can be analyzed in two ways: to say X has an interest in Y may mean (i) that Y, on balance, improves X's well-being (or opportunity for well-being) or (ii) that X desires, wants, or seeks Y. It seems that it is possible for X to be interested in (to desire) something that is not really in

From *Personalist*, 60, [April]: 201–10, 1979. Reprinted by Permission of *The Personalist*.

his interests; and it is also possible for something to be in X's interests regardless of the fact that X is not presently interested in (does not presently desire) it. So X may be interested in eating a bar of soap, even though it does not seem in his interests to do so. X may be interested in the soap for a variety of reasons: he may not know the results of eating it; or he may know the results but not care; or he may know and care but value other ramifications of the act more than the negative consequences of eating it. In the last two instances it is plausible to claim that perhaps eating the soap is not really opposed to X's interests, since X may have no desires which would contravene his desire to eat the soap.

On the other hand an action may be in X's interests and X may not be presently interested in it for a variety of reasons: he may not even be aware of this action; or he may be aware of it but not realize it would serve his interests because he lacks certain knowledge about the nature of the action; or he may simply pass up this particular opportunity to satisfy his interests and ignore the action completely.

But regardless of whether interests are analyzed in terms of some objective criterion or whether they are simply the class of an individual's wants and desires, it seems clear that one important claim we make when we talk about human interests is that desires, wants, and aims are crucial to that concept.

Now the vast majority of us do have wishes, desires, and wants concerning what happens to our corpse, our reputation, and the stipulations of our will after we are dead. These desires transcend the duration of our life in that they can be fulfilled or trangressed after we are dead. A philosopher who maintains that one's interests are merely identical to one's desires and wants should also be willing to concede that not all our desires and wants are confined to events occurring during our earthly lives, and that hence not all our interests are confined to our earthly lives. A philosopher who maintains that some objective criterion is necessary to determine what is in one's interests cannot show that our desires regarding our reputation after we are dead, towards the handling of our corpse, and the disposition of our will are really *against* our interests by applying the objective criterion; nor can he show these desires to be *unrelated* to our interests unless he adheres to one of the unsound arguments which will be discussed now.

II

Some might be tempted to advance what I call the argument from cognitive awareness:

1) Suffering negative sensations is a necessary condition for having one's interests harmed.
2) The dead lack the capacity for experiencing sensations and for cognitive awareness.

Therefore, the dead cannot be harmed.

But this argument confuses (i) being wronged with (ii) knowing that one has been wronged. Surely someone's interests can be harmed without his being aware of that harm and without his suffering negative sensations.

Consider the following example: An officious busybody named Jones would garner a great deal of pleasure from reading the personal diary of his neighbor, Russo. Jones is a bawdy sort, whose greatest joy in life is monitoring the activities of his neighbors, who would never suspect that Jones would be so inclined. While Russo is away Jones enters his home, finds the diary, and reads it. Jones is so successful in his ploy that Russo never discovers that his diary has been read. Meanwhile Jones has gained lascivious delight in learning of Russo's intimate contacts with females, and other peculiar details about Russo's personal habits.

Now Russo is unaware that his diary has been read and suffers no pain or anxiety of any sort because of Jones' action. Surely we would still claim that Russo's interests have been harmed—in this case his interest in privacy—even though Russo is unaware that his privacy has been violated by Jones.[1] It would be extremely odd to say that Jones had done nothing wrong or that Russo would be wronged only if he *learned* of Jones' act. Of course, upon learning of Jones' act, Russo would indeed suffer many negative sensations: humiliation, shame, outrage, and anxiety; but these negative emotions do not constitute entirely the extent of the harm that Jones has done to Russo's interests. These emotions, rather are the *acknowledgment* that Russo's interests have been harmed; they are not the harm *per se*.

This example shows the folly of thinking that one can be wronged only if one experiences negative sensations or becomes cognitively aware that others have transgressed against him. Even if Russo had never learned of Jones' act, his interests would have been harmed by Jones' actions. Clearly, then, it is plausible to claim that neither suffering pain because of another's act, nor becoming aware of that act is a necessary condition of having one's interests harmed by the act.

The general moral principle which would reflect our moral intuitions in this matter would be formulated along these lines: It is morally wrong to contravene the desires of individual X concerning the way others may treat him except in those cases in which complying with X's desires would violate other weightier moral obligations, or unless that treatment which X desires is clearly supererogatory. Clearly Jones has contravened Russo's desires, and Jones can offer no justification for his action in terms of weightier moral obligations, nor can he claim that respecting Russo's right to privacy is supererogatory.

Hence it cannot be said that dead humans cannot be harmed merely because they cannot *know* that others have acted against their interests or because they will not feel negative sensations in response to the noxious acts of others toward them.

In fact, it should be clear that there are some interests of human beings that can only be fulfilled after they die. One's interests concerning the discharge of her will, the treatment of her corpse, and the maintenance of her reputation after she is dead can only be affected after she dies. So not only may humans have interests satisfiable after they are dead, but they have certain interests which are *only* satisfiable after they are dead.

A critic might rejoin that the only interest we really have in these kinds of things is that it is important for us while living to think our desires in these matters will be respected after we die. So on this view, as long as we *think* that others will not malign our reputation, or mutilate our corpse, or discharge wrongly our will, then our interests in these matters are satisfied. I think this view rests upon a confusion between (i) X thinking his interests will be fulfilled after he dies and (ii) X's interests *being* fulfilled after he dies. Our interests and desires are not satisfied merely by our thinking they are. Only if the object of our interests and desires is realized are these interests and desires fulfilled. And I would think that the desires not to be slandered after we are dead and not to have our corpse mutilated are desires that are fulfilled not by our *thinking* that these acts will not occur, but rather by these acts *not occurring*. If our interests and desires were really reducible to our thinking they were fulfilled they could be satisfied by the manipulations of a good hypnotist.

There are other reasons sometimes given as explanations of why we think that certain treatment of dead humans is wrong:

(A) *The Transference Argument*
  (1) The interests/rights of a person are transferred to relatives and survivors upon the person's death.
  (2) Any transgression of these rights is really a violation against the interests of the living.

Therefore, the dead cannot be harmed since they have no interests.

Initially this seems plausible because we know that the wills of the dead usually benefit the dead person's relatives, and that any violation of the dictates of the will surely does infringe upon the rights of these heirs, and violate their interests. And the survivors of the dead person may take umbrage and be harmed themselves if he is maligned or slandered. So the claim that it is wrong to perform certain acts upon a corpse or slander the dead, or violate wills because harm results to the dead person's surviving relatives does have an intuitive appeal. But upon closer examination, it seems to be an incomplete explanation of why we think certain acts are wrong. For, what if the dead person has no surviving relatives? Or, what if these surviving relatives do not care if the dead person is maligned or his corpse mutilated? Or, what if the surviving relatives, themselves, are the ones who do the maligning or mutilating? Would we really think that nothing wrong has occurred?

Suppose someone wrote a book claiming that Rocky Marciano[2] gained fame only because his fights were fixed or because he illegally coated his hands with gauze soaked in plaster of Paris to increase his punching power. Suppose this individual also told lies slandering Rocky's reputation in other, more personal, areas as well. Surely we would think that anyone who did such a thing did something morally wrong. And we would think this, not merely because Rocky's relatives would be insulted. And if Rocky's surviving relatives themselves were the slanderers, we would think *they* did something wrong. All this suggests that it is not merely our aversion to insulting the heirs of the dead that accounts for our thinking that certain acts performed by the living against the dead are morally wrong.

But the transference theorist might reply that he can rescue his theory by giving an alternate account of why we would think Rocky's relatives were morally wrong. The theorist could claim that Rocky's relatives told falsehoods and it is always morally wrong to tell falsehoods, all other things equal, regardless of whether or not anyone is harmed by these statements. Therefore, the transference theorist might assert that it is true that Rocky's heirs did something wrong, but the reason these actions were wrong involves their telling falsehoods, and does not involve any harm done to the dead.

This too has an initial appeal, since it would allow us to account for our feelings that the actions were wrong and allow the transference theorist to salvage his belief that the dead cannot be harmed. But once again a closer scrutiny will find this explanation unacceptable. Suppose someone alleged that Dagwood Bumstead was an alcoholic or that Beetle Bailey had strange sexual preferences or that Hagar the Horrible was a coward. Would any of us seriously think that person had done something morally wrong? Or suppose that person told falsehoods about a stone or a chair. Clearly it is possible to tell falsehoods about cartoon characters (insofar as their real cartoon lives are revealed in the comics) and mere physical objects, but we would hardly consider these falsehoods on the same moral level as falsehoods told about Rocky Marciano.

Falsehoods cannot harm cartoon characters and mere physical objects. And that is why we would feel little, if any, moral disapprobation toward the individual who told these falsehoods, although we might think her somewhat strange. But falsehoods told about Rocky Marciano can harm him: they can harm his interests in a good reputation; they can denigrate and cast aspersions on his achievements and personal comportment. In short, Dagwood Bumstead, Beetle Bailey, Hagar the Horrible, and chairs cannot be slandered; Rocky Marciano, although dead, can be slandered. And this slander is pernicious for reasons independent of the transference theorists claims.

Consider a case of gift giving. If X was to give Y a gift of a certain commodity Z, but W intervened and unjustifiably prevented the transaction as he seized Z for himself, we would think that not only had Y's rights been violated (since he did not receive an item to which he had an entitlement) but also that X's rights had been violated (since he had not intended *merely* to relinquish his entitlement to Z, but had specified legitimately to whom the entitlement to Z was to be transferred). X was wronged in that he had the right to specify to whom the entitlement to Z would pass and W transgressed this right.

Now this is similar to what happens if the stipulations of a dead person's will are ignored; not only are his surviving heirs wronged, but the rights of the dead person are also violated. He had the right to dispose of his property and this right is transgressed if the living, in the absence of overriding considerations, ignore his wishes in this matter. Therefore, ignoring the provisions of someone's will is wrong not only because it violates the interests of his heirs, but also because it violates the interests of the originator of the will.

(B) *The Argument from Offense*
   (1) Acts are wrong (at least sometimes) because people are offended by them.
   (2) The dead cannot be offended; but certain actions toward the dead are wrong.

Therefore, these acts are wrong because they offend the living.

Many think that actions such as necrophilia are immoral and illegal because the living are deeply affronted by such actions. These people would claim that the dead have no moral or legal rights but that these actions ought to be legislated against in deference to the sensibilities of the living.

Now it is true that necrophilia and degradation of corpses clearly offend most of us. Stories about the shameless manner in which morbid medical students treat corpses or of the preferences of certain sexual deviates are surely likely to be offensive to those of us with a more refined sense of the appropriate. So there does seem to be a kernel of truth in the offense theorist's claim.

But is it really true that these actions *are* wrong because we are offended, or are we offended *because* they are wrong? I would think that the offense we take at learning that these acts have occurred is really an acknowledgment that the acts are morally wrong; the repugnance is not what makes the actions wrong. And why are we offended, anyway? Part of the explanation must involve our belief that necrophiliacs and those who mistreat corpses are doing something which the person would not have wished done to her body after death. Would you want your corpse used by necrophiliacs? Would you want your corpse ridiculed by disrespectful sophomoric medical students?

Necrophilia is immoral because it involves the involuntary participation of one of the sexual partners. The corpse cannot enter voluntarily into a contract with a living human. Cases of necrophilia can be considered instances of the rape of dead humans. Now it may seem like corpses are mere objects; certainly they cannot feel pleasure and pain. But are they mere objects in the same way that rocks, tables, and stones are objects? One of the reasons, at least, that we honor death-bed promises, normally take care when handling and displaying the bodies of the dead, and avoid maliciously defaming the reputations of the dead is that we feel some compulsion to respect the wishes in these matters of those now dead. Don't we feel that there is a difference between being buried with dignity and being hung and mutilated after we die? Wouldn't we prefer the former? And the reason we would think this involves the fact that no *mere* object is involved, but rather a human corpse.

This was, in fact, the reason that Italian partisans (the non-Fascists) thought that subjecting Mussolini to degradation after he was dead was harming Mussolini. They assumed he still possessed certain interests which could be harmed by the indignities inflicted.

So although it seems true that most of us are offended by certain atrocities performed upon corpses, this is a *recognition* that these acts are wrong, and not the *reason* that they are wrong.

(C) *The Argument from Sentiment*

   (1) The living have emotional attachments to the dead.

   (2) The living often present posthumous citations to the dead; but the dead cannot be aware of these awards.

   (3) If the dead cannot be aware of these awards, then they cannot benefit from them.

Therefore, posthumous citations are awarded because of sentiment only.

This argument contends that we grant posthumous awards not from a rational desire to avoid harming the interests of the dead, but from an irrational allegiance we feel towards them, which translates into mawkish action.

Once again there does seem to be an element of truth to this contention. Many of our gestures toward the dead *are* merely sentimental. Those who try to talk to their dead spouse, or communicate with the dead by means of spiritualists, or who burn sacrificial offerings, may be labeled sentimental or superstitious. But not all actions toward the dead fall into this category.

Let us consider posthumous citations: Suppose that various rules/conditions which specify who shall receive certain prizes or awards are set forth.[3] It would seem that an individual who satisfied these qualifying conditions would have a claim of entitlement upon the award in question. We would think this unless some more important overriding considerations invalidated the claims of the individual who satisfied the qualifying conditions for the award. But suppose upon fulfilling these conditions the individual, overwhelmed by her achievement, suffers a massive heart attack and dies. Does this mean that no award should be issued? Does this mean that if an award is issued it is only a sentimental gesture? I think not. It seems to me that if an award is not issued when someone has fulfilled its qualifying conditions, in the absence of overriding considerations, an injustice occurs—a denial of that which is the individual's due, since she had an entitlement to it and hence a right to it. The individual who did not receive this award would have been wronged.

But a critic might reply that this does not occur if a dead person is involved. He might say that since the individual died immediately after fulfilling the award's qualifying conditions we cannot wrong her. But I think that a wrong does occur. Even though the dead person herself cannot claim the award to which she is entitled, she *is* entitled to the award simply by fulfilling its qualifying conditions. One need not claim an award, or even be able to personally claim it, to be in fact entitled to it and have a right to it. It is only in the presence of an explicit denial of her claim to it that we can justifiably withhold the award in the absence of other overriding considerations; clearly the dead person has issued no such denial.

Of course if a couple were entitled to a trip to Paris because they won this prize in a sanctioned lottery, but they died prior to embarking on the journey, we need not place them in caskets and carry them around Paris. For even though they have a claim of entitlement to the trip, corpses do not have the ability to benefit from such treatment and this is the kind of overriding consideration that would allow us to withhold the prize justifiably. However I am claiming that the dead do have the ability to benefit from not being slandered and from posthumous awards, since these citations enhance their reputations and we have an interest in a good reputation *simpliciter.*

If all this is true then it would seem not that all posthumous awards are merely sentimental gestures, but they are often requirements of justice. To withhold the award would often be a denial of what is owed, or due, another as a matter of entitlement and right. The mere failure to be sentimental is not an injustice; but the denial of what is owed another, even if she cannot personally claim what is due her, is an injustice. It is not obvious how we can violate morality by not being sentimental. It is clear that morality is violated when we are unjust.

But isn't all this talk of interests after death predicated on the superstition that we might persist in some way or other after death? And isn't this just an irrational hope for wish fulfillment?

I said at the outset that I would not assume the truth of any personal immortality thesis; but I do think that as a matter of fact each of us does persist after death in a sense. Each of us leaves a certain legacy to those who follow us, and, depending upon the kind of life we lead, we shall be remembered as heroic or despicable, or most probably, as somewhere in between these extremes. It is a psychological fact that much of our behavior while we are alive is motivated by a desire to leave some kind of positive legacy to those who remain after we die. Few of us will achieve the monumental status of Socrates or Christ or Da Vinci, but we would surely rather be remembered in that way than as Benedict Arnold or Charles Manson or Bluebeard. Regardless of whether our heirs appreciate what we did, *we* want to be remembered in light of what we accomplish and the kind of person we were. In fact it can be said that we *deserve* this recognition based on our past performances and deeds.

Is our desire to be remembered irrational? Surely if no personal immortality thesis is assumed we shall never be able to experience pleasant sensations or even be aware of the fond remembrances that others have of us; but many of us still want to be remembered fondly even after conceding all this. And this desire may well be grounded upon the principle of desert. One deserves to be remembered in accord with his past deeds. Our desire to be fondly remembered may be a demand that a principle of justice be applied properly when evaluating the life we have led.

Even after we die certain things can happen to our corpses, our reputations, and certain of our desires. Some of these things are morally wrong not because they are offensive to the living or a discomfort to the dead person's surviving relatives, but because they violate two important principles of justice: desert and entitlement. Our desire to be remembered fondly is not, as some may think, an irrational fancy built upon an absurd belief in personal immortality, but rather a demand that the imperatives of justice be acknowledged in dealing with us even after we are dead. This analysis can account for our belief that many things done to the dead are immoral. They are immoral because they violate the demands of justice.

III

Of course arguing for the acknowledgment of the interests of the dead does not entail that their interests or wishes ought to be *absolutely* respected. Their interests and rights may be justifiably overriden by more important considerations, just as the interests and rights of the living are often justifiably overridden. If we could save the life of another human by slandering Rocky Marciano we should not hesitate to do so in most circumstances; but our reaction would probably be the same as if we could save someone's life by slandering another living human.

But what of the relative stringency between the rights of the dead and the rights of the living? Is it *equally* wrong to slander Rocky Marciano and Muhammad Ali? Although it is immoral to slander Rocky Marciano it is probably morally worse to slander Ali. This is due to the logical and empirical possibility of Ali's being *hurt* by the slander in addition to being harmed by it. Remember that Rocky's interests can be harmed by the slanderer, but Rocky cannot be hurt by him since Rocky cannot experience pleasure or pain and he cannot become aware of the slander. Hence the foreseen and actual consequence of slandering Ali may be worse than the foreseen and actual consequences of slandering Marciano. If one believes (and I do) that at least one of the factors constituting the morality/immorality of an action is the foreseen and actual consequences of the action, then he is committed to the view that slandering Ali is the morally worse act.

This concession is not a retreat from the original argument expressed herein, but is only an admission that slander which harms *and* hurts is morally worse, other things being equal, than slander which only harms.

Some people think that paying so much deference to the fulfillment of the desires of the dead results in the subjugation of the interests of the living. For instance, why shouldn't we use the bodily organs of the recently deceased to insure the well-being of those still living who could benefit from these organs? Doesn't the great good which results override any alleged interest of the dead?

It should be clear that one can assert that human beings have interests that can only be fulfilled after they are dead and simultaneously agree that the bodily organs of the dead can be justifiably used for the benefit of the living. These two claims are compatible because the former does not entail that the interests being considered are absolutely inviolable, while the latter *may* only mean that the interests of the living have a higher priority than the interests of the dead. There is a considerable difference between contending that (i) the bodily organs of the dead can be used because the dead have no interests and

(ii) the bodily organs of the dead can be used because the interests of the living override the interests of the dead. The former is incompatible with the main thesis of this essay, but the latter is not. The latter states that, at the very least, we have a *reason* for not using the bodily organs of the dead—it violates the interests of the dead if by using their organs we transgress their wishes—but it concludes that the reasons we have *for* using these organs are more compelling and justify their use.

Those who claim that it is not permissible to use the organs of the dead to benefit the living believe that the interests of the dead override the interests of the living; those who argue in manner (ii) that organ use is permissable are claiming that the interests of the dead are overridden by the needs of the living. So their disagreement is not concerned with whether or not the dead *have* interests, but is concerned with the relative stringency and priority of these interests. Only if someone argued in manner (i) would there be a basic incompatibility with the main thesis of this essay.

Now I am not arguing in defense of tack (ii); I am showing only that it is convenient to agree with my thesis and still conclude that cadaver organs ought to be used for the benefit of the living. Although I am not advocating this position, it is not ruled out by the acceptance of my main thesis. Hence those who feel intuitively that it is correct to use these organs need not think themselves philosophical adversaries of my position on that basis alone.

IV

Of course X's having an interest in the attainment of some commodity Z is not a sufficient condition for saying that X has a right to Z. We have many interests which do not translate into rights; it may be in my interest to be a millionaire or to be a famous writer or to be declared president, but I do not have a right to such things. It is not a matter of injustice that I am not a millionaire or a famous writer or the president. We may have a right to equal opportunity to fulfill these interests, but we surely do not have a right to these things *simpliciter*.

There are several different analyses of what it means to have a right, and the assumption of one, or even a few, of these will exclude some necessary condition of someone's favorite theory of rights. But we should note that it seems *prima facie* wrong to deny certain things to dead humans; and the reason it is wrong involves their interests in these things (e.g., their interests in a good reputation, proper disposal of their worldly possessions, and considerate handling of their corpse); furthermore third parties can justifiably act as agents on behalf of the dead and claim that their interests and desires be respected in these matters: these third parties can also sometimes intervene to prevent a potential violator of these interests from succeeding; and withholding certain things from the dead is an injustice— denial of the dead person's due based on his entitlements and deserts. Since all of these are often cited as necessary conditions of one's having a right to something,[4] it makes perfectly good sense to speak of the rights of the dead.

Although dead humans cannot appear in courts of law or make claims on their own behalf, the living, acting as their agents, may justifiably demand that the interests of the dead be respected. Of course, it is possible for someone who is still alive to assign one of his surviving heirs to act as his agent after he is dead. But even if the dead person does not formally assign one of the living to act as his agent, the living may still assume this role, much as we do on behalf of animals, infants, and the mentally retarded.

It might be objected that the dead cannot have rights because they are not, themselves, moral agents. This view seems to be philosophically unfashionable now, since many do acknowledge generally the rights of infants, the retarded, and animals even though they are not presumably moral agents (i.e., they are not capable of making moral judgments vis-à-vis their conduct towards us); but if one requires some element to reciprocity or some contractual basis for rights, this can be provided. We may all contractually agree to respect the interests of those already dead, and in return expect that our interests will be respected by those who are living when we are dead. In this way the elements of reciprocity and contracts are fulfilled even though humans cease to be moral agents at death. Equally self-interested individuals could easily agree to such a contract.

If we assign rights to the dead we must reject the following as necessary conditions for an acceptable analysis of rights:

(I) Having a right to life at Time T is a necessary condition for having other rights at T.

(II) Having the capacity to experience sensations at T is a necessary condition for having rights at T.

(III) Having the capacity to be hurt by wrongs done at T is a necessary condition for having rights at T.

(IV) Having the capacity to be a moral agent at T is a necessary condition for having rights at T.

(V) Having the ability to make demands on one's behalf at T is a necessary condition for having rights at T.

Perhaps all that is required here is the introduction of different temporal indices which would reflect the fact that the dead person had all these capacities in the past, and that they serve as the basis of his rights to certain things after he dies.

What, then, are the rights of the dead? At the very least, the following are proper candidates:

(A) The right to dispose of property.

(B) The right to the reputation which is merited by deeds performed when alive.

(C) The right to any posthumous award to which a claim of entitlement can justifiably be lodged.

(D) The right to specify the burial procedures and handling of one's corpse.

This may not be an exhaustive list, but certainly represents the most obvious list of possible rights of the dead.

V

But there is an additional problem not easily explained. Many have the feeling, I think, that slandering Rocky Marciano is morally worse than slandering Cicero. It seems that as time passes our abhorrence of offensive acts committed against the dead decreases. Wouldn't we think it worse if someone slandered us six months after we died than if we were slandered two hundred years after our death?

What can account for this? There is an analogous situation involving hurts suffered by the living: suppose X slanders Y and Z discovers this, but Z does not tell X because he knows that X is easily hurt and Z wishes to avoid needlessly hurting X. However thirty years after the initial slander Z does tell X because he feels that enough time has passed that X will not be hurt much, if at all. Z reasons that although the offense against X has not changed, the time factor will tend to alleviate X's hurt. And Z may well be correct in his reasoning.

Is this time element a mere psychological factor which does not translate into a moral difference? That is, is it really *just* as morally pernicious to slander Cicero as Rocky? Or does the time element really make a moral difference? If the time element does make a moral difference then the interests and rights of the dead are not eternal. And if these interests and rights are not eternal then exactly *when* do they vanish? And *why* would they vanish?

Clearly one of the reasons we might think that it was worse to slander Rocky is that we feel a much closer relationship to him than we do to Cicero. Many of us have seen Rocky fight, or met him, or read about him; we can still view films of him pummeling Ezzard Charles and vanquishing Jersey Joe Walcott; and we may have heard our friends and relatives speaking fondly of his exploits. Cicero is a remote historical figure of whom we may have no remembrance at all other than our difficulty in translating his Latin prose into English in high school. But does this psychological difference translate into a moral difference between the two acts of slander?

It has been claimed that we have a special interest, at the very least, in having our reputations not maligned during the lifetimes of those who knew us and those who were our contemporaries.[5] Few of us will be remembered at all after the passage of a century, or even fifty years, after our death. Those who knew us and were our contemporaries are those most likely to slander or remember us at all. Rationally self-interested moral agents might well be content to agree upon some point after death when, although not all lies are permissable, slander would not bear the moral disapprobation it does shortly after death.

I do not find this argument totally convincing, because I am skeptical that the closer personal relationship we feel toward Marciano really translates into a morally relevant feature which dictates that slandering him is worse than slandering Cicero. Suppose that someone slandered a close friend of yours who was still living; the next day this same individual makes the same slanderous remark about someone who is a total stranger to you. Although it is clear that *you* would feel more aversion to the slandering of your friend, it also seems clear that the slanderer has performed two actions of equal moral disapprobation. So even though *you* might be more disturbed about the slanderous statement which was directed against your friend, it does not follow from this that the two acts of slander are not equally bad from a moral point of view. So too the mere fact that we feel a closer relationship to Rocky Marciano than to Cicero does not entail that slandering Cicero is any less noxious than slandering Rocky.

NOTES

1. For a more complete analysis of harm, awareness of harm, and hurt, see Joel Feinberg, *Social Philosophy,* Englewood Cliffs: Prentice-Hall, Inc., 1973, pp. 25–31.
2. Rocky Marciano was the heavyweight boxing champion from 1952–1956. He retired undefeated. He died in an airplane crash in 1969.
3. For the best discussion of the notions of desert and entitlement see Joel Feinberg, *Doing and Deserving,* Princeton University Press, Princeton, New Jersey, 1970, especially chapter 4.
4. Several analyses of rights have been offered in philosophical literature. See D. G. Ritchie, *Natural Rights,* London: Allen & Unwin, 1894; Joel Feinberg, "Can Animals Have Rights?" in *Animal Rights and Human Obligations,* edited by T. Regan and P. Singer, Englewood Cliffs: Prentice-Hall, Inc., 1976, pp. 190–196; H. J. McCloskey, "Rights," *Philosophical Quarterly,* Vol. 15 (1965), pp. 121–124; and Richard Wasserstrom, "Rights, Human Rights, and Racial Discrimination," *The Journal of Philosophy,* Vol. 61 (1964). These four works are a representative cross section of different approaches to the question of rights.

5. Joel Feinberg, "The Rights of Animals and Unborn Generations," in *Philosophy and Environmental Crisis*, edited by
William T. Blackstone; University of Georgia Press, Athens,
1974, pp. 58–60.

MEDICINE IN THE AGE OF HIV

AIDS and Medical Confidentiality

Raanan Gillon

CONSULTANTS in sexually transmitted disease clinics dealing with patients with the acquired immune deficiency syndrome (AIDS) or positive for the human immunodeficiency virus (HIV) "are being over-protective of the confidentiality," a general practitioner and member of the British Medical Association's central ethical committee is reported to have said.[1] On the other hand, the BMA in its third and most recent statement on AIDS says, "The traditional confidentiality of the doctor-patient relationship must be upheld in the case of patients suffering from AIDS and HIV seropositive individuals."[2]

Clearly, the advice from the BMA is disputed by many general practitioners. The Leicestershire Local Medical Committee, representing 400 general practitioners, wrote to the BMA complaining that its guidelines were "very wrong"; as with any other serious illness general practitioners should be informed by specialists who discovered important medical information about their patients, including infection with HIV.[3] In a straw poll three out of the four general practitioners questioned by a medical newspaper on this issue are reported to have opposed the BMA's policy and to have stated that general practitioners should be told.[4] At the BMA's annual representative meeting this year a variety of motions demanded that they shall be told.[5] But in an excellent debate last week the annual conference of local medical committees, which represents all National Health

From *British Medical Journal*, vol. 294, June 27, 1987. Reprinted by permission of the author and the *British Medical Journal*.

Service general practitioners, rejected by 156 votes to 109 a proposal that family doctors had a right to be told if a patient was found to be positive for HIV and decided that patients were entitled to normal standards of confidentiality.

The problem arises when people are found to be positive for HIV in a clinic for sexually transmitted diseases and refuse permission for the information to be passed on, despite advice about why it would be preferable for their general practitioner to be informed. The main justifications stated or implied in favour of breaking confidentiality in such circumstances are (1) that it is normal medical practice; (2) that it is in the interests of the patient by leading to better medical care; (3) that it is in the interests of the general practitioner and associated staff by reducing their risks of accidentally acquiring HIV infection; (4) that it may be in the interests of other patients who might risk becoming infected by the patient; and (5) that it is in the interests of society in general by helping to reduce the spread of the AIDS epidemic.

Normal Medical Practice?

Two questions need to be answered. Firstly, Is it normal medical practice to pass on medical information to other doctors against patients' wishes? Secondly, If it is, what follows?

To agree that specialists normally pass on information to patients' general practitioners in no way means that they normally do so *when the patient refuses to allow such transfer of information about him or her*. The fact that it is normal for specialists to pass on information to general practitioners surely only reflects the fact that in most cases patients agree, or can be reasonably assumed to agree, that it is in their interests for such information to be passed on. But when patients do not agree, or can reasonably be expected not to agree, then is it not also entirely "normal medical practice" for doctors to respect their patients' wishes? The two most obvious categories of such medical behaviour are when a patient is receiving psychotherapy or when a sexually transmitted disease has been diagnosed; the latter instance offers the most clearly relevant example in which it is precisely *not* normal medical practice for specialists to pass on medical information to general practitioners against the patient's wishes.

In any case, even if it were normal medical practice to pass on medical information against patients' wishes, what would follow from this? Certainly not that the practice is therefore right. For it to be accepted right, independent justification would be required, and the example of AIDS, as in so many other contexts, provides a stimulus for re-examining our normal practices. Some might argue (especially perhaps in other European countries) that to urge the breaking of confidentiality in cases of HIV positivity is a regrettable indication of how far we have already travelled down the slippery slope away from the absolute requirement of medical confidentiality demanded in the World Medical Association's international code of medical ethics[6] and also apparently, but equivocally, in the new European guide to medical ethics[7] (equivocally because as well as requiring a guarantee to the patient of complete confidentiality the guide also provides for exceptions "where national law provides for exceptions"). The claim that medical confidentiality is an absolute requirement has been thoroughly presented by one contemporary European medical writer[8] and in the face of erosions undoubtedly has its attractions. But, though I have argued previously that such absolutism is in the end untenable,[9] medical confidentiality clearly remains a strong medicomoral principle and should be broken only if yet stronger moral reasons prevail. A mere claim that overriding confidentiality has become normal medical practice, even if it were true, would not provide moral justification for doing so.

Is Disclosure in the Interests of the Patient?

Given that a patient, because he perceives his own interests to be best served by confidentiality, rejects the view of a clinician in a sexually transmitted diseases clinic that it would be preferable to tell his general practitioner of his disease, it would surely be unusually arrogant for a doctor to persist in assuming that "doctor knows best" and that disclosure is in the patient's best interests. A vital aspect of the medical objective of doing good for one's patients is to discount one's own perception of what is good for them in favour of their own, autonomous beliefs about what is good for them. Even in cases in which we believe that there is a clear discrepancy between what the patient autonomously desires and what is in the patient's best interests we have to be extremely careful in justifying imposing our beliefs on our patients in their interests when they explicitly reject such "help." A poignant example of reluctance to do so, even when death will be the outcome, was given by Sir Richard Bayliss, the patient being a Christian Scientist who refused medical treatment for thyrotoxicosis.[10] Can justification "in the patient's best interests" be offered in this particular context of overriding confidentiality against the patient's will?

Three reported justifications are that if the general practitioner does not know of the patient's HIV positivity he may make wrong diagnoses, not treat the patient properly, or order potentially risky diagnostic tests.[3] Of course there is a higher chance of wrong diagnosis and inappropriate treatment, but patients who are positive for HIV tend to maintain a continuing therapeutic relationship with the clinician at the clinic for sexually transmitted diseases who made the original diagnosis; thus even if the general practitioner does not pick up disorders related to AIDS the clinician at the clinic is likely to do so and treat them appropriately. As for potentially harmful diagnostic tests, I wonder which ones and in what sorts of circumstances. Thinking of the typical diagnostic tests in general practice that I request, such as radiography, blood tests, and urine tests, it is not clear to me how, if the tests were clinically in the patients' interests without my knowing about his HIV positivity, they would be transformed into being against his interests if I did know. In any case patients who did not wish me to know about their HIV positivity would probably consult their clinician at the sexually transmitted diseases clinic before undergoing special tests recommended by me such as contrast radiography. Thus it seems unlikely, from the point of view of the patient's best interests, that diagnostic tests would be a problem, and the problems of imperfect diagnosis and treatment by the general practitioner are likely to be compensated for by the continuing care of the specialist in sexually transmitted diseases.

Like most general practitioners I would regret such lack of confidence by the patient in me, but I do not believe that overriding his wishes for confidentiality is likely to improve matters or to be in his best interests. Even if I did I can certainly see no general justification in "the patient's best interests" for imposing such transfer of information to me against his will.

Insurance Medicals and Patients' Best Interests

In the context of best interests it is worth recalling that benefiting one's patients should also be considered in the context of the harm that a proposed benefit risks: it is net benefit over harm that counts. A patient's interests are not confined to strictly medical interests, and a proposed medical benefit may result in non-medical harms. A single example should suffice to demonstrate this. It is usually the general practitioner who is contacted for medical information when patients want life and health insurance. If the general practitioner knows about his patient's HIV positivity he must, presumably, in honestly and professionally answering the relevant question disclose this information. If, however, the general practioner does not know he can honestly say so. Thus in some cases it may well be in the patient's best interests for the general practitioner not to know.

Here, incidentally, is another example in which our current medical norms—those concerning insurance medicals—are called into stark relief by the AIDS epidemic. It seems clear that when we complete an insurance medical form we use information gathered in the course of a therapeutic relationship for an essentially commercial purpose, and this commercial purpose is in some cases likely to conflict with the best interests of the patient. It is of course done with consent, but the sort of consent that the patient in many cases would prefer not to have to give. Perhaps we ought to change our norms so that in all cases in which there is any doubt in the general practitioner's mind about whether completing an insurance medical questionnaire would be in the patient's best interests (1) the patient should be consulted and (2) if the patient prefers, the general practitioner should return the insurance medical form uncompleted. The company could then arrange for an independent and explicit "non-therapeutic" medical assessment. In addition, the choice of having an independent medical assessment should perhaps be explicitly offered by insurance companies to all applicants for insurance right from the start.

Is Disclosure in the Interests of General Practitioners and Other Members of the Primary Care Team?

This is essentially the argument that confidentiality is too dangerous for general practitioners and other primary care health workers including nurses to respect in cases of HIV positivity. I considered the arguments of danger in a previous article about refusal to treat patients with AIDS and those positive for HIV.[11] In summary, I argued (1) that the medical profession (including "the greater medical profession") accepted a certain degree of risk as part of its professional norms and (2) that the extensive empirical evidence currently available showed that the probability of accidental transmission of HIV to medical staff and families and other close contacts of patients positive for HIV or with AIDS was very low, given normal care with blood and other body fluids.

Is Disclosure in the Interests of Other Possible Patients?

I find this the most difficult of the arguments in favour of breaking confidentiality, though at most it seems to justify disclosure against a patient's will only in exceptional circumstances. Thus if either a clinician in a sexually transmitted diseases clinic or a general practitioner knows or has strong reason to believe that a patient positive for HIV intends to have sexual intercourse with a new and uninfected partner or partners without telling the partner(s), and efforts to persuade the patient to tell have been rejected and there is a reasonable prospect of preventing the event(s), then efforts to inform such contacts do seem justifiable in order to try to prevent them from being infected with what is likely to be a fatal virus. This seems particularly clearly justified if the previously uninfected contact is also a patient of the doctor concerned (because of the special obligations doctors have to their patients), but it might also apply, for example, in the context of tracing contacts of patients with sexually transmitted diseases as part of a general concern to protect others from potentially fatal diseases.

Even against this very limited justification of breach of confidentiality, however, it might be argued, as I do below, that it is still better not to break confidentiality. Thus by being known to maintain a very strict level of confidentiality the medical profession has a better chance of maintaining the trust of high risk groups; it will therefore be better able to influence them and more effectively protect the health of others in general. Although I would agree that it is almost always likely in practice that preserving confidentiality will be the better course for precisely such consequentialist justification, I find it impossible to rule out circumstances in which I, at any rate, would believe it right to break confidentiality. I can imagine, for example, a "psychopath" positive for HIV who makes it clear that he or she does not care about transmitting the virus to others, and indeed intends to do so, and when I know that another of my patients, probably uninfected with HIV, is a likely new partner.

The possible existence of such rare exceptions (for most patients positive for HIV like most other patients and people in general are not psychopaths and do care about others) is simply evidence for my earlier claim that medical confidentiality should not be an absolute requirement, only a very strong one. In the context of a just society strong evidence of likely and preventable death or severe injury to others can afford justification for overriding confidentiality, including the passing on of information between doctors and to new contacts. But such circumstances will be extremely rare. In most cases the probability of preventing death or severe injury by breaking medical confidentiality about HIV state will be low—and every time a doctor does break such confidentiality he or she will further reduce a trust in the profession that while it exists can itself be reasonably expected to help reduce the spread of the disease.

Is Disclosure in the Interests of Society?

The final argument sometimes offered for passing on information about patients positive for HIV is that it is in the interests of society by helping to reduce the spread of AIDS. Justice, it might be added, requires doctors to take into account not only the interests of their individual patients of the moment but of society in general. Though the desire to minimise the spread of AIDS is doubtless shared by all sane people, and though the claim that doctors must include the interests of society in their medicomoral reasoning is one that I would strongly support, it does not follow that overriding the traditional norms of medical practice in the context of AIDS is the best way to achieve those objectives. I hope to return to this theme in a subsequent paper, but, in brief, the spread of AIDS seems most likely to be curtailed and the interests of society best served if the trust and cooperation of those at greatest risk can be obtained and maintained. Thus the consequentialist objective of minimising the spread of AIDS fortunately seems to point in the same direction as the traditional rules of medical deontology, including the norms of medical confidentiality. In the context of this paper it seems particularly implausible to argue that the spread of AIDS will be curtailed if specialists in sexually transmitted diseases are routinely required to break medical confidentiality by passing on to general practitioners information about patients' HIV positivity against those patients' wishes. On the contrary, it seems far more probable that the interests of society will be best served if the medical profession in general, and perhaps specialists in sexually transmitted diseases in particular, can preserve their reputation, especially among those most at risk of infection, for conforming to a very strong—though not absolute—principle of medical confidentiality.

Summary

In summary, I have argued that the arguments offered or hinted at in favour of doctors' breaking medical confidentiality by passing on information about their patients' HIV state to others, including other doctors, when this is against the patient's considered wishes are generally unconvincing. Although in highly exceptional cases there may be justifications for overriding confidentiality, the requirement of medical confidentiality is a very strong, though not absolute, obligation. Patients, their contacts, doctors and their staff, and the common good are most likely to be best served if that tradition continues to be honoured.

NOTES

1. Duncan N. GPs demand to be told results of AIDS tests. *Pulse* 1987; Jan. 3:1.
2. British Medical Association. *Third BMA statement on AIDS.* London: BMA, 1986.
3. Beecham L. Support for confidentiality for AIDS patients. *Br Med J* 1987;294:1177.
4. Kennard N. Should GPs be told AIDS test results? *Pulse* 1987; Jan 17:25.
5. British Medical Association. Agenda of the British Medical Association's annual representative meeting 1987, motions 359–374. *Br Med F* 1987; 294 (insert in issue of 6 June).
6. British Medical Association. *Handbook of medical ethics.* London: BMA, 1984: 70–1.
7. Anonymous. European guide to medical ethics. *IME Bulletin* 1987; No 25:3–7.
8. Kottow MH. Medical confidentiality: an intransigent and absolute obligation. *F Med Ethics* 1986; 12:117–22.
9. Gillon R. Confidentiality. *Br Med J* 1985; 291:1634–6.
10. Bayliss R. A health hazard. *Br Med J* 1982;285:1824–5.
11. Gillon R. Refusal to treat AIDS and HIV positive patients. *Br Med J* 1987; 294:1332–3.

AIDS in Historical Perspective: Four Lessons from the History of Sexually Transmitted Diseases

Allan M. Brandt, Ph.D.

Introduction

It has become abundantly clear in the first six years of the AIDS (acquired immunodeficiency syndrome) epidemic that there will be no simple answer to this health crisis. The obstacles to establishing effective public health policies are considerable. AIDS is a new disease with a unique set of public health problems. The medical, social, and political aspects of the disease present American society and the world community with an awesome task.

The United States has relatively little recent experience dealing with health crises. Since the introduction of antibiotics during World War II, health priorities shifted to chronic, systemic diseases. We had come to believe that the problem of infectious, epidemic disease had passed—a topic of concern only to the developing world and historians.

In this respect, it is not surprising that in these first years of the epidemic there has been a desire to look for historical

Editor's Note: Portions of this article are based on the author's book, *No Magic Bullet, A Social History of Venereal Disease in the United States.* Oxford University Press, 1985, Rev. Ed. 1987

From *American Journal of Public Health,* April, 1988, Vol. 78, No. 4, pp. 367–371. Reprinted by permission of the author and *The American Journal of Public Health.*

models as a means of dealing with the AIDS epidemic. Many
have pointed to past and contemporary public health approaches
to sexually transmitted diseases (STDs) as important precedents
for the fight against AIDS.[1] And indeed, there are significant
similarities between AIDS and other sexually transmitted infections which go beyond the mere fact of sexual transmission.
Syphilis, for example, also may have severe pathological effects. In the first half of the twentieth century, it was both
greatly feared and highly stigmatized. In light of these analogues, the social history of efforts to control syphilis and other
STDs may serve to inform our assessments of the current
epidemic.

But history holds no simple truths. AIDS is not syphilis; our
responses to the current epidemic will be shaped by contemporary science, politics, and culture. Yet the history of disease
does offer an important set of perspectives on current proposals
and strategies. Moreover, history points to the range of variables that will need to be addressed if we are to create effective
and just policies.

In these early years of the AIDS epidemic, there has been a
tendency to use analogy as a means of devising policy. It makes
sense to draw upon past policies and institutional arrangements
to address the problems posed by the current crisis. But we
need to be sophisticated in drawing analogues; to recognize
not only how AIDS is like past epidemics, but the precise ways
in which it is different. This article draws four "lessons" from
the social history of sexually transmitted disease in the United
States and assesses their relevance for the current epidemic.

Lesson #1—Fear of Disease Will Powerfully Influence Medical Approaches and Public Health Policy

The last years of the nineteenth century and first of the
twentieth witnessed considerable fear of sexually transmitted
infection, not unlike that which we are experiencing today. A
series of important discoveries about the pathology of syphilis

and gonorrhea had revealed a range of alarming pathological consequences from debility, insanity, and paralysis, to sterility and blindness. In this age of antibiotics, it is easy to forget the fear and dread that syphilis invoked in the past.

Among the reasons that syphilis was so greatly feared was the assumption that it could be casually transmitted. Doctors at the turn of the twentieth century catalogued the various modes of transmissions: pens, pencils, toothbrushes, towels and bedding, and medical procedures were all identified as potential means of communication.[2] As one woman explained in an anonymous essay in 1912:

> At first it was unbelievable. I knew of the disease only through newspaper advertisements [for patent medicines]. I had understood that it was the result of sin and that it originated and was contracted only in the underworld of the city. I felt sure that my friend was mistaken in diagnosis when he exclaimed, "Another tragedy of the public drinking cup!" I eagerly met his remark with the assurance that I did not use public drinking cups, that I had used my own cup for years. He led me to review my summer. After recalling a number of times when my thirst had forced me to go to the public fountain, I came at last to realize that what he had told me was true.[3]

The doctor, of course, had diagnosed syphilis. One indication of how seriously these casual modes of transmission were taken is the fact that the US Navy removed doorknobs from its battleships during World War I, claiming that they had become a source of infection for many of its sailors. We now know, of course, that syphilis cannot be contracted in these ways. This poses a difficult historical problem: Why did physicians believe that they could be?

Theories of casual transmission reflected deep cultural fears about disease and sexuality in the early twentieth century. In these approaches to venereal disease, concerns about hygiene, contamination, and contagion were expressed, anxieties that reflected a great deal about the contemporary society and culture. Venereal disease was viewed as a threat to the entire late Victorian social and sexual system, which placed great value on discipline, restraint, and homogeneity. The sexual code of that era held that sex would receive social sanction only in marriage. But the concerns about venereal disease and casual transmission also reflected a pervasive fear of the urban masses, the growth of the cities, and the changing nature of familial relationships.[4]

Today, persistent fears about casual transmission of AIDS reflect a somewhat different, yet no less significant, social configuration. First, AIDS is strongly associated with behaviors which have been traditionally considered deviant. This is true for both homosexuality and intravenous drug use. After a generation of growing social tolerance for homosexuality, the epidemic has generated new fears and heightened old hostilities. Just as syphilis created a disease-oriented xenophobia in the early twentieth century, AIDS has today generated a new homophobia. AIDS has recast anxiety about contamination in a new light. Among certain social critics, AIDS is seen as "proof" of a certain moral order.

Second, fears are fanned because we live in an era in which the authority of scientific expertise has eroded. This may well be an aspect of a broader decline in the legitimacy of social institutions, but it is clearly seen in the areas of science and medicine. Despite significant evidence that HIV (human immunodeficiency virus) is not casually transmitted, medical and public health experts have been unable to provide the categorical reassurances that the public would like. But without such guarantees, public fear has remained high. In part, this reflects a misunderstanding of the nature of science and its inherent uncertainty. While physicians and public health officials have experience tolerating such uncertainty, the public requires better education in order to effectively evaluate risks.[5,6]

Third, as a culture, we Americans are relatively unsophisticated in our assessments of relative risk. How are we to evaluate the risks of AIDS? How shall social policy be constructed around what are small or unknown risks? The ostracism of HIV-infected children from their schools in certain locales, the refusal of some physicians to treat AIDS patients, job and housing discrimination against those infected (and those suspected of being infected) all reveal the pervasive fears surrounding the epidemic. Clearly, then, one public health goal must be to address these fears. Addressing such fears means understanding their etiology. They originate in the particular social meaning of AIDS—its "social construction." We will not be able to effectively mitigate these concerns until we understand their deeper meaning. The response to AIDS will be fundamentally shaped by these fears; therefore, we need to develop techniques to assist individuals to distinguish irrational fears of AIDS from realistic and legitimate concerns. In this respect, many have focused on the need for more education.

Lesson #2—Education Will *Not* Control the AIDS Epidemic

Early in the twentieth century, physicians, public health officials, and social reformers concerned about the problem of syphilis and gonorrhea called for a major educational campaign.[7] They cogently argued that the tide of infection could not be stemmed until the public had adequate knowledge about these diseases, their mode of transmission, and the means of prevention. They called for an end to "the conspiracy of silence"—the Victorian code of sexual ethics—that considered all discussion of sexuality and disease in respectable society inappropriate. Physicians had contributed to this state of affairs by hiding diagnoses from their patients and families, and upholding what came to be known as the "medical secret." One physician described the nature of the conventions surrounding sexually transmitted diseases:

> Medical men are walking with eyes wide open along the edge of despair so treacherous and so pitiless that the wonder can only be that they have failed to warn the world away. Not a signboard! Not a caution spoken above a whisper! All mystery and seclusion. . . . As a result of this studied propriety, a world more full of venereal infection than any other pestilence.[8]

Prince Morrow, the leader of the social hygiene movement, the antivenereal disease campaign, concluded, "Social sentiment holds that it is a greater violation of the properties of life publicly to mention venereal disease than privately to contract it."[9]

During this period, the press remained reticent on the subject of sexually transmitted infections, refusing to print accounts of their effects. Reporters employed euphemisms such as "rare blood disorder," when forced to include a reference to a venereal infection. Nevertheless, magazines and newspapers did accept advertisements for venereal nostrums and quacks. In 1912, the US Post Office confiscated copies of birth control advocate Margaret Sanger's *What Every Girl Should Know,* because it considered the references to syphilis and gonorrhea "obscene" under the provisions of the Comstock law.[4]

Enlightened physicians vigorously called for an end to this hypocrisy. "We are dealing with the solution of a problem," explained Dr. Egbert Grandin, "where ignorance is *not* bliss but is misfortune, and where, therefore, it is folly not to be wise."[10] Social reformers viewed education and publicity as a panacea; forthright education would end the problem of sexually transmitted infection. If parents failed to perform their social responsibilities and inform their children, then the schools should include sex education. By 1919, the US Public Health Service endorsed sex education in the schools, noting, "As in many instances the school must take up the burden neglected by others."[11] By 1922, almost half of all secondary schools offered some instruction in sex hygiene.

Educational programs devised by the social hygienists emphasized fear of infection. Prince Morrow, for example, called fear "the protective genius of the human body." Another physician explained, "The sexual instinct is imperative and will only listen to fear." Margaret Cleaves, a leading social hygienist, argued, "There should be taught such disgust and dread of these conditions that naught would induce the seeking of a polluted source for the sake of gratifying a controllable desire."[12]

In this sense, educational efforts may have actually contributed to the pervasive fears of infection, to the stigma associated with the diseases, and to the discrimination against its victims. Indeed, educational materials produced throughout the first decades of the twentieth century emphasized the inherent dangers of all sexual activity, especially disease and unwanted pregnancy. In this respect, such educational programs, rather than being termed sex education were actually anti-sex education.

Pamphlets and films repeatedly emphasized the "loathesome" and disfiguring aspects of sexually transmitted disease; the most drastic pathological consequences (insanity, paralysis, blindness, and death); as well as the disastrous impact on personal relations.

This orientation toward sex education reached its apogee during World War I, when American soldiers were told, "A German bullet is cleaner than a whore." Despite their threatening quality, these educational programs did not have the desired effect of reducing the rates of infection. And indeed, sexual mores in the twentieth century have responded to a number of social and cultural forces more powerful than the fear of disease.

There are, nonetheless, some precedents for successful educational campaigns. During World War II, the military initiated a massive educational campaign against sexually transmitted disease. But unlike prior efforts, it reminded soldiers that disease could be prevented through the use of condoms, which were widely distributed. The military program recognized that sexual behaviors could be modified, but that calls for outright abstinence were likely to fail. Given the need for an efficient and healthy army, officials maintained a pragmatic posture that separated morals from the essential task of prevention. As one medical officer explained, "It is difficult to make the sex act unpopular."[13]

Today, calls for better education are frequently offered as the best hope for controlling the AIDS epidemic. But this will only be true if some resolution is reached concerning the specific content and nature of such educational efforts. The limited effectiveness of education which merely encourages fear is well-documented. Moreover, AIDS education requires a forthright confrontation of aspects of human sexuality that are typically avoided. To be effective, AIDS education must be explicit, focused, and appropriately targeted to a range of at-risk social groups. As the history of sexually transmitted diseases makes clear, we need to study the nature of behavior and disease. If education is to have a positive impact, we need to be far more sophisticated, creative, and bold in devising and implementing programs.

Education is not a panacea for the AIDS epidemic, just as education did not solve the problem of other sexually transmitted diseases earlier in the twentieth century. It is one critical aspect of a fully articulated program. As this historical vignette makes clear, we need to be far more explicit about what we mean when we say "education". Certainly education about AIDS is an important element of any public health approach to the crisis, but we need to substantively evaluate a range of educational programs and their impact on behavior for populations with a variety of needs.

Because the impact of education is unclear and the dangers of the epidemic are perceived as great (see lesson #1), there has been considerable interest in compulsory public health measures as a primary means of controlling AIDS.

Lesson #3—Compulsory Public Health Measures Will *Not* Control the Epidemic

Given the considerable fear that the epidemic has generated and its obvious dangers, demands have been voiced for the implementation of compulsory public health interventions. The history of efforts to control syphilis during the twentieth century indicates the limits of compulsory measures which range from required premarital testing to quarantine of infected individuals.

Next to programs for compulsory vaccination, compulsory programs for premarital syphilis serologies are probably the most widely known of all compulsory public health measures in the twentieth century United States. The development of effective laboratory diagnostic measures stands as a signal contribution in the history of the control of sexually transmitted diseases. With the development of the Wassermann test in 1906, there was a generally reliable way of detecting the presence of syphilis. The achievement of such a test offered a new series of public health potentials. No longer would diagnosis depend on strictly clinical criteria. Diagnosis among the asymptomatic was now possible, as was the ability to test the effectiveness of treatments. The availability of the test led to the development of programs for compulsory testing.

Significantly, calls for compulsory screening for syphilis pre-
dated the Wassermann exam. Beginning in the last years of the
nineteenth century, several states began to mandate premarital
medical examinations to assure that sexually transmitted infections were not communicated in marriage. But without a definitive test, such examinations were of limited use. With a laboratory
test, however, calls were voiced for requiring premarital blood
tests. In 1935, Connecticut became the first state to mandate
premarital serologies of all prospective brides and grooms. The
rationale for premarital screening was clear. If every individual
about to be married were tested, and, if found to be infected,
treated, the transmission of infection to marital partners and
offspring would be halted. The legislation was vigorously supported by the public health establishment, organized women's
groups, magazines, and the news media. Many clinicians, however, argued against the legislation, suggesting that diagnosis
should not rely exclusively on laboratory findings which were,
in some instances, incorrect. N.A. Nelson of the Massachusetts
Department of Public Health explained, "Today, it is becoming
the fashion to support, by law, the too common notion that the
laboratory is infallible."[14] Despite such objections, by the end
of the World War II, virtually all the states had enacted provisions mandating premarital serologies.

Legislation is currently pending in 35 state legislatures that
would require premarital HIV serologies. The rationale for
such programs is often the historical precedent of syphilis screening. The logic seems intuitively correct: We screen for syphilis. AIDS is a far more serious disease, we should therefore
screen for AIDS. In this respect it is worth reviewing the
effectiveness of premarital syphilis screening as well as those
factors that distinguish syphilis from AIDS.

Mandatory premarital serologies never proved to be a particularly effective mechanism for finding new cases of syphilis.
First, physicians and public health officials recognized that there
was a significant rate of false positive tests which occurred
because of technical inadequacies of the tests themselves or as a
result of biological phenomena (such as other infections). As
the concepts of sensitivity (the test's performance among those
with the disease) and specificity (the test's performance among
those free of infections) came to be more fully understood in
the 1930s, the oversensitivity of tests like the Wassermann was

revealed. As many as 25 percent of individuals determined to be infected with syphilis by the Wassermann test were actually free of infection; nevertheless, these individuals often underwent toxic treatment with arsenical drugs, assuming the tests were correct. Beyond this, individuals with false positive tests often suffered the social repercussions of being infected: deep stigma and disrupted relationships. As many physicians pointed out, a positive serology did not always mean that an individual could transmit the disease. Because the tests tended to be mandated for a population at relatively low risk of infection, their accuracy was further compromised. Some individuals reportedly avoided the test altogether.[15]

Many of the difficulties associated with the high numbers of false positives were alleviated as new, more specific tests were developed in the 1940s and 1950s, but the central problem remained. Premarital syphilis serologies failed to identify a significant percentage of the infected population. In 1978, for example, premarital screening accounted for only 1.27 per cent of all national tests found to be positive for syphilis. The costs of these programs were estimated at $80 million annually.[16] Another study in California projected the costs per case found through premarital screening to be $240,000.[17] Moreover, premarital screening for syphilis continued to find a significant number of false positives. As these studies indicated, the benefits of screening programs are dependent on the prevalence of the disease in the population being screened. In this respect, it seems unlikely that premarital screening effectively served the function of preventing infections within marriage that its advocates assumed it would. These data led a number of states to repeal mandatory premarital serologies in the early 1980s.

Compulsory premarital syphilis serologies thus offer a dubious precedent for required HIV screening. The point, of course, is *not* that the test is inaccurate. ELISA (enzyme-linked immunosorbent assay) testing coupled with the Western Blot *can be* quite reliable, but only when applied to populations which are likely to have been infected. Screening of low-prevalence populations, like premarital couples, is unlikely to have any significant impact on the course of the epidemic. Not only will such programs find relatively few new cases, they will also reveal large numbers of false positives. A recent study concluded that a national mandatory premarital screening program would find approximately 1,200 new cases of HIV infection, one-tenth of 1 percent of those currently infected. But it would also incorrectly identify as many as 380 individuals—actually free of infection—as infected, even with supplementary Western blot tests. Such a program would also falsely reassure as many as 120 individuals with false negative results.[18] Moreover, the inability to treat and render non-infectious those individuals who are found to be infected severely limits the potential benefits of such mandatory measures. With syphilis serologies, the rationale of the program was to treat infected individuals.

This, of course, is *not* to argue that testing has no role in an effective AIDS public health campaign. During the late 1930s, a massive voluntary testing campaign heightened consciousness of syphilis in Chicago, bringing thousands of new cases into treatment. AIDS testing, conducted voluntarily and confidentially, targeted to individuals who have specific risk factors for infection, may have significant public health benefits. Compulsory screening, however, could merely discourage infected individuals from being tested. This makes clear the need to enact legislation guaranteeing the confidentiality of those who volunteer to be tested and prohibiting discrimination against HIV-infected individuals.

As a mandatory measure, premarital screening is a relatively modest proposal. During the course of the twentieth century, more radical and intrusive compulsory measures to control STDs, such as quarantine, have also been attempted. These, too, have failed. During World War I, as hysteria about the impact of STDs rose, Congress passed legislation to support the quarantine of prostitutes suspected of spreading disease. The Act held that anyone suspected of harboring a venereal infection could be detained and incarcerated until determined to be non-infectious. During the course of the war, more than 20,000 women were held in camps because they were suspected of being "spreaders" of venereal disease.

The program had no apparent impact on rates of infection, which actually climbed substantially during the war. In sexually transmitted infections, the reservoir of infection is relatively high, modes of transmission are specific, and infected individuals may be healthy. In the case of AIDS, where there is no medical intervention to render individuals non-infectious, quarantine is totally impractical because it would require life-long incarceration of the infected.

Compulsory measures often generate critics because such policies may infringe on basic civil liberties. From an ethical and legal viewpoint, the first question that must be asked about any potential policy intervention is: Is it likely to work? Only if there is clear evidence to suggest the program would be effective does it make sense to evaluate the civil liberties implications. Then it is possible to evaluate the constitutional question: Is the public health benefit to be derived worthy of the possible costs in civil liberties? Is the proposed compulsory program the least restrictive of the range of potential measures available to achieve the public good?[19]

In this respect, it is worth noting that compulsory measures may actually be counterproductive. First, they require substantial resources that could be more effectively allocated. Second, they have often had the effect of driving the very individuals that the program hopes to reach farther away from public health institutions. Ineffective draconian measures would serve only to augment the AIDS crisis. Nevertheless, despite the fact that such programs offer no benefits, they may have substantial political and cultural appeal (see lesson #1).

Because compulsory measures are controversial and unlikely to control the epidemic, there is considerable hope that we will soon have a "magic bullet"—a biomedical "fix" to free us of the hazards of AIDS.

Lesson #4—The Development of Effective Treatments and Vaccines Will *Not* Immediately or Easily End the AIDS Epidemic

As the history of efforts to control other sexually transmitted diseases makes clear, effective treatment has not always led to control. In 1909, German Nobel laureate Paul Ehrlich discovered Salvarsan (arsphenamine), an arsenic compound which killed the spirochete, the organism which causes syphilis. Salvarsan was the first effective chemotherapeutic agent for a specific disease. Ehrlich called Salvarsan a "magic bullet," a drug which would seek out and destroy its mark.[20] He claimed that modern medicine would seek the discovery of a series of such drugs to eliminate the microorganisms which cause disease. Although Salvarsan was an effective treatment, it was toxic and difficult to administer. Patients required a painful regimen of injections, sometimes for as long as two years.

Unlike the arsphenamines, penicillin was truly a wonder drug. In early 1943, Dr. John S. Mahoney of the US Public Health Service found that penicillin was effective in treating rabbits infected with syphilis. After repeating his experiments with human subjects, his findings were announced and the massive production of penicillin began.[21]

With a single shot, the scourge of syphilis could be avoided. Incidence fell from a high of 72 cases per 100,000 in 1943 to about 4 per 100,000 in 1956.[22] In 1949, Mahoney wrote, "as a result of antibiotic therapy, gonorrhea has almost passed from the scene as an important clinical and public entity.[23] An article in the *American Journal of Syphilis* in 1951 asked, "Are Venereal Diseases Disappearing?" Although the article concluded that it was too soon to know, by 1955 the *Journal* itself had disappeared. *The Journal of Social Hygiene,* for half a century the leading publication on social dimensions of the problem, also ceased publication. As rates reached all time lows, it appeared that venereal diseases would join the ranks of other infectious diseases that had come under the control of modern medicine.

Although there is no question that the nature and meaning of syphilis and gonorrhea underwent a fundamental change with the introduction of antibiotic therapy, the decline of venereal diseases proved short-lived. Rates of infection began to climb in the early 1960s. By the late 1950s much of the machinery, especially procedures for public education, case-finding, tracing and diagnosis had been severely reduced.[1]

In 1987, the Centers for Disease Control (CDC) reported an increase in cases of primary and secondary syphilis. The estimated annual rate per 100,000 population rose from 10.9 to 13.3 cases, the largest increase in 10 years. These figures are particularly striking in that they come in the midst of the AIDS epidemic which many have assumed has led to a substantial decline in sexual encounters. Moreover, after an eight-year decline, rates of congenital syphilis have also reportedly risen since 1983. The CDC concluded that individuals with a history of sexually transmitted infection are at increased risk for infection with the AIDS virus.[24]

Despite the effectiveness of penicillin as a cure for syphilis, the disease has persisted. The issue, therefore, is not merely the development of effective treatments but the *process* by which they are deployed; the means by which they move from laboratory to full allocation to those affected. Effective treatments without adequate education, counseling, and funding may not reach those who most need them. Even "magic bullets" need to be effectively delivered. Obviously effective treatments should be a priority in a multifaceted approach to AIDS and will ultimately be an important component in its control; but even a magic bullet will not quickly or completely solve the problem.

No doubt, new and more effective treatment for AIDS will be developed in the years ahead, but their deployment will raise a series of complex issues ranging from human subject research to actual allocation. And while effective treatments may help to control further infection, as they do for syphilis and gonorrhea, treatments which prolong the life of AIDS patients may have little or no impact on the rates of transmission of the virus, which occurs principally among individuals who have no symptoms of disease.

This suggests certain fundamental flaws in the biomedical model of disease. Diseases are complex bio-ecological problems that may be mitigated only by addressing a range of scientific, social, and political considerations. No single intervention—even an effective vaccine—will adequately address the complexities of the AIDS epidemic.

Conclusions

As these historical lessons make clear, in the context of fear surrounding the epidemic (lesson #1), the principal proposals for eradicating AIDS (lesson #2–4) are unlikely to be effective, at least in the immediate future. These lessons should not imply, however, that nothing will work; they make evident that no single avenue is likley to lead to success. Moreover, they suggest that in considering any intervention we will require sophisticated research to understand its potential impact on the epidemic. While education, testing, and biomedical research all offer some hope, in each instance we will need to fully consider their particular effectiveness as measures to control disease.

Simple answers based upon historical precedents are unlikely to alleviate the AIDS crisis. History does, however, point to a range of variables which influence disease, and those factors which require attention if it is to be effectively addressed. Any successful approach to the epidemic will require a full recognition of the important social, cultural, and biological aspects of AIDS. A public health priority will be to lead in the process of discerning those programs likely to have a beneficial impact from those with considerably political and cultural appeal, but unlikely to positively affect the course of the epidemic. Only in this way we will be able to devise effective and humane public policies.

NOTES

1. Cutler JC, Arnold RC: Venereal disease control by health departments in the past: Lessons for the present. Am J Public Health 1988; 78:372–376.
2. Bulkley LD: Syphilis of the Innocent. New York: Bailey and Fairchild, 1894.
3. Anon: What one woman has had to bear. Forum 1912; 68:451–454.
4. Brandt AM: No Magic Bullet: A Social History of Venereal Disease in the United States since 1880. New York: Oxford University Press, 1985, Rev. Ed. 1987.
5. Eisenberg LE: The genesis of fear. AIDS and public's response to science. Law, Med Health Care 1986; 14:243–249.
6. Becker MH, Joseph JG: AIDS and behavioral change to reduce risk: A review. Am J Public Health 1988; 78:394–410.
7. Yankauer A: AIDS and Public Health. (editorial) Am J Public Health 1988; 78:364–366.
8. Willson RN: The relation of the medical profession to the social evil. JAMA 1906;47:32.
9. Morrow PA: Publicity as a factor in venereal prophylaxis. JAMA 1906; 47:1246.

10. Grandin E: Should the Great Body of the General Public Be Enlightened? Charities and Commons, February 24, 1906.

11. US Public Health Service: The Problem of Sex Education in the Schools. Washington, DC, 1919; p 9.

12. Cleaves M: Transactions of the American Society for Social and Moral Prophylaxis 1910; 3:31.

13. Pappas JP: The venereal problem in the US Army. Milit Surg August 1943; 93:182.

14. Nelson NA: Marriage and the laboratory. Am. J Syphilis 1939; 23:289.

15. Kolmer JA: The problem of falsely doubtful and positive reactions in the serology of syphilis. Am J Public Health 1944; 34:510–526.

16. Felman Y: Repeal of mandated premarital tests for syphilis: A survey of state health officers. Am J Public Health 1981; 71:155–159.

17. Haskell RJ: A cost benefit analysis of California's mandatory premarital screening program for syphilis. West J Med 1984; 141:538–541.

18. Cleary PD, Barry MJ, Mayer KH, Brandt AM, Gostin L, Fineberg HV: Compulsory premarital screening for the human immunodeficiency virus. JAMA 1987; 258:1757–1762.

19. Gostin L, Curran W: The Limits of Compulsion in Controlling AIDS. Hastings Center Report 1986; 16(suppl): 24–29.

20. Marquardt M: Paul Ehrlich, New York: Henry Schuman, 1951.

21. Dowling H: Fighting Infection. Cambridge: Harvard University Press, 1977.

22. Brown WJ, Donohue JF, Axnick NW, Blount JH, Jones OG, Ewen NJ: Syphilis and Other Venereal Diseases. Cambridge: Harvard University Press (APHA), 1970.

23. Mahoney JF: The effect of antibiotics on the concepts and practices of public health. *In:* Galdston I (ed): The Impact of Antibiotics on Medicine and Society. New York: 1958; 98–120.

24. USPHS, Centers for Disease Control: MMWR 1987; 36:393

Morality and the
Health of the Body Politic

Dan E. Beauchamp

THE Acquired Immunodeficiency Syndrome (AIDS) is clearly
a public health threat. The view that it is also a threat to
the majority's values is a form of legal moralism.[1] Like public
health, legal moralism relies on the use of law and regulation to
promote community aims. But legal moralism restricts liberty
as a defense against a moral rather than a physical harm. It uses
law to protect the majority's morality from the deviant group.

The classic defense of moralism is found in James F. Stephen's *Liberty, Equality, Fraternity*, published in 1873,[2] a rebuttal to John Stuart Mill's essay, "On Liberty."[3] Stephen argued
that the majority in any society is a moral majority. In the
moralist's view a principal function of the criminal law and
public policy should be to enforce the norms of that shared
morality, punishing whatever is "offensive, degrading, vicious,
sinful, corrupt, or otherwise immoral."[4]

In recent times this view has been most forcefully stated by
Lord Patrick Devlin in his critique of the 1957 British Wolfenden
Report—the Report of the Committee on Homosexual Offences and Prostitution—which recommended removing criminal sanctions for private homosexual conduct between consenting
adults. Devlin said: "What makes a society of any sort is
community of ideas, not only political ideas but also ideas
about the way its members should behave and govern their
lives; these latter ideas are its morals. . . . [W]ithout shared

From *Hastings Center Report*, 1986, vol. 16, no. 5. Reprinted by permission of
the author and the Hastings Center.

ideas on politics, morals and ethics no society can exist. . . . For society is not something that is kept together physically; it is held by the invisible bonds of common thought."[5] Moralism binds the community tightly within a narrow and precise morality. Moralism seeks to purify the community, dividing the citizenry into the wheat and the chaff. (My discussion of "loose-boundedness" and "tight-boundedness" in culture and politics is drawn from Richard Merelman, *Making Something of Ourselves* [Berkeley: University of California Press, 1984]. However, I depart from Merelman's notion of "loosely-bounded" societies in which a sense of group attachment and limits has vanished. I use the term "loosely-bounded" to mean restrictions that, while less all-encompassing and restrictive than the restrictions of tightly-bounded groups, nevertheless limit autonomy and liberty to promote a shared and common good.)

Opposition to moralism is sometimes expressed as: "Law has no business restricting private conduct." But it is using law to restrict private conduct in order to promote a private morality that is the crux of the problem.

The most powerful objections to moralism lie in disputing two claims often made on its behalf. According to the first thesis, if a common morality is shared by a majority, this alone is sufficient justification to include it in the criminal law.[6] The second thesis is that because a common morality holds a society together, legal moralism is justified on the grounds of self-preservation. But to opponents of legal moralism, serious restrictions on liberty cannot rest solely on appeals to tradition, even when backed by majority approval. Furthermore, there is no evidence that violations of the majority's moral norms, like homosexuality, threaten the existence of society.

The most potent challenge to legal moralism is its frequent collision with a more widely shared value—public health. Restrictions on liberty to promote the public health— paternalism— are today more widely accepted than legal moralism. The trend seems to be, at least over the long run, toward rejecting tightly bounded moral codes in favor of loosely bounded restrictions that promote the public health as a common good. By permitting the majority the right to enforce legally its traditional prejudices, particularly in the sexual realm, the health and safety of the public can be directly threatened.

AIDS mainly strikes two groups—gay men and intravenous

drug users—who under normal circumstances are shunned by the larger society. According to the Centers for Disease Control (CDC), the number of cases of heterosexual transmission is rising, but the percentage of all cases due to heterosexual transmission remains very low, roughly 1 percent, and shows no sign of change.

Our best weapon against AIDS would be a public health policy resting on the right to be different in fundamental choices and the democratic community as "one body" in matters of the common health. This new policy would mean the right of every individual to fundamental autonomy, as in abortion and sexual orientation, while viewing health and safety as a common good whose protection (through restrictions on liberty) promotes community and the common health. The public health policy would reject moralism as a threat to the right of each individual, including gays, to fundamental autonomy and also as a threat to the common health.

AIDS, at least in developed countries, does not seem to behave like a typical infectious disease, which spreads rapidly or easily. Until a vaccine is developed, AIDS will resemble drunk driving or cigarette smoking more than diphtheria or malaria; that is, mortality will rise to a high and stubborn level, which will prove very difficult to reduce. And, as in drunk driving, we will be strongly tempted to use the criminal law to punish the offender rather than to explore the roots of the disease, because the roots of the problem lie in American practices generally.

AIDS policy must begin with a realistic admission that, given the poor prospects for developing a vaccine in the immediate future, there is little hope for elimination of the disease. We can only hope to control the rate of increase among high-risk groups, and to prevent the spread into other groups. By how much we can't say for sure, but reducing the incidence of AIDS by one-half seems an almost utopian goal. Hence, neither quarantine nor isolation can be the principal path to conquering AIDS. Education is our only hope for prevention, and here we confront the barrier of societal practices regarding homosexuality.

The Public Health Service guidelines to reduce the risk of contracting or transmitting AIDS stress eliminating sex with strangers and anal intercourse, and urge the use of condoms at all times.[7] Gay groups have strongly criticized these guidelines, because their global character seems to imply that the main sexual activities of gay men are, by definition, risky. Discouraging anal intercourse, sex with strangers, or almost any sexual activity that is stimulating with those suspected of being exposed to the HIV virus, does seem unrealistic. In many states and localities the publication of such guidelines might provide grounds for criminal charges. Sodomy statutes and other laws against homosexuality serve as a powerful brake on the most potent weapon we have against AIDS—the use of a vigorous public education campaign.

Societal discrimination against gay people slows up the battle against AIDS in two ways. It threatens their health directly, and it impedes changes in gay sexual practices that heighten the risk of AIDS.

The laws against homosexuality in about half the states, as well as continuing social prejudice, prevent public health agencies from developing and aggressively carrying out frank and open sex education campaigns for safer homosexual sex, as well as frustrating prompt medical attention as a part of an overall prevention strategy. We already have ample evidence that this will occur. In the case of the federal government's recent solicitation for "Innovative Projects for AIDS Risk Reduction," the federal government requires that a program review panel, the majority of whom are not the members of at-risk groups, should review program materials to determine that the general public is not offended by sexually explicit material.[8] Federal officials obviously became jittery that successful applicants might draw the ire of opposed groups and even lawsuits, based on state sodomy statutes.

Many might conclude that, because some media and some locales permit rather extensive and public discussion of gay sexuality, these statutes are not a serious problem. While some media carry rather explicit information about "safe sex," the details of such practice are not widely publicized. It is very difficult in many areas in the U.S. to assure that these data are widely disseminated and that homosexuals can freely debate and discuss critical changes in their practices. Where openness is the rule, evidence seems to show a dramatic decline in at-risk sex.

The sodomy statutes also contribute to the poor health of many gays by discouraging their seeking prompt medical advice and treatment for many sexually transmitted diseases (STDs).

The high rate of STDs among homosexual males may increase the risk that those who become infected will develop symptoms or become full-blown AIDS cases. The same might well be true for gay men using drugs of various kinds to increase sexual stimulation. Antisodomy statutes and fear of prosecution or exposure discourage prompt medical attention and limit opportunities for communicating clear advice about safer sexual practices. Indeed, the antisodomy statues may encourage prejudice among the medical community toward homosexual patients.

The antisodomy statutes and other restrictions on gay men may also make it more likely that the sexual practices of some such individuals remain high-risk for veneral disease and AIDS. If the sexual practices of many gay men are to change, and if homosexual sex is to occur in the context of more stable relationships, the larger society will have to permit permanent forms of gay association and civil liberties that encourage such stable relationships. While societal discrimination is not the whole story behind gay liberation, gay sexual practices may have been shaped in part by societal pressures and laws forcing gay men to associate secretly in bars and bathhouses out of view of the majority community, while at the same time proscribing gay association by cohabitation and marriage. Gay people cannot now marry and are denied many other legal and social privileges of straights. The freedoms to live where one wants and with whom one wants; to make contracts; and to obtain employment in a normal manner are likely linked in subtle ways to encouraging enduring relationships, which lower the risk of exposure to STDs.

Success in the battle against AIDS depends on replacing old images of the tightly bound community based on sodomy statutes—"us" and "them"—with a more complex public health policy that combines the right to be different with the view that in matters of the common health and safety we are "one body" with a common good. This complex vision, combining equality and community, rests on a double movement; the health of the body politic depends on mutual trust and a willingness to accept the burdens of citizenship; these burdens are accepted because a narrow moralism is rejected and all are equal partners in the body politic, free to pursue their own ultimate ends.

Therefore, health education against AIDS should involve far more than disseminating explicit sex education materials. Health education means building and strengthening both equality and community, challenging traditional superstitions and defending the legitimate rights of homosexuals. Health officials should actively—albeit prudently—seek the repeal of state laws proscribing homosexuality as major barriers to this public education, laws whose continued existence threatens the public health. Public health groups should also support efforts to broaden the civil liberties of gay people and eliminate laws that permit employers, landlords, the military, or commercial establishments to discriminate in employment, housing, insurance, or military service.

While public health and the rights to citizenship are a cornerstone in any community, removing centuries of prejudice and discrimination dictates caution and political prudence. The prejudices against homosexuality are deep-seated and not likely to give way easily.

Of course, the moralist sees laws against homosexuality as ordained by God and tradition. In this view, laws forbidding sodomy among males and females or partners of the same sex are a vital bulwark against AIDS. If homosexuality were to decline sharply, the number of AIDS cases would fall in turn. Guidelines for safe sex are, accordingly, guidelines for safe sodomy and are, as such, patently repugnant.

Similarly the moralist is reluctant to distribute sterile needles to intravenous drug users as a strategy to stop the spread of AIDS. Drug use, to the moralist, is not just a health problem; it is a vice.

There are many parallels between AIDS and abortion. In *Roe v. Wade,* legal abortion was justified not on grounds of privacy alone (equality) but also on public health grounds (the common good); Justice Blackmun justified his decision in significant part because legal abortions were much safer for the mother than pregnancy and illegal abortions.[9] Securing the right to abortion strengthened the public health by removing the barriers to safe abortions.

Understandably, health officials might want to avoid another issue as contentious as abortion. But it is unlikely that they will be able to do so. The same groups that object, in the name of religion, to abortion, to sex education, and to teenage contraception also object to eliminating the sodomy laws and to expanding the right of privacy in matters of sex, as well as strengthening the rights of homosexuals to decent medical care, to employment, housing, and military service. Public health cannot ignore the blunt truth that society's restrictions on sexual freedom are a fundamental public health issue. Legal moralism has always been concerned at its core with sexual practices believed to hold together and strengthen the traditional family unit.

This is not to say that the majority has no legitimate interest in regulating gay sexual practices on the grounds of morality. Many of these practices may give deep offense to members of the community, much as many features of heterosexual practices placed on public display are offensive. The public peace surely demands reasonable regulation of public sexual practices. The majority seems especially fearful regarding the relation of homosexuals and the young, despite the evidence that sexual molestation seems largely a crime of heterosexual males. Yet prudence seems to indicate that with repeal of sodomy statutes, statutes against child abuse need to be strengthened where necessary.

Moralists believe that certain forms of behavior must be observed if society's central orders—religion, work, family, and relations between the sexes—are to be upheld. Honor to parents, devotion to family, chastity, hard work, and the fear of God are in themselves valuable and should be preserved. But religious morality often becomes a triumph of form over substance. Like those who demythologize superstitions and myths in the Bible, replacing these with the timeless ethic of love and community, the health official must seek to transcend a traditional morality and focus debate on the link between the common good and the equal rights of our fellow citizens who are gay.

In the case of the Bible, John Boswell's exhaustive study of the issue of homosexuality suggests that Sodom was destroyed not because of the abomination of homosexuality, but because the Sodomites refused hospitality to strangers.[10] In fact, homosexuality is explicitly forbidden in only one place in the Old Testament and there for reasons of ritual impurity (like the eating of pork), and not as a fundamental sin.

In the New Testament, Jesus did not mention homosexuality at all; and his ministry to prostitutes, thieves, beggars, and the poor constituted a scandal to the moralists of his time. In fact,

Jesus's reference to the story of Sodom's fall in Matthew 10:14 refers to the Sodomites' lack of hospitality: "Whosoever shall not receive you, nor hear your words, when ye depart out of that house or city, shake off the dust of your feet. Verily I say unto you, it shall be more tolerable for the land of Sodom and Gomorrah in the day of judgment, than for that city." Jesus's attack on religious moralism and his elevation of a gospel of love and community were the principal reasons for his being put to death.

Even Paul, who had some harsh things to say about homosexuality (references which John Boswell persuasively argues may refer more to male prostitution than to homosexuality per se) struggled mightily to rescue Christianity from a narrow religious moralism (witness his attack on religious superstitions surrounding circumcision), and to place it on the foundations of community and love for the neighbor.

Republican Rome, like Golden Age Greece, tolerated homosexual practices. Until the late Middle Ages, the secular authorities largely ignored homosexuality, leaving the regulation of this behavior to the Church. As persecution began to build, Aquinas seems to have condemned homosexuality and other sexual deviations less on theological grounds than as a concession to changing political values. But by the sixteenth century in England, Henry VIII (in part because of his quarrel with Rome) made sodomy or "buggery" a matter of criminal law, to reduce the authority of the Church. The American colonists incorporated the English statutes, making homosexuality a capital offense. Apparently, in the years before the American revolution, only one person was put to death under this law.[11] Nineteenth-century England was another story. According to one authority, "[M]en were regularly hanged for homosexual relations in nineteenth-century England—sixty in the first three decades of the century and another score under naval regulations."[12]

In our times, the trend has been to remove the ancient prejudices and superstitions perserved in the antisodomy statutes in the states—twenty-six states have done so. And some locales have passed gay civil rights ordinances to protect against discrimination. Recently in Georgia, a homosexual male entered federal court arguing that charges of sodomy brought against him for acts committed with a consenting partner in his own home were unconstitutional.[13] While the federal district court ruled against him, the federal circuit court reversed, arguing that these cases demanded a more strict scrutiny if they were to pass the constitutional test. In other words, the state had to demonstrate that it had a compelling interest in legislating against homosexuality, and that this legislation was the most limited means available to achieve its purpose.

The Supreme Court, for the time being, has rejected this view.[14] By a 5 to 4 move in *Bowers v. Hardwick,* the Court upheld the right of the majority to legislate against homosexual acts, committed even in private, on the grounds that repugnance for homosexuality is an ancient and deeply rooted community sentiment. In an earlier decision, the future Chief Justice compared these laws to public health legislation to prevent the spread of communicable diseases. Justice Rehnquist, in 1978, said that laws controlling homosexuals are constitutionally akin to "whether those suffering from measles have a constitutional right, in violation of quarantine regulations, to associate together and with others who do not presently have measles."[15] Rehnquist echoes James F. Stephen in the nineteenth century when he said, "Vice is as infectious as disease, and happily virtue is infectious, though health is not. Both vice and virtue are transmittable, and, to a considerable extent, hereditary."[16]

The decision of the Supreme Court is a threat to the entire advance of the privacy decisions of the past two decades. The work of the Court in trying to untangle the claims of moralism, and the claims of public health, by forging a new equality that combines the common good and the right to be left alone in new ways, has been left dangling. If the Court's ruling is to be reversed, the thesis that legal moralism threatens the public health as well as the rights of all citizens, including gays, must be pressed even more vigorously.

Sexual Practices and Paternalism

A sound public health policy depends on both loosening and tightening the bonds of community. Rejecting moralism does not mean that society can have nothing to say about sexual practices. Sex per se, and that includes homosexual sex, is not the business of the community. But sexual practices that threaten the common health are.

Sexual practices can have many consequences for the public health. Private conduct, even sexual conduct, which threatens compelling community interests like health and safety, is not beyond the reach of regulation, even if the individuals involved are consenting adults. Of course, there are overwhelming practical limits to this principle, but affirming it is important nonetheless.

Human sexuality is an imperative drive like hunger or safety, and sexual practices, at least in private, are likely very resistant to legal prohibition or regulation. Nevertheless, the public health official cannot ignore sexual practices that are unsafe, dangerous, and a threat to all. Public health information campaigns must not flinch from promoting a standard of sexual conduct that is safe and prudent from everyone's standpoint.

The sexual practices of male homosexuals have become a central controversy in the AIDS debate. According to investigators, many AIDS patients report 1,000 sexual partners over a single lifetime,[17] a notorious statistic overshadowing discussion of AIDS prevalence. It is not surprising that those most widely exposed to the risk of infection should become the first AIDS cases.

An authoritative survey of gay sexual practices reveals that this kind of strenuous sexual activity remains confined to a minority; nevertheless, one third of all male homosexuals surveyed nationally reported that they had more than 50 to 70 sexual partners in the previous year.[18] Gay men report that they participate in sexual contact with persons unknown to each other "very frequently" or "fairly frequently." Favorite cruising places for casual sex have included parks and public restrooms, as well as the back rooms of bars where the owners permit such liaisons. Another site for casual sex is the bathhouse, which many gay men prefer because so little effort is required to make contacts.

Another index to the sexual practices of male homosexuals is sexually transmitted diseases. Individuals who are exclusively homosexuals for a considerable part of their lives constitute 5 to 10 percent of the adult male population, according to Kinsey's estimate. If the statistics are reliable, this group accounts for a third of all cases of infectious syphilis, a high rate of gonorrhea, and an increasing rate of hepatitis A and B. Gay males are also at much greater risk for bacterial and enteric diseases like amebiasis and giardiasis. The risk of herpes and other dermatologic disorders is also much greater among gay males.[19]

In 1977, in New York City, 55 percent of all reported cases of syphilis occurred in homosexual males, even though syphilis, among heterosexuals nationwide, has been declining at a remarkable rate. Homosexual men are reported to be ten times more likely to contract syphilis than heterosexuals.

The epidemic of sexually transmitted diseases among homosexual males is in significant part a result of sexual liberation. Gay liberation meant far more than sexual liberation, but a heavy price has been paid for some of the forms sexual liberation has taken in the gay community. The freedom to have multiple sexual contacts with strangers in one evening, and to continue this practice over a period of years, has exposed hundreds of thousands, perhaps one to two million individuals, to a deadly virus. If recent reports are borne out, exposure to the virus may bring the full-blown AIDS disease to as many as 25 to 40 percent of those infected, a much higher risk than originally thought. The spectre of as many as 250,000 to 400,000 cases (the current level of deaths is 15,000), will dramatically increase societal pressures to blame the victim.

As the toll of the disease among homosexuals mounts, the deadly risks associated with homosexual sex are likely to have the greatest impact in reshaping homosexual life. Words like "promiscuity" are regarded by gays with deep suspicion as covert attacks on homosexuality itself. To minimize suspicion we should observe the distinction between restrictions for sexual standards protecting the common life and restrictions promoting an official sexual morality. Frequent sexual activity is of no interest to the law and the community unless it escalates the risk of serious disease. When the disease is AIDS, the community interest becomes paramount, and official educational campaigns should discourage high-risk sex with strangers. Even if such practices as oral and anal sex are presently beyond the law, informed self-interest should help work to bring sharp declines in free-wheeling sex with strangers.

Should public officials go beyond education? Should, for instance, police monitor gay "cruising" for sexual liaisons where there is a high likelihood of contacts between strangers and where the risk of spreading infection is very high? Here the potential for abuse by the police is very great, and the boundaries between controlling homosexuality per se, versus protecting health and safety, are extremely blurred. The likely outcome will be only to make heterosexuals feel (falsely) reassured and the gay community discriminated against.

The major debate has concerned closing or regulating public places such as bathhouses where dangerous sex is practiced. San Francisco took such steps, but the New York City health authorities took a different position. While the state health officials ultimately overruled them, New York City officials argued that the impact of such closings would be minuscule in terms of the overall threat. Still, the public health official is not required to demonstrate that the closings or regulation will result in containing the epidemic. But at the same time, officials should take steps to assure all concerned that the aim is to regulate the public health, not homosexuality, tipping the scales toward regulation versus outright closing. It may well be that regulation, and in the worst cases outright closings, could be a potent symbol for community action.

On the other hand, some argue that these commercial establishments ought to be used to promote safer sex. This tactic has a familiar ring, something like getting the liquor industry to promote "responsible drinking." An industry that has an interest in promoting casual sex—whether bathhouses or bars—is unlikely to be seriously interested in a health education campaign. Realism should guide our regulatory policy. The goal is to restrict commercial establishments that have an interest in unsafe sex—places where sex between strangers is promoted as a commodity. The fact that some hotels, incidental to their doing business, have couples among their guests practicing high-risk sex, is not an adequate argument against closing bathhouses or bars where casual sex is a main feature.

The lead in any public discourse about gay sexual practices must come from the gay community itself. Such a change can only come from a full and extensive dialogue, which should be open, frank, and based on as much careful and dispassionate research as is possible. At all times the participants should remind themselves that the discussion is about public health, not moralism.

Gay people who object that the majority community ought

not control the private behavior of consenting adults forget that membership in the community—which is the ground of public health protections against AIDS—carries obligations as well as benefits. Paternalism to defend the common life protects the health and safety of sexual partners and helps solidify the norms of the shared community. At the present time, frequent sexual activity among strangers promotes spread of a deadly disease. Until this disease is controlled we all share a common interest in a more conservative and restrictive standard for sexual morality.

For their side, homosexuals need to take the leadership and to call for self-imposed restrictions. This is already happening. Also, health statistics in San Francisco and New York City suggest that thousands of gays are altering their lifestyles. Many gay leaders have begun publicly to repudiate the fast-lane life. Political prudence suggests that if gay people want gains against discrimination in housing, employment, medical care, and insurance, then their leaders should speak out against dangerous sexual practices within their community.

I have devoted very little attention to intravenous drug users, a high-risk group that will likely grow more important in the AIDS epidemic. There are many parallels between the problems of preventing AIDS among drug users and homosexuals, not the least of which is that many drug users are homosexual. It is unclear which activity—unsafe sex or contaminated needles—is the primary mode of transmitting AIDS for many individuals. Both activities are illegal, at least in many places, and both groups are the target of deep societal fears and prejudices. The biggest difference is that drug use itself presents a strong health risk for the addict whereas homosexuality per se does not.

Society will certainly have to reevaluate the restrictions in many states on availability to addicts of sterile needles and syringes. Also, as the disease spreads through heroin users, we may have to reopen the controversial question of whether heroin addicts should be registered and furnished safe supplies of heroin by physicians as the most practical way to control the spread of AIDS in the population.

Above all else, for both these groups we should keep our eyes on the central issue—the many ways in which centuries of religious and social superstitions and prejudice stand in the way of improving the public health. Modern public health rests on a complex equality that replaces traditional restrictions with limits rooted in protection against actual harms. Equating the public health with simplistic restrictions on homosexuality per se will only result in fruitless debates over matters like quarantine and isolation, public health strategies that have little role in this epidemic. Hoping for a technological shortcut in the form of a vaccine is not realistic and can cost tens of thousands of lives, especially if this hope keeps us from facing the task of public education and reform of our laws against homosexuality. These reforms can help prepare the way for altering sexual lifestyles among the gay community. The public health community should take the lead and, state by state, demand the repeal of harmful statutes and restrictions on gay life. The health of the body politic depends on rejecting the communal disease of sexual prejudice.

NOTES

1. For a good discussion of "moralism," see Hugo Adam Bedau's discussion in Edwin M. Schur and Hugo Adam Bedau, *Victimless Crimes* (Englewood Cliffs, NJ: Prentice-Hall, 1974). See also Joel Feinberg, *Social Philosophy* (Englewood Cliffs, NJ: Prentice-Hall, 1973) and H.L.A. Hart, *Law, Liberty, and Morality* (New York: Vintage Books, 1963); Ronald Dworkin, *Taking Rights Seriously* (Cambridge: Harvard University Press, 1977), Chapter 11; and A.D. Woozley, "Law and the Legislation of Morality," in *Ethics in Hard Times*, Daniel Callahan and Arthur Caplan, eds. (New York: Plenum, 1981).
2. James Fitzjames Stephen, *Liberty, Equality, Fraternity*, R.J. White, ed. (Cambridge: Cambridge University Press, 1967).
3. John Stuart Mill, "On Liberty," in M. Cohen, ed., *The Philosophy of John Stuart Mill* (New York: Modern Library, 1961), pp. 155–319.
4. Bedau, p. 90.
5. Lord Patrick Devlin, *The Enforcement of Morals* (Oxford: Oxford Univeristy Press, 1959).
6. See H.L.A. Hart, "Social Solidarity and the Enforcement of Morality," *The University of Chicago Law Review* 35 (1967), 1–13, for one of the best critiques of the thesis that society is held together by a specific moral practice.

7. "Prevention of Acquired Immunodeficiency Syndrome (AIDS): Report of Interagency Recommendations," *Morbidity and Mortality Weekly Report* 32:101–103, March 4, 1983.

8. See Barry Adkins, "GMHC Accepts Grant from CDC for Sex Education Research," *The New York Native,* February 10–16, 1986, p. 8. For a good discussion of the potential for an anti-AIDS campaign to serve as cover for a campaign to control homosexuality, see "AIDS—A New Reason to Regulate Homosexuality?" *Journal of Contemporary Law* 11 (1984), 315–43.

9. *Roe v. Wade,* 410 U.S. 113, (1973).

10. The source of this history of Roman and Christian attitudes toward homosexuality is John Boswell's *Christianity, Social Tolerance, and Homosexuality* (Chicago: The University of Chicago Press, 1980).

11. See Robert Oaks, "Perceptions of Homosexuality by Justices of the Peace in Colonial Virginia," in *Homosexuality and the Law.* (A Special Double issue of *The Journal of Homosexuality*) 5 (1979/80), 35–42.

12. These data are found in Bernard Knox's book review, "Subversive Activities," *The New York Review of Books,* December 19, 1985, p. 3. Knox was reviewing Louis Crompton's *Byron and Greek Love, Homophobia in Nineteenth-Century England* (Berkeley: University of California Press, 1985).

13. Kenneth R. Wing, "Constitutional Protection of Sexual Privacy in the 1980s: What *is* Big Brother Doing in the Bedroom?" *American Journal of Public Health* 76 (February 1986), 201–04. The Georgia case is *Hardwick v. Bowers* 760 F.2d, 1202 (1985) reh'g denied. 765 F2d 1123 (11th Circ. 1985).

14. *Bowers v. Hardwick,* 478 U.S.——, 92 LEd2d 140 (1986).

15. See David A.J. Richards, "Homosexual Acts and the Constitutional Right to Privacy," and "Public Manifestations of Personal Morality: Limitations on the Use of Solicitation Statutes to Control Homosexual Cruising," in *Homosexuality and the Law.* (A Special Double Issue of *The Journal of Homosexuality*), 5 (1979/80), 43–66. The 1978 case is *Ratchford v. Gay Lib,* 434 U.S. 1080, 1082, reh'g denied, 435 U.S. 981 (1978).

16. Stephen, p. 146.

17. See Mary E. Guinan, et al., "Heterosexual and Homosexual Patients with the Acquired Immunodeficiency Syndrome:

A Comparision of Surveillance, Interview, and Laboratory data." *Annals of Internal Medicine* 100 (1984), 213–18; and H.W. Jaffe, K. Choi, and P.A. Thomas, et al., "National Case-control Study of Kaposi's Sarcoma and *Pneumocystis Carinii* Pneumonia in Homosexual Men: Part 1. Epidemiological Results," *Annals of Internal Medicine* 99 (1983), 145–51.

18. Karla Jay and Allen Young, *The Gay Report* (New York: Summit Books, 1977).

19. Terry Alan Sandholzer, "Factors Affecting the Incidence and Management of Sexually Transmitted Diseases in Homosexual Men," in *Sexually Transmitted Diseases in Homosexual Men: Diagnosis, Treatment, and Research.* Ed. David G. Ostrow, Terry Alan Sandholzer, and Yehudi M. Felman (New York: Plenum, Medicae Book Co., 1983), pp. 3–12. The estimates of the numbers of gay males in the adult population is from *Sexual Behavior in the Human Male* by Alfred C. Kinsey, Wardell B. Pomeroy, and Clyde E. Martin (Philadelphia: W.B. Saunders Co, 1948) (The Kinsey Report).

The HIV Epidemic in the Age of Medical Scarcity

Nancy F. McKenzie, Ph.D.

Introduction

The HIV [Human Immunodeficiency Virus] epidemic is one that will test our medical ingenuity as well as our ethical commitments.[1] HIV is a largely fatal disease that is incurable; it is global and its control is nowhere in sight. Public health models of catastrophic financial, behavioral, social, ethical, and political impact are appropriate to understanding the epidemic but they often leave out how the epidemic itself is influenced by our current systems of response—health care, education, and employment. This paper will examine our current system of health care and its relationship to the epidemic.

Many articles about the relationship between medicine and HIV highlight the ways in which medicine—the social, institutional, and ethical practice of medicine—is greatly affected by the HIV epidemic. Everything from issues of health care allocation and distribution to the desire of people to become doctors; from confidentiality to the question of the duty to treat, indicates that the epidemic will change medicine for years and possibly decades to come. I have entitled this article "The HIV Epidemic in the Age of Medical Scarcity" because I wish to highlight the connection between our present health care system, which rations medical resources,[2] and the medical exigencies of being HIV-affected. In my argument I will try to display a set of relationships that obtain between health care and the epidemic in America which discloses conditions that have been almost completely neglected in the social commentary on the epidemic. I will look at three features of our health care system. The first two features—our public health care system and the system of primary care—are institutional features and influence the third, discrimination, which is social. The interrelationship between the health care systems, the organization of care-giving itself, and the social attitudes toward HIV infection serve to show how complicated the obstacles are to an effective response to the epidemic.[3]

I. Public Health

Public health medicine has various meanings. One meaning is evaluational and relates to the health of the society as a whole. As medical response, public health agendas are those designed to prevent conditions of medical vulnerability, whether of a microbic or an environmental nature. This view and its response is predicated on the moral position that there are some health stratagems that are out of the reach of some individuals who cannot acquire or maintain them without the help of public agencies and/or without accommodating some change in the public arena itself. In a completely privatized health care system as we have in America, public health medicine essentially sets the floor for those who cannot compete in the market of medical goods. In the most general sense public health medicine is the medicine designed to target those persons who cannot buy themselves out of risk by individually purchasing a healthy environment. This environment may consist of periodic sets of medical advice about prevention; regular and individualized medical intervention for personal health; the parks and green of the suburbs; non-criminal, non-knife-wielding neighbors; a drug-free peer group for one's self and one's child; or a clean, non-toxic work space. "*Public health*" in the first sense is a relative term. It relies for its definition upon a comparison between the level the most well-off can accomplish for themselves *versus* those who are at various levels of physical or mental jeopardy. It applies to that changing set of health matrices, especially in a full market economy, that put certain people at health risk through no actions of their own yet allow others to purchase the common "health space" of work, neighborhood, and environment for their own use and/or profit. Public health strategies provide a public safety net for those vulnerable enough to be put at health risk merely by being born into an unprotected economic class. In the 1980s, we are witnessing the consequences of our economy. The racial and economic reality of HIV infection magnifies the neglected areas of public health. The indicators of America's lack of a public health care system are a soaring rate of infant mortality, tuberculosis, syphilis, and drug dependency.

Under conditions of scarcity where there are very few resources for responding to various levels of health crisis, a paradoxical thing occurs. In an economic period of market entrenchment when medical care and health knowledge are contracting, as is the case now and was also in the 1930s Depression, a second definition of public health, as it pertains to contagious and infectious diseases, becomes visible and emphasized. During a period when there is a present crisis in the health of a large segment of the population, especially when infection is involved, public health in the full sense of a safety or welfare net is the first form of medicine to disappear, to be replaced by public health as *containment* or protection. In an epidemic, this could be neither more predictable, nor more catastrophic since those most vulnerable in an epidemic are those most vulnerable economically. So far, in the United States, we have only discussed the later sense of the public health. The first meaning, however, is the crucial issue.

The present lack of a public health *medical* system in America has some obvious collateral epidemiological consequences. While we have a highly developed epidemiologically, statistically oriented public health sector, we have little else that allows us to confront the public health emergency that is upon us. We have no national form of medical education, no national apparatus for disseminating public health information, and must rely on school districts and local media, with their political factionalism, to educate the public about the disease, preventive strategies and effects. Lacking a governmental structure for reaching the individual through education (many of the affected populations are not literate or are not connected to the public school system) or medically (most medical care for the affected

populations is marginal medicine—part of research and education in urban settings where a patient never sees the same
student-physician twice and only the most skeletal medical staff
is operative),[4] there is really no way in which to reach the
people most in need of a response to their HIV-affection.

It is not only present public health education and public
health thinking that is inadequate to this epidemic. The most
insidious aspect of the epidemic is who is getting it. Poverty,
like homelessness, although not a medical problem in itself,
rapidly becomes one. The indigent of America are also the
medically homeless from both a public health perspective and a
primary care perspective (more on this in Section II). In the last
twenty years the poor of America have become (ideological)
symbols of a voluntarist or social-condition poverty: "the homeless," "the drug dependent," "the child-parents," "the non-
literate," "the institutionalized," and "the *de*-institutionalized."
What these groups share, besides their poverty and their stigmatized objectification, is chronic vulnerability. If the condition
of devastating poverty (which does not occur to this extent in
any other developed country of the world except South Africa)
does not lead to malnutrition and, hence, to an immuno-
compromised state via lack of education, or money for food,
medical care, pre- and postnatal care, or a stable home, then
there is *no* relationship between social/economic conditions and
health. If there *is* a relationship between poverty and disease,
this lack of a system of preventive care, community health care,
and education makes *poverty a pre-existing condition for the
HIV virus* and an entré into a rebounding spiral of further
disease, homelessness, and joblessness.[5] And an even greater
inability to pay for medical care.

Because public health in the resource sense has been sharply
dismantled since the end of the 1970s, the medical response to
the epidemic has come through private organizations. Many
kinds of communities of care currently exist—but on the same
bases that soup kitchens and shelters for battered women exist
for the fully disenfranchised, i.e., primarily without government
acknowledgment or support. Very few communities have been
effective in their response to the epidemic except GMHC [Gay
Men's Health Crisis] in New York City and the Shanti Project
in San Francisco. These particular projects have been enor-

mously effective in setting up true health care options and in lowering the transmission rates among the populations they serve because their organization emerged out of the community.[6,7]

II. Primary Care

Whatever is true for the individual who, in urban settings, attempts to purchase primary care medicine, is ten-fold true for the HIV-affected person. In New York City there has been a reversal of thinking about medical shortage. Initially it was predicted that the existence of HIV infection would take a great toll on the health care system. Now health policy wisdom seems to be that the primary care system itself has a nursing shortage, a shortage of beds, and a significant rise in patient population that is "sicker and much more difficult to manage." This situation predates the epidemic.[8]

Middle-class Americans don't, for the most part, get infectious diseases that require long periods of hospitalization. This is due to preventive strategies long integrated into American communities through private physicians (education, vaccines, inoculations, diet; a wholly "private health system") and the introduction of antibiotics. Although chronic disease is still the focus of American medicine, the medical university, the central headquarters of American health care, relies most markedly upon replacement surgery and technological therapies. The general practitioner has, in fact, almost been eliminated from health care due to the proliferation of subspecialty medicine across the board. As the most developed health care system in the world, we know more about heart transplants than about prenatal care.

Enter infectious diseases in great numbers—not merely HIV-related conditions but new and virulent outbreaks of syphilis, tuberculosis, resistant strains of pneumonia, and pelvic inflammatory disease among women. Not only are many city hospitals without beds and facilities for these populations, they are, more importantly, without a medical orientation to primary care; without the ability to treat and care for the suffering who are essentially helpless and without social, economic, or even inter-personal resources.[9]

Treating the clinical manifestations of AIDS and ARC (AIDS Related Complex) is much like practicing medicine prior to the introduction of antibiotics; much like doing medicine in nine-teenth-century Dickensian England. This is not only because of the inability of medicine to cure infections that largely affect indigent and socially vulnerable populations, but also because of a critical lack of facilities for chronic care in general and a dearth of primary care providers.

The alleviation of suffering is not an American medical agenda, and most physicians do not possess the training, the interper-sonal skills, or the patience to treat such helplessness on a daily basis. Physicians are finding HIV-related conditions the chal-lenge of their careers. They are unaccustomed to treating long-term illnesses and are unused to treating acute illness without a "magic bullet." Prior to the HIV epidemic there were patients who were uneducated, uninformed about medicine, economi-cally helpless, and without resources outside the hospital. With the onset of the epidemic, we have all of that *and* patients infected with an often fatal, largely untreatable virus. Add to this physicians' attitudes about poverty, the existence of racism and homophobia, and a numbing lack of respect for the intrave-nous drug user, and we naturally find debates like that in the *New England Journal of Medicine* over whether physicians have a duty to treat the person with AIDS ("There is a Duty to Treat the AIDS Patient," January, 1988.) Of six letters of response to the editor printed together, not one agreed with the article.[10]

The HIV epidemic is not *bringing about* a crisis in primary care in America, it is disclosing it.[11] HIV-affected people are now the socially visible group that knows what it means to negotiate their health through emergency rooms in our urban cities. They know that in this arena services are, by and large, denied them. The HIV-affected person encounters the palpable consequences of only having access to poverty-medicine.

III. Discrimination

The New York City Commission on Human Rights calls the social climate of the HIV epidemic the "second epidemic." If public health care and primary care are vital to a humane outcome for the HIV-affected, an equally necessary component is a strict antidiscrimination law. This latter necessity is the one least talked about by health professionals, yet this is an absolutely indispensable adjunct to the medical necessities of the epidemic. Quite simply understood is the fact that sick people require a support system that begins with partners and radiates out through the echelons of family, friends, neighbors, churches, community organizations, public services, and medical and legal institutions. This support system—extending from the patient on out through larger social units and passing the barrier from the purely private domain of self and family to the public domains of education, housing, employment, transportation, medical institutions, and the justice system—is a continuum of support that one takes for granted and simply knows is in place when one is ill. The assumption is not merely a psychological one. It is a *tenet* of health care to the extent that, as sick individuals, we call each level into play as we navigate from acute or chronic disease to recovery and then to health. Individuals do not survive debilitating illness without a truly comprehensive health care system, involving both accommodation and support in the private and public arenas of their lives.[12] In the time of HIV, this system, though already limited by the strata of racism, sexism, economic deprivation, or homophobia, is entirely negated. The stigma associated with the disease requires the sick to withdraw their reliance on any system of support. The fact that one cannot tell one's partner, family, neighbor, church or social club, employer, teacher, bus driver, storekeeper, landlord, or even doctor or dentist that one has an HIV-related condition without the expectation of *reprisals* completely changes the expectation of "being ill in America."[13] A not unimportant consequence is that this makes public health strategies in the *containment* sense almost impossible to accomplish. Prevention of contagious disease requires the visibility of information about who is infected—something that can only be accomplished in a climate of mutual trust. The assumption of truth and knowledge are built into our modalities of care, of research, of health practice. They are the expectations of trust and reliance without which we cannot give or receive good medical care, do the research necessary to study the epidemic, or proceed with the smooth running of any public agency. Being hated and feared for being sick is, in fact, entirely destructive of attempts to control the virus or of efforts to ameliorate its suffering. Currently, secrecy and invisibility about one's HIV status are required at every level.

The main officials who could stop the "second epidemic" from occurring are health professionals. The American Medical Association, the National Institutes of Health, the American Dental Association, and others could, in fact, declare that both epidemics cannot be addressed without effective antidiscrimination legislation, and they could recommend that such legislation be instituted where needed and applied where already existent. The Center for Disease Control could make such recommendations today.[14] Such legislation would increase the use of federal disability antidiscrimination law to protect the HIV-affected person. This would essentially eliminate material reprisals for being ill and would put back in place the apparatus of support and information so necessary to treatment and research for the medical epidemic. The fact that this has not occurred and that health professionals, even in the face of finding themselves HIV-affected, have not required tough use of such legislation indicates that discrimination is itself a very complex phenomenon.

The current social attitude toward the HIV-affected person *is* a nasty blend of racism, sexism, heterosexism, and voluntarism[15] and, like most social bias, begins or is sanctioned from the top down—from leadership down to the individual. But it is equally fueled by social institutions, particularly those that are in economic crisis.[16]

Bias against the HIV-affected originates with medicine. We often forget this. It is fueled by the current state of health care delivery.[16] The stigma connected to HIV-infection emerges out of the demedicalization of chronic diseases and the resocialization of illness that has been occurring in a somewhat chaotic fashion for twenty years. The easiest way to see the relationship between this stigmatization and medical scarcity is to look at the history of drug addiction.

The health care delivery system is not a monolithic institution. But it is capable of conferring definition upon human suffering and of doing so with a connotation of patient culpability. What has occurred in America in the change from private to for-profit medicine has been the neglect of many kinds of medical vulnerability as well as their redefinition.[18] The neglect has not only resulted in barring the medically indigent from access to health care goods, it has done so through the *redefinition* of their plight as a socially or individually induced plight. For instance, America in one decade (the 1970s) treated drug addiction as a medical condition and offered public programs to fund and treat it, even going so far as to pass two kinds of federal legislation to protect the addicted from discrimination and unemployment.[19] In the present decade, addiction is treated as a "criminal from within" and enormous medical energy is spent devising tests to insure a "drug free" work space.

There is no absolute definition of health. It is always relative to social or class function. Hence, cosmetic surgery can in one era be considered frivolous; in another, a psychological necessity. In the last forty years, medicine has reduced its urban involvement, organized itself corporately, and literally "moved out of town" to offer for-profit franchise medicine in affluent sectors of America.[20] The social measure of this economic reorganization is the change in the definition of illness. Medicine has effectively stigmatized certain conditions and has made them components of larger social problems or reduced them to individual responsibility.[21]

In consequence, the health care needs of many Americans have not only been neglected, they have become invisible. We spend a great deal of energy on social discourse about drug addiction without talking about its medical requirements. This invisibility not only fails to acknowledge the medical need of a great many people, but it has lulled the medical profession itself into complacency about suffering, which puts into stark relief the plight of the person with HIV-related illnesses. Not only does medicine no longer relate to the indigent poor, it is alarmed if one multiply afflicted person graces its door.

Health, mental health, and substance abuse now require different specialties whose interaction is often an obstacle to the delivery of services. The distribution of medicine into components of disease, each with different funding streams, has made it difficult for the health professional to confront the truly powerless patient.

The structure of medicine has done to the HIV-affected person what it has done to the mentally ill and to the victim of homelessness. The intern or student doctor trying to treat a multiple diagnosis in a homeless or deinstitutionalized person, or a person with an HIV-related illness, finds a blur of conflicting agendas. In the end, he or she regards that person as one representative of a social condition that it is not his or her job to treat. (Sometimes all three—homelessness, drug addiction, and HIV conditions—converge in the same individual. In fact, this is becoming quite common.)

Recently someone in New York said, "Homelessness is a housing problem." What should have been tautological all these years has finally surfaced as the economic problem that it is. Once it dawns on the American public that this is the case, homelessness will no longer be a stigmatized social condition. It will be treated as the economic context of some very real physical and mental struggles.[22] The same is true of drug addiction and, finally, of being HIV-affected. Drug addiction is a medical condition that, because of neglect, has become a way of life—thus, by definition, a social condition. It must be retrieved from that status.

The medical conditions of HIV-infection require a multidisciplinary approach and one that can, indeed, pull apart various aspects of the disease and its accompanying social crises for the individual. But this is difficult to do. HIV is additionally an infectious disease. Because of the scarcity conditions of our public hospitals, is it any wonder that medical professionals are wary of treating the HIV-affected patient? If instruments cannot be sterilized and one has no home to discharge patients to, no beds, a five-day wait for full laboratory work-ups, or one glove per floor per shift, is it any wonder that a discriminatory climate emerges?[23] This is not an individual attitude problem. It is structural discrimination that will not be eliminated merely through training or education. This is not to say that training and orientation to HIV-related illness and HIV-related discrimination wouldn't be a help to caretakers. It is to say that the conditions of our health care system are such that health goods are severely limited. Insofar as that is true in myriad HIV arenas, it is easy to see that the remedies of more money for beds, or more or better testing techniques, or more research into "high risk populations" will not solve the health crisis that is upon us.[24]

Conclusion

The crisis of the HIV epidemic is not simply one of access to health care or of the lack of quality in primary care or a problem of discrimination. It is a crisis formed by all *three* conditions. Two-class medicine, high-tech medicine, and social marginalization all interact to eclipse an effective response to HIV-related conditions.

Recommendations

I. The HIV epidemic cannot be dealt with financially at local levels. Only a federal strategy can begin to confront the needs that the HIV epidemic discloses. We will not be able to stop the epidemic. Although that should certainly be one of our public health goals, more important is a response to the differential effects that the epidemic is having upon communities. The needs for education, financial organization, medical care, child care, drug rehabilitation centers, crisis intervention, and housing differ with each community. Public health in the community sense must be a national priority. This will require infusions of money directly to communities for their own preventive agendas, research, and responses. The current methodology of public health without community leadership and input will result in very little information and little true intervention. Public health programs at university centers should be organized as neighborhood advocacy programs. Students and professors would work not on research but upon empowerment at the community level through self-organized and self-run research units; making recommendations to the community; setting up resources; monitoring responses. Only community-run public health medicine is public health medicine.

II. A national health program must be instituted. This cannot be a program organized merely for economic change—one in which the federal government is the third-party payer. The health care system must itself be revamped. While guaranteeing health care to everyone (and this includes preventive care), the health care system must be designed to decentralize medicine from university headquarters. Health care should be housed in community clinics with expanded backup of hospices and residential facilities for acute illness, employing members of the communities as paraprofessional and homecare personnel. If business colleges and unions can offer credentialing programs for homecare workers and nursing assistants, why not communities in conjunction with clinic facilities? The current expanse of HMO and other prospective payment programs could be easily reorganized as community-owned and community-run medical facilities (particularly those that could include rehabilitative programs for substance and alcohol addiction) and expanded to do preventive care. Housing and employment for the HIV-affected, particularly as they suffer progressive debilitation, as well as provisions for their children, both with them and in foster care agencies, would cut down upon the severe physical, economic, psychological, and emotional problems the HIV-affected undergo from the current lack of these resources.

III. HIV discrimination, like most bias, enters the picture when there is too little of some necessary social good—too few jobs, too little health care, too few apartments. If we can solve the material health, housing, and employment needs of Americans by focusing upon community endeavors, bias against the HIV-affected will slowly dissolve. In the interim, federal prosecution of discriminatory practices against people with disabilities would send a clear and consistent message that America is a nation that will not tolerate bias against people who are ill. In addition, merely the visible antidiscrimination stand by national leaders with respect to HIV-affection would alleviate many of the attitudes of professionals who still deny treatment or services to the HIV affected.

NOTES

1. The years ahead promise to strain our social fabric, for the health care system reflects the true existence of our economic health. As Karen Davis and Diane Rowland point out:

   Unemployment levels today are the highest since the Great Depression. With unemployment, the American worker loses not only a job but also health insurance protection. As unemployment rises and the numbers of the uninsured grow, fewer and fewer resources are available to fill the gaps in health care coverage.

   (*Milbank Memorial Fund Quarterly*/Health and Society, Vol. 61, No. 2, 1983.) Given this economic picture, the HIV epidemic, in effect, merely crushes an already crippled health care delivery system.

2. One component of this rationing is the DRG—the Diagnostic Related Group—a criterion for Medicare and Medicaid payment which restricts the length of hospital stay connected to specified illnesses. Much of the criticism of DRGs points out that there really cannot be a predetermination of hospital need defined through type of illness. Hence, to provide a criterion for payment based upon such predetermination merely puts an immutable cap upon treatment, depriving mainly the poor of therapy appropriate to their illness. DRGs are but the federal form of prospective payment programs—programs that restrict the type of care given by predetermination of need. HMOs are also programs that provide such minimal care. The effect on patients with chronic illnesses and upon preventive care is obvious. For the effect on mortality rate of such programs see "Changes in Location of Death After Passage of Medicare's Prospective Payment System: A National Study," Mark Sager, et al., *New England Journal of Medicine,* Vol. 320, No. 7, February 16, 1989. The general trend of the prospective payment system is to eliminate the difficult case (the seriously ill) from treatment as a way in which a hospital can operate in a cost-effective manner. Such difficult cases are called "outliers." See Allen Meadors and Nick Wilson, "Prospective Payment System for Hospital Reimbursement, Part II" in *Hospital Administration Currents,* 29:1 (1985), 3, for a five-step plan on how to "Avoid Outliers As Much As Possible." No one is more of an "outlier" than an AIDS patient.

3. For a more historical, complex, and not so political analysis of the interdependence of the three areas of neglect by American health care policy, see Daniel Fox's "AIDS and the American Health Polity: The History and the Prospects of a Crisis of Authority," *Milbank Quarterly,* Vol. 64, Suppl. 1, 1986. I am thankful to David Willis, editor of the *Milbank Quarterly,* for pointing me to Fox's article. Would that I had found it prior to the writing of this piece.

4. Barbara and John Ehrenreich gave an excellent description of this marginal care in 1969:

> But today's resident of slums like Brooklyn's Bedford-Stuyvesant, or Chicago's south side, is as effectively removed from health services as his relatives who stayed behind in Mississippi. One region of Bedford-Stuyvesant contains only one practicing physician for a population of one hundred thousand. ("Introduction," *The American Health Empire,* Random House, 1969, p. 4.)

5. I am aware that this is an unorthodox view of the etiology of what we have come to know as the medical condition of AIDS. My reasoning depends upon the fact that malnutrition accounts for most acquired immuno-suppression in the world (which therefore might exacerbate the receptivity to the virus) and the fact that the collateral effects of poverty: lack of education; the use of one's body for money; and drug and alcohol addiction are, after all, "high risk behaviors" for the epidemic. A recent anonymous study of HIV infection of non-AIDS related complaints in emergency room visits in the South Bronx resulted in a finding of a 23 percent rate of HIV infection. Dr. Jerome Ernst, who supervised the study, said of the South Bronx: "Anybody who lives here is in a high risk group." (*New York Times,* Feb. 15, 1989.)

6. "Preventing AIDS Among Women: The Role of Community Organizing," Nancy Stoller Shaw, *Socialist Review,* 100, Fall, 1988. "Because AIDS is a socially transmitted and socially preventable disease, the best way to contain it is probably *not* through health department flyers, television messages by celebrities, or doctors' entreaties, but through changing the patterns of interaction within communities. . . . In fact, until there is a vaccine, this may be the most promising way to halt the epidemic." [p. 77]

7. The success of the Gay Men's Health Crisis and the Shanti Project has not been emphasized enough. See "New York City, Gay Men's Health Crisis," *AIDS: Public Policy Dimensions*, United Hospital Fund, 1986; "The Nonprofit Sector's Response to the AIDS Epidemic: Community-based Services in San Fransisco," Peter Arno, *American Journal of Public Health*, 1986, Vol. 76, No 11.

8. "Hospitals Overwhelmed as Poor in New York City Search for Care." *New York Times*, December 8, 1988. "Building Primary Care in New York City's Low-income Communities," forthcoming from the Community Service Society, New York. In that report, CSS documents the existence of 22 fully functioning physicians for the 1.7 million residents of New York City's nine lowest income communities.

9. "The people in charge of training programs run almost feudal baronies in the clinics where their services get delivered. Their priority is running a world-class program with all its esoterica and attracting research money. Primary care is probably somewhere around the bottom of the list of priorities." [*Ibid.*]

10. Correspondence, *New England Journal of Medicine*, "Do Physicians Have an Obligation to Treat Patients with AIDS?" 320, No.2, pp. 120–121. Cf. also "Health Benefits: How the System Is Responding to AIDS," *Clearinghouse Review*, the National Health Law Program, Los Angeles, 1988.

11. Cf. "Uninsured and Underserved: Inequities in Health Care in the United States," Davis and Rowland, *Milbank Quarterly*, Vol. 61, No. 2; "Access to Medical Care for Black and White Americans: A Matter of Continuing Concern," Robert J. Biendon, et al., *Journal of the American Medical Association*, 1989; 261: 278–281, which gives some telling comparisons: ". . . black Americans continue to have a 1½ times higher death rate than whites of the same age, and the infant mortality rate for blacks is twice that of whites." (p. 278); as well as the new study by the Fund for New York published by the Citizens Commission on AIDS entitled "The Crisis in AIDS Care: A Call to Action," released April 1989. This study shows clearly what the systemic crisis in health care provision in New York City contributes to the crisis presented by the epidemic.

12. Cf. *Homelessness, Health and Human Needs*, National Academy of Science Report, 1988.

13. HIV shares a lot of things with other catastrophic diseases, but one thing it does not share is the requirement that it be

kept a *complete* secret. Rather than compare HIV with leprosy to make this point, we should compare HIV and its related conditions to cancer. Imagine having cancer and not being able to let anyone know for fear of reprisal. Then imagine dying of cancer and struggling to get medical care where there isn't any, while attempting to control people's attitudes as you attempt to negotiate your way through public entitlement programs for therapy and medicine. I am describing a continuum because cancer patients do encounter a variation of these difficulties.

14. The President's commission on the HIV epidemic made such a recommendation in wholly emphatic and urgent terms. There has been no action on its recommendation.

15. The HIV epidemic is ordered by race, class, sexual practice, and gender. This is because, as Nancy Stoller Shaw points out, it is transmitted through intimate activity in a society made up of various communities "subject to varying degrees of separation, segregation and boundary-crossing," p. 76, *Socialist Review, op.cit.* Cf. "AIDS Conference Reports: Education for Women in Short Supply," by Janis Kelly, *Network News,* National Women's Health Network, Sept./Oct. 1988. But the epidemic is also ordered by the ideology of voluntarism—that people "choose their lot in life"—a philosophy that is entirely self-serving for the rich in cultures with great race and class stratifications.

16. This is not the place to go into the social and economic origins of bias. Suffice to say, discrimination is not an arbitrary attitude born solely of "ignorance" or "lack of understanding." Social bias targets particular groups at particular times, in particular social relations, fueled by political and economic causes. Bias is precisely *social* and not individual in origin.

17. We are just emerging out of a twenty-year experiment in the corporatization of health care in America which failed due to the fact that, as it turns out, owning hospitals is not the easiest way to make a profit. This corporatization has created scarcity medical conditions for many Americans. In recent years, the crisis has grown. Rising poverty, employment layoffs and cutbacks, and dismantling of public health programs have left 35 million Americans—"33 percent of whom are children and two-thirds of whom have family incomes below 200 percent of the federal poverty level—uninsured." ("Providing Health Care for Low-income Children: Reconciling

Child Health Goals with Child Health Financing Realities," Sara Rosenbaum and Kay Johnson, *Milbank Memorial Quarterly,* Vol. 64, No. 3, 1986.

18. *Op.cit.* Barbara and John Ehrenreich, *The Health Care Empire,* Random House, 1969; Paul Starr, *The Social Transformation of Medicine,* Basic Books, 1982.

19. The Drug Abuse Office and Treatment Act of 1972 provides that the "drug addicted who are suffering from medical conditions shall not be discriminated against in admission or treatment, solely because of their drug abuse . . . by any private or public general hospital." The Rehabilitation Act of 1973 is the federal civil rights law which accords people with handicaps the status of a protected class. In 1977 this law was interpreted to include drug abuse or addiction.

20. "For-Profit Medicine: A Reassessment," Eli Ginzberg, *New England Journal of Medicine,* Vol. 319, No. 12, 757–760.

21. The individuation of human action into behavior components is fallacious in general and especially with respect to HIV-infection. It is designed to apportion blame rather than look at etiology. There are too many socio/economic factors that interweave with HIV-infection for such analysis to be helpful. Medically, "AIDS will resemble drunk driving or cigarette smoking more than diphtheria or malaria; that is, mortality will rise to a high and stubborn level, which will prove difficult to reduce. And, as in drunk driving, we will be strongly tempted to use the criminal law to punish the offender rather than to explore the roots of the disease, because the roots of the disease lie in American practices generally." ("Morality and the Health of the Body Politic," Dan Beauchamp, *Hastings Center Report,* Vol. 16, No. 5, December, 1986.)

22. *Homelessness, Health and Human Needs, op.cit.*

23. Not one *pair* of gloves but one glove to be reused. This story was related to me by Katherine Franke, an attorney with the Human Rights Commission, who is dealing with the myriad difficulties nurses are having due to their fear of HIV-infection and the fear others have about their becoming HIV-infected.

24. The scarcity of primary health care goods is a "natural" scarcity only to the extent that we accept that the current organization of medical care in America is optimal for filling our health care needs—a premise that is not only difficult for anyone looking at our primary care system to accept but one

that is now met with increasing skepticism by the health care system itself. Cf. "For-profit Medicine: A Reassessment," Eli Ginzberg, *op. cit.*

Acknowledgments: I am most grateful to the following people who offered detailed and substantial help on earlier versions of this paper: Edna McCown; Keith O'Connor, Director, AIDS Discrimination Unit, New York City Human Rights Commission; Katherine Franke, Attorney, AIDS Discrimination Unit; Wendy Sarvasy; and Dawn McGuire, M.D. The mistakes are my own. I am indebted to the 21 people I work with in the AIDS Discrimination Unit for their unending stimulation and care.

About the Authors

Dawn McGuire, M. Div. M.D., is a resident in Neurology.

SECTION I

Karen Davis, Ph.D., is Professor and Chairman of the Department of Health Policy and Management at Johns Hopkins University, School of Hygiene and Public Health.

Diane Rowland, Ph.D., is Professor in the Department of Health Policy and Management at Johns Hopkins University, School of Hygiene and Public Health; and Senior Staff Associate, Subcommittee on Health and the Environment, U.S. Congress.

Barbara Ehrenreich, Ph.D., is with the Institute for Policy Studies, Washington, D.C.

John Ehrenreich, Ph.D., is Professor of American Studies, State University of New York, Purchase, New York.

Harold S. Luft, Ph.D., is at the Institute for Health Policy Studies, San Francisco, California.

SECTION II

Nancy McKenzie, Ph.D., is Director of the Health Unit, Community Service Society, New York City.

Carleton B. Chapman, M.D., M.P.H., LL.D., is Visiting Professor, Institute of the History of Medicine, Johns Hopkins School of Medicine; former Dean, Dartmouth Medical School; former President and Vice-President, Commonwealth Fund; former President of the American Heart Association.

John M. Talmadge, M.D., is in private practice and Associate Professor, Graduate Faculty, Texas A&M Medical School.

Robert M. Veatch is Professor of Medical Ethics at the Joseph and Rose Kennedy Institute of Ethics, Georgetown University.

Morris F. Collen, M.D., is former Chairman of the Executive Committee of The Permanente Medical Group, Oakland, California.

SECTION III

Onora O'Neill is Professor in the Department of Philosophy, the University of Essex, Colchester, England.

Anthony Shaw, M.D., is Professor of Surgery, the Pediatric Surgery Division of the Department of Surgery, University of Virginia Medical Center, Charlottesville, Virginia.

Dr. Michael H Kottow was a physician at the Olga Children's Hospital, Stuttgart, Federal Republic of Germany, and is currently practicing in Santiago, Chile.

SECTION IV

Hans Jonas is Professor Emeritus, the Graduate Faculty, the New School for Social Research.

Paul Ramsey, Ph.D., is Professor of Religion, Princeton University.

John C. Fletcher, Ph.D., is Professor of Medical Ethics at the University of Virginia School of Medicine.

Joseph D. Schulman, M.D., is Professor of Human Genetics and Pediatrics, the Medical College of Virginia.

Marc Lappé, Ph.D., is Professor and Director of Humanistic Studies, Center for Educational Development, University of Illinois at Chicago.

SECTION V

Anne R. Sommers is Adjunct Professor in the Department of Environmental and Community Medicine, College of Medicine and Dentistry, Robert Wood Johnson Medical School, New Jersey.

H. Richard Lamb, M.D., is Professor of Psychiatry, University of California School of Medicine, Los Angeles, California.

Sara Rosenbaum, J.D., is Director, Programs and Policies, Children's Defense Fund, Washington, D.C.

Kay Johnson, M.Ed., MPh, is Director, Health Division, Children's Defense Fund, Washington, D.C.

SECTION VI

Antony Flew is Professor of Philosophy, University of Reading, England.

Richard L. Trammell is Professor of Philosophy and Religion at Grove City College, Grove City, Pennsylvania.

Gregory E. Pence, Ph.D., is Professor of Philosophy, School of Medicine, University of Alabama, Birmingham, Alabama.

David A. Peters, Ph.D., is Professor of Philosophy, Department of Philosophy, University of Wisconsin, River Falls, Wisconsin.

Joel Feinberg, Ph.D., is Professor of Philosophy, University of Arizona, Tucson, Arizona.

Raymond A. Belliotti, Ph.D., is Professor of Philosophy, Virginia Commonwealth University, Richmond, Virginia.

SECTION VII

Raanan Gillon, MB, MRCP, is Director, Health Center, Imperial College of Science and Technology, London; and Editor, *Journal of Medical Ethics*.

Allan M. Brandt, Ph.D., is Professor of the History of Medicine and Science, Harvard Medical School.

Dan E. Beauchamp, Ph.D., is Professor of Health Policy and Administration, School of Public Health; and Professor of Social and Administrative Medicine, School of Medicine, University of North Carolina, Chapel Hill, North Carolina.